Best Remedies

Best Remedies

Breakthrough Prescriptions That Blend Conventional and Natural Medicine

MARY L. HARDY, M.D., AND DEBRA L. GORDON

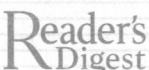

The Reader's Digest Association, Inc.
Pleasantville, New York | Montreal

Project Staff

Editor
Marianne Wait

Designer
Rich Kershner

Cover Design
George McKeon

Contributing Writers
Sarí Harrar
Alisa Bauman

Copy Editor
Jeanette Gingold

Indexer
Nan Badgett

Reader's Digest Health Publishing

Editor in Chief
Neil Wertheimer

Managing Editor
Suzanne G. Beason

Creative Director
Michele Laseau

Production Technology Director
Douglas A. Croll

Manufacturing Manager
John L. Cassidy

Marketing Director
Dawn Nelson

President, U.S. Books & Home Entertainment
Dawn Zier

Reader's Digest Association, Inc.

President, North America Global Editor in Chief
Eric Schrier

First printing in paperback 2008

Library of Congress Catalog-in-Publication Data
Best remedies : breakthrough prescriptions that blend the best of conventional and natural medicine / editor in chief, Neil Wertheimer; managing editor, Suzanne Beason; editor, Marianne Wait.
    p. cm.
Includes index.
ISBN 0-7621-0721-9 (hardcover)
ISBN 978-0-7621-0899-2 (paperback)
  1. Therapeutics--Popular works. 2. Integrative medicine--Popular works. I. Wertheimer, Neil. II. Beason, Suzanne. III. Reader's Digest Association. IV. Title.

RM122.5.B47 2006
615.8'8--dc22

2005033555

We are committed to both the quality of our products and the service we provide to our customers. We value your comments, so please feel free to contact us.

The Reader's Digest Association, Inc.
Adult Trade Publishing
Reader's Digest Road
Pleasantville, NY 10570-7000

For more Reader's Digest products and information, visit our Web site at:
www.rd.com (in the United States)
www.readersdigest.ca (in Canada)

Printed in the United States of America

1 3 5 7 9 10 8 6 4 2 (hardcover)
3 5 7 9 10 8 6 4 (paperback)

Note to Readers
The information in this book should not be substituted for, or used to alter, medical therapy without your doctor's advice. For a specific health problem, consult your physician for guidance. The mention of any products, retail businesses, or Web sites in this book does not imply or constitute an endorsement by the authors or by the Reader's Digest Association, Inc.

Acknowledgments

Writing this book has been a tremendously fulfilling experience for me, and I would like to thank the people who made this possible. First, all my patients, who have presented me with unique challenges and then insisted that I learn to treat them creatively and holistically—they have always been my best teachers. Next, my professional colleagues who are developing this new field of integrative medicine—I hope our work returns all of us to the arts of medicine that I first saw in my grandfather's practice.

A special thank-you to my coauthor, Debra Gordon, a talented writer and a great sport. She has a real gift for taking complex material and turning it into lively, comprehensible text. I valued this collaboration as much for her personal good cheer as for her excellent work. We are both indebted to our editor, Marianne Wait, whose vision gave this project shape and whose attention to detail kept the book on track without sacrificing quality.

Finally, I wish to thank my family and friends, who have always been unstinting in their love and support. My husband, Jim, and son, Chris, put up with a deadline-crazed maniac with their usual good humor. I also think now of my father and grandfather, who are no longer with me, but showed me what a great doctor should be well before I ever went to medical school, or even grammar school. A special thank-you to my mother, who always encouraged me—she's more excited about this book than I am!

It is my intention that this book helps the readers and their loved ones to find the most effective, least toxic, and most creative path toward healing and fulfillment.

—**Mary L. Hardy, M.D.**

Best Remedies has truly been a team effort. Mary Hardy's sense of humor, immense knowledge of medical and natural remedies, and incredible patience made the writing of the book both a pleasure and a fabulous learning experience. Meanwhile, our editor, Marianne Wait, provided her usual eagle-eye approach to ensure that everything we wrote was not only razor-sharp accurate, but met and exceeded our readers' needs and expectations. I also want to thank Jeanette Gingold, a copy editor who takes no detail for granted, Alisa Bauman for her backup support, and, as always, my husband, Keith, for being about as close to the "perfect husband" as any man could ever get.

—**Debra L. Gordon**

Contents

PART 4

Integrative Cancer Care

PART 5

Resources

Introduction

Since the dawn of modern medicine, healers pretty much split themselves into two camps. One camp, made up of conventional white-coat doctors, healed with prescription drugs and surgery, the "big guns," the "quick fixes." The other camp, made up of natural healers, believed in using herbs, oils, diet, and techniques like massage and acupuncture to help the body heal itself—which usually took longer but caused less collateral damage to the body. Both camps had a lot to offer, but patients had to choose one or the other because the two camps weren't on very friendly terms.

Finally that's changed. A "meeting of the minds" has resulted in a whole new way of healing, called integrative medicine because it integrates the approaches of both camps. The result is the best possible healing strategies for what ails you.

Integrative medicine has lots of advantages, which you'll discover for yourself when you start using the "best remedies" in this book. If your condition's not too serious, we'll show you gentle, natural healing methods that can help you avoid the side effects of drugs. (We'll also tell you your drug options.) If you're dealing with something like heart disease or diabetes, we'll steer you toward the right drugs, but we'll also show you steps you can take on your own that will help your body heal—and maybe allow you to lower the dose of the drug you're taking.

In Part 1, "The Best Path to Total Health," you'll find out how integrative medicine finally came about and read some of the new proof behind natural healing techniques. You'll also learn how to use this book. In Part 2, "The Ultimate Anti-Aging Prescription," you'll discover the six Super Threats behind most age-related diseases and exactly how to combat them, thereby reducing your risk of many of the ailments we cover in Part 3, "The Best Remedies," which tells you in depth how to treat more than 100 common ailments with an integrative approach.

You'll notice we give you lots of options—more than you'll want to actually use. One of the tenets of integrative medicine is that doctors and patients work closely together to determine the right course of action. So go ahead and try some of the remedies on your own (especially the ones we give in the "Do This Now" prescription for fast relief), but work with your doctor to put together the best combination of treatments for you.

In Part 4, "Integrative Cancer Care," we'll show you natural ways to alleviate the side effects of cancer treatment, and tell you about the foods and herbs that may prove helpful in preventing cancer.

Finally, in Part 5, "Resources," we list major integrative medicine centers and other places you can go for treatment or information. There's also an important section that lists cautions for herbs and supplements we recommend. Take them seriously—and remember, always let your doctor know what you're taking. If he or she practices integrative medicine (and we suggest you find someone who does), you'll get the support and guidance you need.

Wishing you total health and well-being.

—The Editors

PART I

The Best Path to Total Health

Integrative Medicine: The Future of Healing

This year, more than one in three Americans will use some form of natural medicine. Maybe they'll get a massage to ease back or neck pain, take some echinacea to ward off a cold, visit an acupuncturist to ease their irritable bowel syndrome (IBS) symptoms, or brew a cup of chamomile tea to help them get to sleep.

Of course, they could have taken an entirely different approach: muscle relaxants for the neck or back pain, antihistamines and decongestants for the sneezing and sniffling, prescription drugs for the IBS, and sleeping pills to force slumber.

Such is the fork in the road people often reach when looking to solve a medical problem: Down one path, the path of "natural" medicine, lie gentle and often age-old treatments—like acupuncture, yoga, massage, herbs, and supplements—designed to help the body heal itself. Down the path of "conventional" medicine lie potent drugs and procedures based on modern science and the notion of the all-powerful physician as the dispenser of health and healing.

Both paths have their merits. In fact, in an ideal world, we'd choose the best treatment or combination of treatments—regardless of which discipline they belonged to—for optimal results with the fewest possible risks and side effects. *Best Remedies* brings that world to you.

Natural vs. Conventional Medicine

It's interesting that Western medicine is often referred to as "traditional" medicine, while other forms of healing that are centuries old are called "alternative" or "complementary." After all, you don't get much more traditional than practices dating back thousands of years.

The story of how we got from natural healing to today's multibillion-dollar medical-industrial complex is a fascinating one. The origins of medicine lie in the herbs and concoctions that were the first "medicines," in the shamans and other healers who used everything from touch to music to prayer to heal. Those early healing traditions were inextricably bound up with religion, with healers given godlike attributes and revered for their supposed ability to communicate with spirits.

Science, Please

With Hippocrates, however, came the beginning of the scientific method. Now physicians were trained to observe the physical world, and to make predictions based on what they saw. It was the start of the split between the rational and nonrational aspects of healing—a split that continues to this day.

In the 1600s a British doctor named William Harvey identified the heart as the organ responsible for pumping blood. His "radical" theories on anatomy laid the groundwork for modern physiology—and married us to the view of man as machine. Just as clockmakers took apart a timepiece to discover why it wasn't ticking, anatomists began exploring the human body, taking it apart, examining the parts.

Unfortunately, while they began to understand how our bodies worked, they didn't have many tools at their disposal to cure the sick. Their treatments were barbaric, relying mainly on purging, bleeding, and poisons like arsenic and mercury. But in the late 1800s and early 1900s, with the discovery of ether, sterilization, and insulin, medical treatments became increasingly effective. With the first two, doctors could now painlessly, and with less risk, cut into a person to "fix" him. And with the third, they could, for the first time, put something *back* into a person to make him healthy again. Illnesses that once involved drastic treatment or carried a certain death sentence could now be "cured" in a way that seemed miraculous to both doctor and patient.

Medicine had changed. Instead of coaxing the body back into its natural equilibrium, healing now meant replacing a defective part in a broken machine. The shift made the slow, careful restorative work of the traditional herbalist look ineffectual and risky, particularly if it delayed or prevented access to "real" medicine.

What Is Integrative Medicine?

Integrative medicine is based on certain philosophies about health and healing. It aims to:

- reaffirm the importance of the relationship between the practitioner and the patient

- focus on the whole person

- make use of all appropriate treatments, health-care professionals, and healing disciplines to achieve optimal health and healing

- try the least invasive and least toxic treatments first

- help the body heal itself

- engage the mind, body, and spirit to facilitate healing.

Where Science Stops Short

And so Western medicine developed as a science. While this has paid off with the very advanced medical technology of the 20th and 21st centuries, we can't help feeling that we've lost something along the way.

It didn't become clear just what we'd lost until the second half of the 20th century. After all, prior to that time, most people died in their 50s or early 60s; few lived long enough to develop chronic diseases like high blood pressure, diabetes, heart disease, and cancer. But as life span lengthened (thanks first to better sanitation and nutrition, then to better drugs and treatments) and health issues became more complex and less easily "fixed," we realized that the modern health-care system simply wasn't meeting all of our needs.

The system rewarded intervention, generally ignored prevention, and viewed healing as coming from the physician, not the patient. It did a pretty good job of getting rid of *disease*, but an overall lousy job when it came to focusing on *health,* which, according to the World Health Organization, is not simply the absence of disease or infirmity but "a state of complete physical, mental, and social well-being."

So in the late 1980s, Americans began looking outside the conventional medical system for a better approach.

Bridging the Divide

Integrative medicine represents the culmination of a trend that has been under way for more than a decade. It began in earnest in 1993, when Harvard researchers published the results of a 1990 survey in the *New England Journal of Medicine* on the use of complementary and alternative medicine (CAM). The paper shocked the medical world: The researchers found that an estimated one in three Americans had used CAM during the past year, making an estimated 425 million visits to alternative practitioners and spending over $30 billion—out of their own pockets—on the treatments.

Four years later, another survey by the same authors found the prevalence of CAM use had grown by 25 percent, while the number of visits to alternative practitioners had increased nearly 50 percent. Interestingly, patients were not ditching conventional medicine in favor of alternative therapies; rather, they were pursuing both, often at the same time.

There were several reasons millions of Americans sought alternative treatment approaches: frustration with modern medicine's inability to treat and prevent chronic disease, erosion of the traditional patient-physician relationship thanks in part to the rise of managed care, and a desire to maintain more control over their health and limit

the increasingly greater risks associated with modern medicine.

But surprisingly, the primary reason turned out to be something other than dissatisfaction with the health-care system. Even among people who said they were highly satisfied with conventional medicine, 4 out of 10 still sought alternative remedies. Instead, it was a desire to see practitioners who shared a similar view of health and healing, who believed that the health of the body, mind, and spirit were related.

Initially these practitioners were considered "alternative." They'd been eliminated as economic competition by the conventional medical system earlier in the 20th century, and were now viewed as "quacks," entirely separate from "real" medicine. This, of course, was a silly way to treat patients, with neither side talking to the other and the poor patient caught in the middle. In fact, study after study found that despite the large numbers of Americans seeking alternative care, only a small number ever told their doctors what they were doing.

The Birth of Integrative Medicine

The shift toward merging the two approaches began in Great Britain, where the idea of "complementary" medicine had caught on. Now, instead of treatment A or treatment B, you could have both, sometimes provided by the same doctor, more often via a referral from your conventional doctor. Conventional medicine still came first, however, with the alternative system playing a supporting role. For instance, a doctor might recommend an acupuncturist for chronic back pain—after trying anti-inflammatories, physical therapy, and, possibly, surgery. Acupuncture became just one more thing to try on a laundry list of available treatments, rather than part of a healing art that depended on an overall evaluation of the patient to determine diagnosis and guide treatment. Western doctors were focusing on treating symptoms and ignoring the larger view.

Enter Andrew Weil, M.D. In 1994 Dr. Weil, a faculty member at the University of Arizona's medical school in Tucson, founded the university's Program in Integrative Medicine, a two-year fellowship for physicians who had completed a residency in a primary care specialty such as internal medicine, pediatrics, family practice, or obstetrics/gynecology. His goal was to offer alternative training to doctors who didn't want to turn their backs on all the good Western medicine offered, but who recognized that the current focus on disease rather than wellness didn't work very well when it came to many chronic conditions.

A Perfect Marriage

Although they are very different, approaching health and disease from opposite perspectives, conventional and natural medicine make a wonderful match. Just consider their strengths and weaknesses.

Fixing Broken Parts

Conventional medicine focuses on disease, responding to illnesses and injuries by isolating a problem—be it a germ, torn ligament, plaque deposit, or cancerous cell—and waging a strong, focused attack against it (or removing it altogether). It views individuality as distracting, and creates protocols that, when followed properly, effectively treat the disease in the greatest number of people possible.

If you're in a car accident, you develop a bacterial infection, or you break your leg, conventional medicine shines. It is best at treating acute illnesses and injuries, particularly self-

Although they approach health and disease from opposite perspectives, *conventional and natural medicine* make a wonderful match.

contained ones that can be repaired or cured. That's why most internists would rather see a patient with pneumonia than one with diabetes. The first patient can be treated and sent on his way; with the second, there's no simple fix.

Conventional medicine seeks to break down disease into the smallest or most fundamental part that can be identified and changed. Here, the thinking goes, if we can figure out which enzyme is responsible for a certain disease, we can fix the disease by modifying that enzyme. This reductionist view is the reason there are more than 90 different medical specialties today. It's why patients can sometimes wind up seeing five or six doctors, all specialists treating various conditions in the same person, often without knowing what the others are doing.

Not only do we have cardiologists, we have interventional and preventive cardiologists. There are regular gynecologists, oncologic gynecologists, and reproductive gynecologists. Need surgery on your nose? You'll need to decide if you should see a plastic surgeon (probably one that specializes in head and neck surgery), a head and neck surgeon, or an otolaryngologist (ear, nose, and throat specialist, or ENT). If you have back pain, you could see your primary care doctor, a general orthopedist, an orthopedist certified in spinal medicine, a neurologist, or a rheumatologist.

Healing the Whole Person

Natural medicine, on the other hand, views the body as more than the sum of its parts. It sees those parts as inextricably connected into a unified system. Instead of focusing on one broken part, it examines the whole person—physically, emotionally, and spiritually—to understand and treat problems. The therapies, ranging from herbs to aromatherapy to chiropractic, focus on bolstering the body's own natural healing processes. At the core of the various philosophies lies a belief in the body's ability to repair itself.

Alternative practitioners tend to spend a good deal of time with patients (an initial assessment can take more than an hour) developing the kind of relationship often lacking with conventional healers. They stress nonmedical treatments first, particularly for conditions that are lifestyle oriented. So, for instance, instead of immediately putting you on a statin drug to control your high cholesterol, a naturopath or integrative medicine physician might first develop a program of diet, exercise, and stress reduction to try to reduce your cholesterol naturally.

Another big difference: The patient is the center of care. Unlike with conventional medicine, it is not up to the practitioner to cure you. Only *you* can cure you. The alternative practitioner or integrative physician is there to encourage you to adopt a healthier lifestyle and help determine the most effective and least toxic solution to any health problem. Notice that we said *help* determine. What a patient believes will work and is willing to try are important factors. When was the last time a doctor asked you how you felt about taking a certain drug? Physicians writing prescriptions usually expect you to take the pills regardless of your attitude. Given that more than half of all medications aren't taken as directed, if they're taken at all, you can see the

Integrative medicine is flexible: The focus can shift depending on your condition and how serious it is.

advantage of considering the patient's own wishes in any treatment plan.

Alternative medicine, however, isn't as good at treating acute problems. While it may serve well when used along with conventional cancer treatments like radiation, chemotherapy, and surgery, these treatments still do a better job at destroying cancer cells than any alternative approach. And if you injure your spleen and are bleeding internally, all the herbs, acupuncture, and meditation in the world aren't going to fix it. But herbs to bolster your immune system and acupuncture for pain relief can limit postoperative complications and speed your recovery.

As you can see, these two approaches don't conflict at all; in fact, they combine like yin and yang, two sides of the healing process that together are much stronger than either one alone.

What You Need, When You Need It

One of the advantages of integrative medicine is that it is flexible: The focus can shift depending on your condition and how serious it is.

If you break a bone, at first you're going to be relying heavily on the Western end of the treatment spectrum—perhaps surgery, for instance. But you could also add other approaches to help both body and mind heal. You might consider hypnosis before surgery, which has been shown to help with wound healing; herbal remedies to strengthen your immune system to fight off infection; mind-body therapies to help you manage the stress that comes from a serious accident and hospitalization; or magnet therapy to speed bone healing.

Integrative medicine also considers your emotional well-being. Western doctors are trained to be in charge of the body. But when an illness occurs, it affects a patient's life, spirit, and mood. That's probably why prayer is the most common method of alternative healing used in serious illnesses.

At the beginning of every patient visit, integrative practitioners should ask: Why do you think this happened to you? What do you need to get well? The answers provide important clues as to what motivates the patient and, therefore, how best to tailor treatment for the individual.

Tending to a patient's emotional well-being isn't just a nice gesture; it's good medicine.

Science is gaining a better understanding about the complex interactions between mind and body—for instance, how stress compromises health and affects the ability to heal. In fact, a whole new field, called psychoneuroimmunology, has sprung up to study those mind-body interactions. Consider the strength of the placebo effect—30 percent of patients get better even if you give them a fake treatment—and you can understand the power of the mind to heal.

If an integrative approach to medicine is better for the patient, it's also better for the doctor. Instead of rushing through visits and viewing the patient as the enemy (got to get him out of here so I can see the other six patients scheduled for this hour), doctors can take their time, get to know the person, form a partnership. They can treat the person and not just the disease. And in that way, they help their patients heal themselves.

New Evidence, New Thinking

Are you taking any prescription drugs? Do you have any fears about their side effects? One reason more people are turning to alternative therapies is the gradual erosion of our previously unshakeable confidence in the safety and efficacy of Western medicine.

Take hormone therapy, for instance. For half a century, doctors handed out estrogen prescriptions as if they were mandatory passes to the second half of a woman's life, assuring patients the drugs would stem their hot flashes and also protect them from the most common cause of death in women—heart disease—without increasing the risk of the disease they dreaded most—breast cancer. In this climate of certainty the Women's Health Initiative (WHI) was launched. It was the first major study designed to confirm the benefits of hormone therapy on everything from a woman's brain to her bones.

The initial shocking results were announced in the summer of 2002, when the first part of the trial was abruptly halted: The most commonly prescribed estrogen/progesterone therapy in the world not only didn't protect women's hearts, but increased the risk of heart disease, stroke, breast cancer, and blood clots. The findings overturned just about everything doctors had been telling their patients about hormone replacement.

The results sparked a revolution among menopausal women. Millions quit taking hormone therapy cold turkey, and a week after the results were published, sales of herbal remedies for menopausal symptoms skyrocketed.

Since that time, other common drugs have taken major hits to their safety records. In September 2004 the U.S. Food and Drug Administration (FDA) added black box warnings (the strictest warning available) to the most commonly prescribed antidepressants, cautioning that they could increase the risk of suicide, especially in children. Later that month, pharmaceutical giant Merck pulled its blockbuster pain reliever Vioxx (rofecoxib) from the market after study results found it could significantly increase heart attack risk. A few months later, Bextra (valdecoxib), another pain-relieving drug, was pulled from the market, and the FDA called for new warnings on numerous other pain relievers, including over-the-counter ibuprofen (Advil, Motrin) and naproxen (Aleve).

Safety issues with pharmaceuticals aren't the only problems facing conventional medicine. Consider medical errors. Overall, government studies find, between 44,000 and 98,000 Americans die from medical errors every year, more than from breast cancer, AIDS, and motor vehicle accidents combined.

We're not saying there are no risks attached to CAM therapies. But fewer patients are harmed in a year using these therapies than are hurt using much stronger conventional medical treatments. Problems with herbal products usually involve mix-ups in ingredients, contamination of ingredients, or use in the wrong type of patient—not an intrinsic problem with the active ingredient. And while there are isolated reports of patients contracting hepatitis from unclean acupuncture needles or nerve damage from an improperly performed chiropractic adjustment, these events are very rare.

If CAM therapies are safe, do they work? Is there proof? The issue of clinical studies becomes a major bone of contention when we try to get the conventional medical world to accept or prescribe or pay for alternative therapies.

The Proof Is in the Pudding

Many conventional physicians point to poorly designed studies, inconclusive results, small study samples, and outcomes that can't be reproduced as "proof" that alternative therapies don't work.

In some instances, they're right. But in truth, there is no "proof" that numerous conventional medical therapies work either. For instance, surgical techniques are rarely evaluated to prove their effectiveness before they are routinely used on patients. In fact, it may only be after thousands of operations that we learn a particular procedure, such as surgery for lower back pain, isn't very effective. Or that one surgery, such as open-heart cardiac bypass surgery, may be a better option for some patients than the more commonly performed angioplasty. Or, for that matter, that either of these surgeries may not be as effective as aggressive drug therapy.

Additionally, many large, drug company sponsored studies of conventional medications provide positive results, but have design flaws that should invalidate the findings.

Which leaves us where?

With the need for compromise and flexibility on both sides. We definitely need more well-designed studies of CAM therapies. But we also need to remember that these therapies operate under a very different set of ideas than the conventional medical model, and that sometimes the only "proof" we'll have that they work are the results we see in patients or the observations of generations of healers over time. Although there may not be dozens of carefully controlled, double-blind studies showing the benefits of herb A over placebo, or herb B over prescription medication C, most traditional systems of healing do have evidence behind them; it's just a different kind of evidence, one based on experience over time.

That said, more "proof" of CAM therapies is on the way. Of 17,712 clinical trials published in major medical journals in 2004, just 1,900, or about 11 percent, were on complementary therapies. But that's an improvement over 1999, when the percentage was a little over 7 percent. And

Between 44,000 and 98,000 Americans die from *medical errors* every year, more than from breast cancer, AIDS, and motor vehicle accidents combined.

more studies are coming. Today the National Center for Complementary and Alternative Medicine (http://nccam.nih.gov), part of the National Institutes of Health (NIH), funds research into CAM approaches for everything from arthritis, heart disease, and menopause to better understanding the underlying mechanisms of herbs and energy medicine. In 2004 the center funded 279 research projects, investigating everything from alternative therapies for alcohol and drug abuse to the effect of Chinese herbal medicine on food allergies to the power of compounds in green tea to lower cholesterol.

Funding is coming from other sources as well, as more conventional doctors begin investigating alternative therapies. For instance, in 2005 the National Cancer Institute (NCI) awarded researchers at Wake Forest University Baptist Medical Center a $1 million grant to study the properties of turmeric and bee propolis. Why? Because population studies find dramatically reduced rates of colon cancer in people whose diets are rich in curcumin. The NCI has been developing curcumin as an anticancer agent since 1988; the grant to Wake Forest was to better understand just why this bright orange spice seems to work so well.

As for propolis, it's been used since ancient times as an antibacterial and anti-inflammatory remedy. But more recent studies find that at least one component in propolis protects mice against radiation-induced inflammation and skin damage, and protects rats against certain forms of heart muscle damage following chemotherapy. So a combination of observed evidence and Western science could lead to a new medication that could help millions of people.

Although we try to provide supporting data for most of our recommendations in *Best Remedies*, in some instances the studies just aren't there. We're still recommending the treatment, however, based on tradition of use and success with patients.

New Evidence For...

The growing evidence that does exist for some CAM therapies is enough to excite even skeptics. Take a peek at some of the most exciting research and discover the latest thinking on everything from herbs to acupuncture.

Herbs and Supplements

Given the growing availability of a staggering array of herbal, vitamin, and other supplements, it's no surprise that the use of these remedies is one of the largest areas of complementary medicine. There are more studies on these treatments than any other alternative therapy.

It's difficult to study herbal remedies because we don't know what chemical or active ingredient (or ingredients) are responsible for their effects. And sometimes the benefits depend on the individual. For instance, there's good evidence that a daily multivitamin can help people with diabetes reduce their blood pressure, while supplementing with certain minerals can improve their levels of "good" HDL cholesterol, evidence we haven't seen quite so strongly in healthy people.

Still, well-designed studies on certain remedies have turned up positive results. These remedies include ginkgo to slow the progress of dementia, glucosamine for arthritis of the knee, saw palmetto for enlarged prostate, vitamin E and selenium for preventing prostate cancer, black cohosh for menopause symptoms, and St. John's wort for minor and moderate depression.

We're finding that supplements like CoQ_{10} can protect the heart during chemotherapy, that fish oil should be a part of everyone's daily supplement regimen for its valuable anti-inflammatory properties, and that folic acid is a white knight when it comes to preventing certain birth defects in babies and reducing high levels of homocysteine, a risk factor for heart disease.

The Challenges of Clinical Trials

Why aren't there more clinical studies on CAM approaches? Many reasons.

Money

Clinical trials often cost hundreds of thousands, even millions, of dollars to conduct. Because most CAM therapies can't be patented as a new drug can, it's difficult to get funding.

Part vs. whole

Evidence-based medicine typically requires testing one standardized element against another. But with CAM therapies it can be difficult to break out just one element. For instance, Traditional Chinese Medicine relies on a complex interaction of herbal remedies, not to mention treatments like acupuncture. Even individual herbs may derive their benefits from interactions between many of the constituents of the plant. In other words, the treatment is greater than the sum of its parts.

Individuality

Western research is designed to be reproducible and broadly applicable; in other words, we want the treatment to be as consistent and effective as possible for as many people as possible. CAM therapies, however, are often designed specifically for an individual, with the understanding that what works for one person may not work for another. They also rely to a certain extent on a person's belief in the treatment. If you don't think acupuncture might help you, it probably won't.

Specificity

Many of the treatments tested in CAM trials are innately variable. For example, take a chiropractic adjustment. There are more than 300 different adjustments used by chiropractors. With herbs, the exact product may vary based on how and where the plant was grown, which part is used, and how it was prepared.

Reproducibility

In standard drug trials, you should be able to reproduce the results of a given study using the same dose and frequency. But that's hard to do with therapies like massage or chiropractic, in which the practice patterns and training of the practitioners providing the therapy may be different. Plus, if an herbal combination or multitherapy approach is not described specifically enough in the study, the results may not be reproducible, either by other experts or by patients trying the same methods.

Placebos

The gold standard clinical trial relies on placebos, or sham treatments, tested against the real thing. But it's hard to "fake" a massage, chiropractic adjustment, or yoga.

You'll read much, much more about useful supplements in the ailment entries in Part 3.

Diet

Although nutritional supplements fill every pharmacy and health food store, the evidence regarding the power of nutrition to protect health and prevent disease is strongest when it comes to diet. While most people know the definition of a healthy diet—lean protein, lots of fruits and vegetables, plenty of fiber, not too much fat, etc. (more on this in Part 2)—many probably don't realize the profound impact the food you consume has on your overall health.

But thanks to several major, long-term studies over the past 20 years, we have amassed a wealth of information about the benefits of overall diets and individual foods. For instance, who would have thought that dark chocolate could protect your heart? Well, we now know it can, thanks to compounds called catechins that serve as powerful antioxidants in the coronary arteries. Those same chemicals are thought to be responsible for green tea's cancer-preventive properties. For instance, studies find that men who regularly drink green tea are much less likely to develop cancer. For nearly every fruit and vegetable, someone, somewhere, has found a powerful component within the plant that can have significant effects on your health. Here are a few examples:

Cruciferous vegetables. Diets high in these vegetables, which include broccoli, cauliflower, and cabbage, seem to protect against lung cancer.

B vitamins. High levels of these vitamins in your diet (found in legumes, dark green vegetables, and whole grains) can reduce women's risk of colorectal cancer.

Wine. Not only are you more likely to live longer if you drink a glass or two of wine a day, but you're also less likely to develop heart disease, osteoporosis, diabetes, ulcers, and memory loss than people who abstain.

Fish. People whose diets are rich in omega-3 fatty acids, found in fatty fish, have a lower risk of everything from depression to dry eye syndrome to heart disease.

Milk. Studies find women with high levels of vitamin D and calcium in their diet are less like to have premenstrual syndrome.

Raisins. One study found compounds in raisins help reduce bacteria in the mouth that cause dental problems.

The scientific paradox comes when we try to translate the benefits of real food into supplements. Too often, the supplement just doesn't convey the same protection.

For instance, numerous population studies found that people who ate diets high in beta-carotene had much lower rates of lung cancer than people whose diets were lower in the vitamin. But when scientists conducted large, long-term cancer prevention trials in which participants received either beta-carotene supplements or a placebo, the results were, to say the least, disappointing. Researchers had to halt the trials early when they learned that beta-carotene supplements not only didn't prevent lung cancer in people at high risk for the disease, but appeared to *increase* rates of the disease, particularly among smokers.

Now, that doesn't mean that there still isn't some protective benefit of beta-carotene, but it's quite likely that, as with so many things in integrative medicine, the nutrient works as part of a whole, in association with other antioxidants, and the best place to get it is in its natural state—through vegetables and fruits.

So save supplements for situations in which you can't eat enough food to get the nutrient (calcium and omega-3 fatty acids are good examples) and/or when specific benefits have been proven for a given product or combination of ingredients.

Aromatherapy

Although aromatherapy seems to be everywhere today—in candles, body lotions, even dishwashing soap—true aromatherapy is the use of essential plant oils in healing.

Aromatherapy is one of the fastest-growing complementary therapies in this country. It's also one of the oldest. Even the Bible describes numerous instances in which scented oil was used for mental, physical, and spiritual healing.

Although we are just beginning to see clinical studies on aromatherapy in this country, it is a well-established form of healing in other countries.

The philosophy behind the use of essential oils relies not only on their chemical properties—they

The philosophy behind the use of *essential oils* relies not only on their chemical properties, but also on the power scent has over our emotions.

penetrate the body well, whether through the skin or the nose, and they have proven antifungal and antibacterial actions—but also on the power scent has over our emotions. That's why essential oils are particularly beneficial for relaxation and stress reduction. If you train yourself over time to deliberately relax when you smell lavender, for instance, eventually just a whiff will automatically trigger that relaxation response.

Although aromatherapy research is still in its infancy, some interesting studies are appearing. One, conducted in mice, found that geranium essential oil applied to the skin suppressed inflammation and swelling after injury by reducing inflammatory chemicals called neu-trophils. There are plenty of studies in humans too. One found that using aromatherapy during labor decreased women's need for medication. A Korean study found that postpartum episiotomies healed better with less bacterial infection when women used a sitz bath or soap infused with a mix of essential oils.

Studies also found that elderly people with Alzheimer's disease whose hands were massaged with a lavender-scented oil showed significantly less aggressive behavior than those who received no treatment or a massage with unscented oil. In fact, aromatherapy has been shown to be effective in numerous conditions affecting the elderly, including constipation and insomnia.

The therapy has been used to treat arthritis patients, with one study of 40 patients finding that a mixture of lavender, marjoram, eucalyptus, rosemary, and peppermint oil added to a carrier oil and massaged into the painful joint signifi-cantly reduced levels of pain and depression compared to a control group.

Homeopathy

Conventional medicine has scoffed at homeop-athy ever since its introduction to the United States in the 19th century. The theory behind homeopathy simply made no sense: Homeopathic solutions are so dilute that no molecule of the original substance can be found. Since there was no plausible mechanism of action, conventional doctors believed any benefits had to be related to the placebo effect. Keep in mind, however, that we still don't know how or why numerous approved drugs (including Tylenol) and well-respected therapies work in the body either.

The first inkling that homeopathy was more than quackery came in 1991 with the publication of a review article in the *British Medical Journal*. The authors evaluated 107 clinical studies on homeopathy and found 81 trials whose positive results couldn't be attributed to placebo. Six years later, the renowned British journal *Lancet* pub-lished another analysis of 89 placebo-controlled clinical studies. After subjecting the studies to rig-orous scientific analysis, the researchers concluded that people who received homeopathy had twice the therapeutic benefit of those who received a placebo.

Since then, three other major reviews have been published, and two came to the same con-clusion: Homeopathy seems to work. One of those studies, published in the *Annals of Internal Medicine* in 2003, concluded that while more and better research is needed, "it is important that physicians be open-minded about homeopathy's possible value and maintain communication with patients who use it."

Consumers seem to agree. Today Boiron's homeopathic flu remedy Oscillococcinum is the best-selling flu medicine in drugstores, while Hyland's Teething Tablets are the top-selling oral pain reliever for children.

So just what is homeopathy best for? Some of the better-designed studies find that Oscillococcinum is effective for the flu, that *Galphimia glauca* works to treat hay fever, and that arnica can help reduce pain and improve healing after trauma and surgery. Other trials find that classical homeopathy—that is, individually mixed preparations—can reduce the duration of diarrhea in children and improve asthma symptoms.

While we recommend several commercially available homeopathic remedies in *Best Remedies,* overall we believe that custom therapies prescribed by a homeopathic healer work better than premade remedies, which may be why there isn't more positive evidence of homeopathy's benefits in the scientific literature. See page 33 for information on finding a homeopathic healer.

Traditional Chinese Medicine and Acupuncture

Traditional Chinese Medicine (TCM) is based on the view that the body is organized along functional, not anatomical, principles and that the state of disease or health depends on the flow of energy, or chi (pronounced "chee"), in the body. It encompasses a wide range of treatments, including acupuncture and herbal therapies, t'ai chi, a particular kind of abdominal massage, and nutrition—all focused on enhancing or balancing the flow of energy in the body.

Practitioners will tell you that much of TCM's benefits come from herbal formulations, which can be quite complex. That's why we rarely suggest you use TCM herbal remedies on your own. See page 31 for more on finding a TCM healer in your area.

Although there are studies in the literature on individual TCM preparations, they are few and far between, and are often published in Chinese. The majority of Western-based research on this form of healing focuses on acupuncture, which is one of the most studied forms of CAM in the United States.

Acupuncture was introduced to the West in the 16th century by French priests who traveled to the Orient. However, as China re-isolated itself, the West forgot about it. Its dramatic reintroduction came in 1972, when then-President Richard M. Nixon opened up China to the rest of the world. A member of his diplomatic party needed his appendix removed, an event that made front-page news when we learned acupuncture was the only anesthesia he received.

It was another 25 years before acupuncture started to receive serious scientific attention. In 1997 the NIH hosted a conference that found that acupuncture was being "widely" practiced by thousands of acupuncturists, physicians, dentists, and others for pain relief or prevention and various other health conditions. Conference organizers also wrote that acupuncture had "potential clinical value" for nausea/vomiting and dental pain.

Since then, the evidence behind acupuncture has become much stronger, with thousands of published studies. In 2005 an overview of more than 500 clinical studies concluded there was "good evidence" for acupuncture's use to prevent and treat postoperative and chemotherapy-related nausea and vomiting, and dental pain, and "promising evidence" for its role in treating migraine and other headaches, low back pain, temporomandibular joint disorder (TMJ), osteoarthritis, and asthma.

We're also starting to see more studies comparing acupuncture to conventional treatments. A Duke University Medical Center study found that electroacupuncture (in which the needles are attached to a device that generates continuous electric pulses) worked better to reduce nausea

Traditional Chinese Medicine encompasses a wide range of treatments, all focused on enhancing or *balancing the flow of energy* in the body.

and vomiting after breast surgery than the leading drug, as well as decreasing postoperative pain.

One study in patients with arthritis of the knee even found that an integrated approach incorporating acupuncture along with the nonsteroidal anti-inflammatory drug Cataflam (diclofenac) worked better at relieving pain and restoring motion than the drug alone. Researchers are also exploring acupuncture's ability to improve a patient's condition after a stroke. And, in an early indication of what may be to come, studies in rats find that acupuncture can lower blood pressure.

Look for more well-designed studies on acupuncture; studying the technique has become much easier since a "sham" form was developed in which researchers use needles or electrical impulses on sites that are not true acupuncture points.

Ayurveda

Along with Traditional Chinese Medicine, this Asian/Indian form of healing is one of the oldest continuously documented medical practices on the planet. Ayurveda (meaning "science of life") places equal emphasis on body, mind, and spirit, and strives to restore the innate harmony of the individual. Primary Ayurvedic treatments include diet, exercise, meditation, herbs, massage, exposure to sunlight, and controlled breathing.

More than 1,250 herbs are used in Ayurvedic medicine. Treatments include herbs designed to address the primary condition as well as others to aid in the digestion and absorption of the therapeutic remedy and balance any negative side effects.

This doesn't mean you have to see an Ayurvedic practitioner, however (there aren't that many of them around); many companies and Indian stores in the U.S. sell Ayurvedic products. Just make sure you purchase those that document good manufacturing practices (GMP), which should be stated on the label.

There are very few published clinical trials on Ayurvedic herbal remedies in humans. One well-designed study comparing standard medical treatment for irritable bowel syndrome (IBS) with Ayurvedic herbal medicine or a placebo in 169 patients found that 64 percent of those receiving an Ayurvedic herbal remedy reported their symptoms improved compared to only about a third receiving placebo. Standard medical treatment worked best, however.

Another small study found that the Ayurvedic remedy Liv. 52, which contains six different herbs, improved the condition of the livers of 19 people with hepatitis or cirrhosis.

Meanwhile, a few studies attest to the cardiovascular benefits of several Ayurvedic herbal remedies including hawthorn, pushkarmoola (*Inula racemosa*), *Terminalia arjuna,* and astragalus root. For instance, in one small trial of nine men with angina, those who received powdered pushkarmoola had less chest pain and fewer breathing problems than those who received nitroglycerin.

In the United States, Ayurveda has hit the mainstream in the form of yoga. Today about 5 percent of the adult population practices yoga every year. However, if your yoga instructor focuses only on the physical postures without explaining yoga's philosophical underpinnings, you may be getting a good workout but you're not getting the full benefits of traditional yoga.

Most studies on yoga focus on its benefits for stress reduction and stress-related conditions, such as high blood pressure and heart disease. For instance, numerous studies show that yoga, along with a low-fat diet and other lifestyle changes, improves coronary artery function more than diet and lifestyle changes alone.

Now we're beginning to see the practice evaluated for other chronic conditions, including carpal tunnel syndrome, chronic insomnia, arthritis, asthma, and chronic low back pain, with good results. One study of 149 patients with type 2 diabetes even found improved blood glucose control after 40 days of yoga in 70 percent of participants.

Mind-Body Medicine

In recent years, doctors and other experts have become more and more attuned to the fact that our emotions affect our immune systems and our overall health. In fact, an entirely new field of study, called psychoneuroimmunology, has sprung up to examine the connection. Mind-body medicine uses the power of the mind to help the body heal. It encompasses numerous therapies, including:

Meditation. Meditation is the self-regulation of attention. There are various forms, including the most studied, transcendental meditation (TM), which was developed in India and brought to the United States in the 1960s. Numerous studies attest to the benefits of TM for a variety of health conditions, including high blood pressure and cholesterol, substance abuse, and chronic anxiety. Additionally, a vast body of work exists examining the underlying physiological effects of TM. For instance, MRI studies find that longtime TM practitioners show meditation-like changes in their brain-wave patterns even when they're not meditating. The result? Greater alertness and increased mental efficiency.

Hypnosis. Forget magic shows and parlor tricks; hypnosis, or hypnotherapy, has entered the medical mainstream. Well-designed studies find it works for everything from pain management to allergy and asthma control, even helping surgical wounds heal faster. Even that most conservative bastion of medicine, the American Medical Association, approved its use as early as 1958, and today physicians can be board-certified in clinical hypnosis.

The idea behind hypnosis is to harness the power of the mind to affect the body. Today, thanks to sophisticated imaging systems, we're beginning to see just how hypnotherapy works in the brain. For instance, researchers at Virginia Polytechnic Institute in Blacksburg, Virginia, found that during hypnosis for pain, the prefrontal cortex, which controls concentration, directs other areas of the brain to reduce or eliminate their awareness of pain.

Guided imagery. This form of mind-body therapy, which might be considered a first cousin to hypnosis, uses the imagination to affect your physical or emotional state. Generally you're asked to imagine a specific scene, incorporating all your senses in the vision. For instance, a colon cancer patient might be asked to imagine immune cells attacking cancer cells in a specific part of his colon.

The greatest body of research finds good evidence for guided imagery's use in managing chronic pain. Studies also find good results using the therapy to help patients manage postsurgical pain, and many pain clinics incorporate it as part of their menu of treatments.

Biofeedback. In biofeedback, you learn to consciously control an involuntary physical function, for instance, lowering your blood pressure, dilating blood vessels to prevent headaches, or tightening the bladder muscle to keep urine from leaking out. One sign of biofeedback's acceptance: Medicare, the national health insurance program for the elderly and disabled, covers it as a treatment for urinary incontinence.

The best evidence for biofeedback probably comes in the area of gastroenterology, particularly its use to treat constipation and incontinence. But there are also some convincing studies on its use to treat attention-deficit hyperactivity disorder in children, as well as headaches and other pain.

Progressive muscle relaxation (PMR). This is a good one to try when you can't fall asleep. With PMR, you tighten, then relax, different sets of muscles, one at a time, until your entire body is relaxed. When the NIH assessed the therapy, it concluded there was "strong evidence" for its use in reducing chronic pain.

Other analyses find that PMR can help with tension and migraine headaches, side effects of chemotherapy, and tinnitus (ringing or buzzing in your ear). When compared to the antianxiety medication Xanax (alprazolam), one study found that PMR worked just as well to reduce anxiety, although the drug worked a bit faster.

We'll address each of these mind-body therapies in more detail in Part 2 when we talk about stress, and explain how to use or access them.

Bodywork and Bioenergetics

These therapies include such well-researched techniques as chiropractic, osteopathy, and massage, as well as less understood ones, including the Alexander Technique (in which you learn to improve your posture and movement and to use your muscles more efficiently) and Feldenkrais (in which you learn to improve your overall coordination). Also under this subheading: energy and healing touch, Reiki, and reflexology (massaging particular points on the feet, hands, or ears that are thought to correspond with specific body parts and systems).

The majority of studies focus on chiropractic, or spinal manipulation. Today the NIH estimates that more than 75 percent of insurance companies provide at least some reimbursement for chiropractic care, a clear sign of its acceptance as a mainstream treatment.

More than 43 well-designed clinical trials show good benefits from chiropractic in treating lower back pain. There's also good evidence that it may be as effective as some medications for migraine and tension headaches, and may offer short-term benefits for neck pain.

Clinical studies on massage also find significant effects on the body. For instance, massage can alter various neurochemical, hormonal, and immune markers, such as substance P in patients who have chronic pain, serotonin levels in women who have breast cancer, cortisol levels in patients who have rheumatoid arthritis, and natural killer (NK) cell numbers and CD4+ T-cell counts in patients who are HIV-positive.

Studies have found that massaging preterm infants can improve weight gain, possibly by stimulating the release of more hormones for more efficient food absorption. There are also good results in studies exploring the use of massage as an adjunct treatment for substance abuse, anorexia, and smoking cessation, as well as numerous pain-related conditions.

Putting It All Together

You don't need to know everything about all of the therapies we've just talked about in order to incorporate some of them into your treatment. Most important is that you have a skilled provider to help you sort through what's best for you in your individual situation. You'll learn how to find that provider starting on page 30.

Plus, we promise you much more information on the benefits of these therapies and others as you read through *Best Remedies*. We even list some of the best studies behind them in the references section in the back of the book so you can look them up yourself or share them with your health-care provider.

Using This Book

So now that you have the background, it's time to explain how to use the advice in *Best Remedies*. You may have already peeked ahead at your own particular medical conditions, but we also want you to take time to read Part 2. There we show you how to prevent or reduce the six Super Threats to health: inflammation, oxidative stress, insulin resistance, stress hormones, toxins, and immune impairment. Think of the information in this section as the underpinnings of both prevention and healing.

Now let's talk about the ailment entries in *Best Remedies* and how to use them. First, understand that the information in this book is intended for reference only. It is designed to help you and your health-care providers make comprehensive, informed decisions about your medical care. It is not a prescription to be followed, nor is it intended to replace any treatment your doctor has already prescribed. In fact, we urge you *not* to change any medical treatment you're currently receiving without first talking with your doctor. That includes adding treatments, as well as stopping any medications.

The Ailment Entries

Most entries contain four primary sections: Do This Now/Our Best Advice; Why It Works; Other Medicines and Other Approaches; and Prevention.

Do This Now. This section provides a handful of approaches you can take immediately, either on your own or with your doctor's help, to bring you some relief during the acute stage of the condition. These recommendations are for symptom relief—they're not cures. They provide you with things you can do to buy yourself some time while you make lifestyle adjustments or, in some instances, arrange to see a conventional, complementary, or integrative healer.

Understand that if we'd asked 15 different integrative physicians to come up with the "Do This Now" section, you'd have 15 different recommendations. That's the art of medicine. The approaches we recommend come from both realms of research and years of experience working with patients.

Our Best Advice. This heading replaces "Do This Now" for chronic conditions, like high cholesterol, that don't have an acute phase. Here we offer you the top treatments/lifestyle changes for this condition, the "if you're only going to do a few things, do these" recommendations.

Why It Works. This section provides you with the background as to why we're making the recommendations we do for "Do This Now" and "Our Best Advice."

Other Medicines and Other Approaches. These two sections complete the "treatment" section of each entry. They offer second-line approaches to treating the acute or, in most instances, chronic phase of your condition. "Other Medicines" includes herbs and supplements, over-the-counter drugs, and prescription drugs. In "Other Approaches," we include non-pill approaches such as diet, aromatherapy, Traditional Chinese Medicine, and surgery.

We don't expect you to pick one from every category, nor do we expect you to focus only on one category. Together with your doctor or other health-care providers, you should use these options as a kind of menu to consider when designing a plan that works best for your situation.

For instance, if you really hate taking medicine, you might want to start with an herbal therapy; if you don't get relief, you can then move on to a drug. In some instances, you'll combine two or more treatments. Maybe an aromatherapy steam treatment for your sinus infection along with an over-the-counter decongestant.

One thing we don't expect you to do is try *everything,* or try to treat your condition using *only* our advice. In some instances—for a short-term bout of diarrhea, for example—that might be fine, but most of the conditions we describe here are fairly serious and require support from a professional. *Best Remedies* is not designed as a home remedies book, even though many of our recommendations can be done on your own.

You'll also see times when we recommend that you consult with a specific practitioner. For instance, while you can purchase many patent homeopathic remedies at pharmacies and health food stores, we prefer that you see a homeopathic healer who can prescribe an individual formula designed for your diagnosed condition.

That's why we don't have very many specific recommendations under Traditional Chinese Medicine (TCM) or Ayurveda. These healing traditions require interaction with a trained professional. Occasionally we suggest acupuncture or TCM herbal formulations, but, in general, if you have a qualified TCM or Ayurvedic practitioner in your area, it's worth making an appointment, particularly for chronic, long-term conditions.

The same is true for chiropractic care—it's hard to adjust your own back. Massage therapy is a bit different, however; while you'll get the greatest therapeutic benefit with a professional, loving family members or friends can also impart a good deal of benefit.

Remember: A key component of integrative medicine is first understanding the underlying issues in your life and spirit, as well as body, that may be contributing to your condition, then devising the best possible approach for *you.*

Prevention. Don't skip over this section. It has two goals: to help you avoid an acute episode or flare-up of a chronic condition, and to help you avoid developing the condition in the first place.

You'll see that most of these recommendations are focused on lifestyle changes—diet, exercise, stress reduction. We don't go into a lot of detail on exactly what to do—you'll find that information in Part 2. Our advice in Part 2 is critical to any preventive remedies we suggest.

Generally you *can* do everything we recommend in the "Prevention" section. Combining certain supplements with a change in your diet, regular exercise, or even yoga classes all work together to strengthen the underpinnings of your immune system, mental health, and spirit.

Stocking Your Medicine Cabinet

While most households have a medicine cabinet stocked with ibuprofen, aspirin, Tylenol, bandages, and a topical antibiotic, how many also contain peppermint oil and cramp bark? That's what we thought.

We've put together a list of additional items we recommend you pick up at your local drugstore, health food store, or, if necessary, online. (See "Your Natural Medicine Cabinet," page 29.) These aren't the only at-home remedies we recommend throughout the book, but they'll provide a good start. You'll also want to stock whichever remedies we recommend for the conditions you experience most often. The chart includes a sampling. For more details, see the individual ailment entries in Part 3.

Most natural remedies have a shelf life of about a year with proper storage in a cool, dark place. Some vitamins and herbs as tinctures could last longer, so check for the expiration dates. Once a bottle is opened, the product is exposed to air and may start to spoil more quickly than the expiration date suggests. Sniff your natural medicines when you open them so you know what they should smell like. Later on, if they don't smell right or they look different, they're probably not worth taking. They usually won't harm you, but they're generally less effective.

Using Supplements Safely

Herbal products, vitamins, minerals, and other nutritional supplements are considered dietary supplements, which means the FDA regulates them in a different and much less rigorous manner than it regulates drugs. For instance, it does not require manufacturers to prove the efficacy or safety of their products before marketing them. However, manufacturers cannot make specific claims about their products' ability to treat medical conditions. So, for instance, you won't see a label on a bottle of saw palmetto claiming to treat enlarged prostate, but one noting the herb improves or maintains prostate health. And if the FDA determines that a product isn't safe, as it did with ephedra, it has the right to order it removed from the market.

The FDA also doesn't oversee the manufacturing of these products as strictly as it does drugs. This can lead to some issues with quality control. That's why it's important to stick with well-known, well-respected manufacturers who follow their own standards for quality control or even industry standards.

To ensure the quality of your supplements, only buy products with third-party certification, which means that an independent body, such as ConsumerLab.com, the National Nutritional Foods Association (NNFA) TruLabel Program, the NSF Certification Program, or the USP Dietary Supplement Verification Program, has verified that the product complies with certain standards. Those could range from manufacturing standards to purity to the level of active ingredients in the product.

Another thing to remember: Natural doesn't necessarily mean safe. Even a seemingly benign multivitamin, if taken inappropriately or in combination with certain other supplements or drugs, can be harmful. We learned that in 2004, when the FDA took the highly unusual step of banning the sale of all products containing ephedrine alkaloids, components found in the Chinese herb ephedrine (except those found in Traditional Chinese Medicine formulations) because of deaths related to its use.

See pages 369-370 for cautions about using specific supplements.

Your Natural Medicine Cabinet

Here are the natural medicines we recommend you stock in your medicine cabinet:

Herbal Remedies

- Peppermint, green, and chamomile teas
- Valerian extract
- Aloe vera gel
- Ginger in some form (tea, fresh gingerroot, capsules, or ginger candy)
- Andrographis pills or echinacea tincture

Vitamins and Nutritional Supplements

- Multivitamin/mineral
- Vitamin C with flavonoids
- Vitamin B complex supplements
- Calcium/magnesium/vitamin D supplements
- Fish oil and/or flaxseed oil supplements
- Probiotics (beneficial bacteria) supplements such as *Lactobacillus*

Aromatherapy

- Lavender, peppermint, eucalyptus, tea tree, and ginger essential oils
- Castor oil as a carrier oil to dilute the essential oils

Homeopathic Remedies

- Arnica for pain and inflammation
- *Anas barbariae* (a flu remedy sold under various brand names, including Oscillococcinum)

Other

- Capsaicin cream for pain
- Willow bark tablets for pain
- Aveeno oatmeal or Domeboro for soothing baths
- Bromelain for swelling and bruising

You should also stock remedies for the conditions you experience often. Here's a sampling. Check the ailment entry in Part 3 for more information.

Condition	Recommended Supplements
Allergies	Bee pollen, butterbur, nettle,* quercetin, zinc
Arthritis (osteo)	Boswellia, devil's claw, glucosamine,* willow bark extract
Cold sores	Lemon balm ointment,* lysine,* quercetin, vitamin C with flavonoids
Colds	Andrographis,* eucalyptus oil, fenugreek, slippery elm (for coughs and sore throat), zinc lozenges and Zicam*
Constipation	Magnesium, psyllium seed and/or husk
Flu	Fenugreek (for coughs), elderberry extract (Sambucol),* Oscillococcinum or Flu Remedy*
Headache	Magnesium,* peppermint oil*
Heartburn	Artichoke leaf extract, chamomile or slippery elm tea, Iberogast, peppermint oil capsules (enteric coated), red pepper capsules
High blood pressure	Fish oil, folic acid, hibiscus flower, potassium
Insomnia	Calms Forté, chamomile tea, melatonin, valerian extract
Menstrual cramps	Chaste tree berry extract, cramp bark tincture, fennel oil, fish oil, ginger oil, magnesium pidolate, valerian tincture
PMS	Calcium and magnesium,* chaste tree berry,* evening primrose oil, ginger (for nausea), ginkgo, nettle or dandelion (for bloating), St. John's wort, vitamin B_6
Prostate enlargement	Bee pollen, beta-sitosterol (if you also have high cholesterol), saw palmetto,* possibly combined with African plum or nettle

*Highly recommended

Finding the Right Healer

Looking for an integrative medicine practitioner? The possibilities can be confusing. Everything from a single acupuncture practitioner to a comprehensive academic medical center program can call itself an integrative medicine clinic.

Today at least 27 medical centers have integrative medicine programs that serve as both training and treatment facilities. These include some of the top names in medicine, such as Columbia, Duke, Georgetown, Harvard, and the University of California (at Los Angeles, Irvine, and San Francisco). Their centers go by all sorts of names, from the obvious—Center for Integrative Medicine—to the not-quite-as-clear (the University of Massachusetts Center for Mindfulness, for instance). Some offer a plethora of services ranging from conventional medical treatment to acupuncture and homeopathy; others focus more on stress reduction or lifestyle interventions and really operate in more of a complementary approach to conventional medicine than a truly integrated effort.

Just what *is* an integrative medical clinic? It's a team of health-care practitioners from different disciplines working cooperatively to provide you with the broadest range of appropriate therapies possible. The majority of these clinics have a "lead" practitioner, usually a physician (M.D.) or an osteopath (D.O.). After an initial evaluation, typically aimed at confirming the diagnosis, you'll be involved in helping create a treatment plan. If you have an urgent medical problem, this may require immediate referral for conventional medical treatment. But for most patients, this means outlining a series of lifestyle modifications, supplements, and treatments to help you cope with and improve your health condition.

An integrative medicine clinic may have all or most of the services provided on-site, or may coordinate with a group of outside providers for care. Coordination of services usually occurs during sessions in which all providers involved in your care meet to review your case.

What to Look For in an Integrative Practice

Our recommendation when it comes to finding a quality program? Start at the top. The core of an integrative clinic, program, or practice should be, as we noted earlier, a conventionally trained M.D. or D.O., board-certified in internal medicine, family practice, ob-gyn (if the program focuses on women's health), or pediatrics (if the program focuses on children). If you're looking for a specialty integrative care clinic in areas such as cardiology or cancer, make sure the physicians on staff are board-certified in that particular specialty.

You want a physician who can prescribe all medications, perform surgeries within his or her scope of practice, and has privileges at a quality hospital. What you don't want is a doctor who graduated from medical school, never finished a residency, and now decides this form of medicine might make a nice "fallback" position. Integrative medicine is a calling on its own, just like surgery or obstetrics. It also requires additional training beyond what one receives in medical school and through a conventional internship and residency.

Ideally, look for a physician who has completed a fellowship or residency in integrative medicine, such as the ones offered by the University of Arizona and other medical schools. However, these are relatively new programs. So many physicians who developed an interest in integrative medicine earlier may have received less formal training. Don't write them off; they've typically been doing this work for years, attending ongoing training programs, and even providing training for some of the new residency and fellowship programs.

From there, however, evaluating the quality of an alternative provider becomes more difficult, although checking with professional societies, many of which we've listed below, can help. That's because certification and licensing regulations for practitioners depend on what state you live in. For instance, although all states license chiropractors, licensing regulations for most other specialties, including acupuncture, Traditional Chinese Medicine, massage therapy, and naturopathy, are all over the map. Even when states do

Integrative medicine is a calling on its own, just like surgery or obstetrics. It also requires additional training beyond what one receives in medical school and through a conventional internship and residency.

require licensing, what one state allows a practitioner to do may be different from what another state allows. For instance, some states allow acupuncturists to recommend herbal therapies, while at least one state specifically prohibits it.

You should always be prepared to ask about the training, licensure, and professional memberships of any integrative medicine provider. Most will provide you with a résumé or biography that includes this information. If they don't, think carefully about whether to use this person to provide your care. After all, the health-care provider-patient relationship needs to start from a foundation of honesty and trust.

Evaluating Complementary Medicine Practitioners

If there is no integrative medicine clinic near you, you may need to cobble together your own integrative medicine team. How do you know what to look for in a practitioner? Here's our best advice.

Traditional Chinese Medicine practitioner. Ideally, every integrative medicine clinic should include this practitioner, who should have completed a traditional four-year college, then another three years of training at an accredited

TCM program. Don't get a TCM practitioner confused with an acupuncturist. While all TCM practitioners learn acupuncture, not all acupuncturists learn about the herbal side of the practice.

When it comes to licensing, the picture is murky. At least 42 states and the District of Columbia require a license to practice acupuncture, but training requirements are generally minimal. Additionally, some states have separate boards of acupuncture or Oriental medicine, while others oversee these specialties via the board of medical examiners or even their commerce or health departments.

We recommend seeking out practitioners certified by the National Certification Commission for Acupuncture and Oriental Medicine (NCCAOM) in acupuncture, Chinese herbology, and/or Oriental bodywork therapy, which ensures that they have met strict training and testing criteria. If your state licenses this type of practitioner, make sure you see a copy of the license or check with the state to make sure the person is licensed.

Another good source: The American Academy of Medical Acupuncture, which has an online database at www.medicalacupuncture.org.

Chiropractor. If the physician involved with an integrative medicine program is not an osteopath, we like to see an on-site chiropractor so someone is available to provide spinal manipulation for musculoskeletal injuries.

All states license chiropractors and most require that they take and pass the National Board of Chiropractic Examiners' standard national certification examination. Also look for a chiropractor who trained at one of the 14 U.S. chiropractic colleges accredited by the Council on Chiropractic Education; you'll find a list of colleges at www.cce-usa.org. A good source to find a chiropractor in your area is the American Chiropractic Association at www.amerchiro.org.

Massage therapist. Today 35 states regulate the practice of massage therapy and require licensure, and the American Massage Therapy Association (AMTA) is working to get that number up to 50. The AMTA is also a good place to find a qualified massage therapist (www.amta-massage.org). Most states require that massage therapists have at least 500 hours of in-class training, pass the National Certification Board of Therapeutic Massage and Bodywork exam, maintain continuing education credits, and carry malpractice insurance.

You Say Osteopath, We Say Physician

Whether the initials after your doctor's name are M.D. or D.O., rest assured that he or she has attended a traditional four-year medical school and completed all the required postmedical school training and credentialing prior to licensing.

An M.D. or a D.O. are identically trained in all ways except one: Osteopaths, who attend a college of osteopathic medicine, receive extra training in the musculoskeletal system (nerves, muscles, and bones) so they can better understand how an injury or illness in one part of the body affects other parts.

They also receive variable amounts of training in the manual manipulation of the musculoskeletal system. Some will be as comfortable with manual manipulation as a chiropractor, while others will have only somewhat more training in this area than the average M.D.

Osteopaths may have a more holistic view of health and the human body than many M.D.'s. This, of course, makes them particularly well suited to participating in an integrative medicine program.

Also look for a massage therapist who graduated from a program accredited by the Commission on Massage Therapy Accreditation (COMTA) or from a school that is a member of the AMTA, and ask about any training the therapist has in specific massage techniques. For instance, if she hasn't received any special training in Rolfing, she shouldn't be offering that service.

Naturopathic physician. Naturopathic physicians (N.D.'s) receive training in many of the same areas as medical doctors, such as anatomy, physiology, and pharmacology. While naturopathic doctors don't receive the same depth of information on conventional medical subjects as medical doctors, they do receive many additional hours of training in preventive medicine, diet, herbal medicine, hydrotherapy, and musculoskeletal techniques. They may also take additional training in Traditional Chinese Medicine, homeopathy, or midwifery, and become certified in those areas, as well as in naturopathy.

As of this writing, just 13 states, four Canadian provinces, the District of Columbia, and the U.S. territories of Puerto Rico and the U.S. Virgin Islands had licensing laws for naturopathic doctors. State licensing laws typically require that naturopathic doctors graduate from a four-year, residential naturopathic medical school, pass the Naturopathic Physicians Licensing Examinations, complete regular continuing education, and follow the specific scope of practice (outlining what they can and cannot do) regulated by their state. These scopes of practice differ from state to state, with some states, like Oregon, allowing N.D.'s to prescribe some drugs and give immunizations.

Unfortunately, in states that don't license N.D.'s, anyone can hang out a shingle and call himself a naturopath. So look for a naturopath who graduated from one of the four naturopathic schools accredited by the Council on Naturopathic Medical Education (CNME): Bastyr University in Kenmore, Washington; the Canadian College of

What to Expect During Your Visit

The job of an integrative physician at your first meeting is not only to make or confirm a diagnosis if you're having a health problem, but also to thoroughly assess your situation in order to create an individualized treatment plan. In addition to asking you about your medical history, your family's medical history, and any drugs and supplements you take, the physician may ask you about other issues that affect your health and well-being, such as:

- What foods you tend to eat
- Whether you drink or smoke
- Your exercise habits
- Your sleep habits
- Your relationships
- Causes of stress in your life
- Your hobbies and interests
- What you do to relax

Naturopathic Medicine in Toronto; the National College of Naturopathic Medicine in Portland, Oregon; and the Southwest College of Naturopathic Physicians in Tempe, Arizona. Additionally, the Boucher Institute of Naturopathic Medicine in British Columbia and the University of Bridgeport College of Naturopathic Medicine have been granted candidacy status from the CNME. Stay away from anyone who received a degree via a correspondence or online course.

Naturopaths should also have passed the Naturopathic Physicians Licensing Examination, the standard examination used by all licensing jurisdictions for naturopathic physicians in North America.

Homeopath. Although an estimated 6,000 people practice homeopathy in the United States, just three states license them (Arizona, Connecticut, and Nevada), and then only if the practitioners also have medical licenses. Some states include homeopathy within the scope of practice of other specialties, such as chiropractors or naturopaths, even veterinarians!

Your best bet is to find an M.D. or a D.O. who is also board-certified in homeopathy through the American Board of Homeotherapeutics, or an N.D., since naturopaths receive extensive training in homeopathy as part of their education. While other boards offer certification for nonlicensed and licensed health professionals, they lack recognition by the U.S. Department of Education (a sign of credibility). Our recommendation? Don't go looking for a homeopath on your own. Get a referral from your physician or naturopath to someone she trusts.

Hypnotherapist. Anyone can call himself a hypnotherapist. Your best bet is to find a licensed M.D. or D.O. also trained in hypnotherapy through the American Society of Clinical Hypnosis or the Society for Clinical and Experimental Hypnosis.

Biofeedback provider. There is no national license required to practice biofeedback, although some states require that practitioners be licensed psychologists, nurses, psychotherapists, or other medical professionals. However, biofeedback technicians without those credentials may practice under their employers' license. Look for practitioners certified by the Biofeedback Certification Institute of America, and ensure that they've received certification in their specialty area: general biofeedback, which covers electromyography (EMG) and thermal therapies; electroencephalogram (EEG) or neurofeedback; or pelvic muscle dysfunction biofeedback, which helps control urine and fecal incontinence and pelvic pain disorders.

PART 2

The Ultimate
Anti-Aging
Prescription

Stopping Disease in Its Tracks

Long before the first bottles of high-priced and questionable "anti-aging" supplements hit the shelves, humans were already seeking the secret to longer life. Consider Adam and Eve, the River of Immortality, the Taoist immortal masters, and Ponce de León and the Fountain of Youth (a.k.a. Florida). But the truth is, there's no way to thwart death. Our bodies have a built-in timer—and eventually it goes off.

That's okay. Few of us really want to live forever anyway. What we want is to live as long as possible and stay healthy while we do it. No one wants to spend his last 20 years in pain from arthritis or diabetic nerve damage, stooped over from osteoporosis, demented from Alzheimer's, or fatigued and breathless from heart failure.

The ills we just listed aren't unrelated. In fact, you'll be amazed to learn how very much they have in common. In recent years we've come to understand that many or even most ailments and diseases develop as a result of a small handful of disease processes. Let one or more of them go on too long, and you're almost certain to get sick.

Fortunately, every one of these processes can be reversed—think of it as pressing the biological rewind button. Of course, you won't *be* younger as a result (no one's invented the time machine yet, after all), but by undoing accumulated damage you'll feel younger and be more resistant to age-related chronic diseases. And in our minds that's almost as good.

In this section, we've focused on the six disease processes that cause the most trouble. We've coined them Super Threats, for that is what they truly are—the ultimate threats to your health and well-being at the most basic level.

To understand how the Super Threats contribute to disease, picture how a really bad day typically unfolds. It's not usually one doom-and-gloom thing that goes wrong, but a series of problems that build on the one before. Say you went to bed too late, which caused you to oversleep in the morning; as you sped to work, you got in a fender bender, which made you late for a meeting, which lost you an important client. Losing the client is the end result of a chain reaction that started with a lack of sleep. Likewise, most chronic diseases result from chain reactions involving the six Super Threats. Reverse even one of these Super Threats, and you change the whole outcome for the better.

At this point you may be wondering, Isn't my fate already sealed by my genes? Certainly your genes play a role in your health—but they don't operate in a vacuum. If you have a genetic risk for colon cancer, for instance, it's the foods you eat and other everyday habits you choose that determine whether that risk becomes a reality or just a note for your medical record. Research has proved that in most cases, especially by middle age, your lifestyle plays a much bigger role in your health than your genes do.

Our goal with this section is to show you how the six Super Threats are intimately connected with the health problems that plague us as we age, and how you can combat each one with simple lifestyle changes. In the process you'll slash your risk of just about every major ailment from heart disease and stroke to diabetes, certain cancers, and Alzheimer's disease and other forms of dementia. Follow our advice here and you'll also feel better, have more energy, and live longer (most likely). You'll also slow the aging-related processes that contribute to less serious conditions such as wrinkles.

We've devoted a separate chapter to each Super Threat. Each chapter includes a description of the Super Threat, a list of tests that can help you determine your own risk level in that area, a list of conditions directly related to the Super Threat, and most important, our best strategies for combating the threat. Finally, we help you start using these strategies in our 7-Day Super Protection Plan. Follow it and you'll begin to reduce all six Super Threats in just one week.

The 6 Super Threats at a Glance

1. Chronic inflammation

Inflammation is a natural part of the immune response to illness, injury, or other threats, but it can cause damage throughout the body if it goes on too long.

2. Oxidative stress

Unstable molecules called free radicals damage healthy cells in the process known as oxidation, similar to rusting. Oxidation speeds aging and contributes to diseases.

3. Insulin resistance

When cells are resistant to insulin, the body can't process blood sugar properly. Glucose and insulin build up in the blood, increasing inflammation and oxidative damage.

4. Immune stress

When your immune system is overwhelmed or weakened by internal or external forces, your health suffers. Immune stress also taxes your body's detoxification system and increases inflammation and oxidative damage.

5. Elevated stress hormones

When you are under chronic stress, your body releases large amounts of stress hormones that can damage your health, trigger inflammation, increase the risk of insulin resistance, and create oxidative stress.

6. Toxin exposure

Toxins are anything that the body needs to break down or detoxify. Your body's ability to get rid of toxins is critical to overall health. Otherwise, inflammation and oxidative stress increase and the immune system suffers.

Chronic Inflammation

If there is one main villain to point to in the cascade of events that age us, it's inflammation. "Inflammation is probably the background and driving force behind all major age-related diseases," said Claudio Franceschi, M.D., to a *Time* magazine reporter in 2003. Franceschi, scientific director at the Italian National Research Center on Aging in Ancona, coordinated a major study on people ages 100 and older.

Franceschi was one of the first scientists to emphasize the importance of inflammation, or "inflam-aging" as he called it, as a major contributor to numerous chronic diseases of aging. When he first put forth his groundbreaking theory in the early 1990s, it raised eyebrows for sure. But today a mounting pile of compelling evidence reveals the role of inflammation in everything from Alzheimer's disease to osteoporosis, from heart disease to cancer, rheumatoid arthritis, allergies, and asthma. In other words, it looks like Franceschi was right.

But what the heck *is* inflammation? And why is it implicated in so many diseases?

Answering the Alarm

In short, inflammation is a side effect of the immune system at work.

Whenever there's any challenge to your body—a cut from a kitchen knife, invasion by a cold virus, even emotional stress—your immune system sets off an alarm, a cry for help, initiating a cascade of events. Various cells rush to the damaged site to deal with the perceived injury or irritation. Inflammatory chemicals flood the system, performing various roles—increasing blood flow to the area under attack, making blood vessels "leaky" so help can get to the trouble spot faster, and making blood stickier and more ready to clot (to stem the bleeding from that cut, for instance).

Think of this process as the first response to potential disaster. As with any disaster response, the normal rules and regulations are relaxed (think of a fire truck bombing down the road at way past the speed limit, running red lights and possibly even endangering other motorists in the process) to get the greatest help to the most people as quickly as possible.

RELATED AILMENTS

Inflammation is both a cause and a consequence of a host of diseases. Following the anti-inflammatory diet and the recommendations outlined here will help you manage and/or prevent the following:

- Acne
- Allergies
- Alzheimer's disease
- Asthma
- Bursitis and tendinitis
- Cancer (some)
- Carpal tunnel syndrome
- Congestive heart failure
- Coronary artery disease
- Dandruff
- Diabetes (type 2)
- Diverticulitis
- Eczema
- Endometriosis
- Fibromyalgia
- Gum disease
- Hepatitis
- Herpes
- High blood pressure
- High cholesterol
- Hives
- Inflammatory bowel disease (IBD)
- Lupus
- Menstrual cramps
- Obesity
- Osteoporosis
- Parkinson's disease
- Peripheral vascular disease
- Premenstrual syndrome
- Psoriasis
- Rheumatoid arthritis
- Rosacea
- Sinusitis and sinus infection

Things usually return to normal after the disaster is over, but not so with chronic inflammation. The response to the fire never stops. Now, instead of solving problems, the response team is just creating new ones.

The "fire" can be just about anything. Sometimes an infection you don't even know you have can trigger low-level, chronic inflammation. One culprit is *H. pylori*, the bacterium linked to most ulcers. Another is the bacterium that causes gum disease. And it's not just bacteria that trigger inflammation. Anything that irritates the body, such as smoking, or the blood vessels, such as high blood pressure, also leads to inflammation.

Lingering Havoc in the Body

Chronic inflammation wreaks all sorts of trouble throughout the body, even if you don't know you have it. That's partly because even while inflammation serves a purpose, the process can also damage healthy cells. If inflammation strikes your arteries—maybe in response to bacteria that don't belong there, or even to assaults from cholesterol particles attempting to burrow into artery walls—it can eventually damage the arteries, making them more prone to heart disease.

Once you have heart disease, inflammation makes it worse. It makes the sticky plaque lining arteries less stable and more likely to break off. Small pieces can lodge in a narrow artery and block blood flow to the heart. Rupturing plaque also triggers yet more inflammation as your immune system seeks to repair the injury. This can lead to blood clots on top of the plaque, further narrowing the artery and possibly causing a heart attack.

It turns out that inflammation plays such a strong role in heart disease that it is actually just as dangerous as—or even more dangerous than—traditional risk factors like high cholesterol.

Once the inflammation becomes established or escapes normal controls, it doesn't necessarily stay where it started, but may spread throughout your system. In the liver, uncontrolled inflammation can cause scarring, or cirrhosis. We also think inflammation is behind many brain diseases in the elderly, like Alzheimer's. When researchers tracked 1,050 men over 25 years as part of the Honolulu-Asia Aging Study, they found that men with the highest levels of C-reactive protein (CRP), a protein that indicates inflammation, were three times more likely to develop dementia than those with the lowest levels.

Chronic inflammation is also linked to certain cancers. For instance, people with a history of inflammatory bowel disease have a much higher risk of developing colorectal cancer. And certain other cancers, such as gallbladder, stomach, and ovarian cancer, appear to be associated with bacterial or viral infections that trigger ongoing inflammation.

Inflammation gets worse as you get older because your body starts producing more hormones that promote inflammation and fewer hormones that keep it in check.

If it seems like inflammation is a process that's simply out of your control, take heart. Although there's not much you can do to protect yourself from a rogue virus or bacteria, there is much you can do to protect yourself from the kind of chronic, low-level inflammation that is most likely to lead to the diseases of aging.

Three Common Causes of Inflammation

Remember, the six Super Threats are closely interrelated. Many of the five Super Threats you have yet to read about, like oxidation and chronic stress, also contribute to inflammation. By combating them, you'll also combat inflammation. But there are three triggers of inflammation we want to point out here.

Belly Fat

Abdominal fat, the kind that gives men their "beer belly" and women their "apple" shape, isn't like other fat. Unlike the stuff that pads your hips or thighs, this fat actually secretes hormones and inflammatory chemicals. In other words, it actively contributes to inflammation.

Inflammation triggered by abdominal fat may be the reason overweight people are more likely to develop heart disease, arthritis, and high blood pressure, among other conditions. It's probably also why studies find that extremely low-calorie diets seem to extend longevity in humans and

---

Inflammation and Smoking

Smoking wreaks havoc in numerous ways, but inflammation may be one of the most devastating. Experts now think smoking does its dirty work in large part by inflaming artery walls. One study found that when smokers quit, markers of inflammation remained elevated even after other health numbers, such as cholesterol and blood pressure, went down. But eventually the inflammation does subside. In the study, inflammatory markers returned to normal within five years after the smokers quit.

---

animals—fewer calories means less abdominal fat, which means less inflammation.

Want to know if your belly fat is within the "safe" range? Take a tape measure and, starting at your belly button, wrap it around your waist. A measurement of less than 30 inches is considered ideal for women, less than 35 inches is good. Less than 35 inches is ideal for men, less than 40 inches is good. For an even better sense of your level of risk, figure your waist-to-hip-ratio. Divide your waist measurement by your hip measurement to get your ratio. For men, a ratio of .95 or less is best; for women, .80 or less is best.

You already know the formula for managing your weight—eat fewer calories and exercise more. You can find specific approaches to weight loss in Obesity on page 291. Remember, when you lose weight, you lose it from your belly first—a good incentive to start.

Inflammatory Foods

Your diet contributes to inflammation in more ways than one. Yes, if you eat too much you'll develop belly fat that, as you've just read, triggers inflammation. But certain foods cause inflammation more directly. The main culprits are saturated fat (the kind in meat, poultry, and dairy), most vegetable oils, and trans fat (man-made stuff that keeps processed foods like crackers, cookies, and cakes shelf stable). These contain or promote the production of inflammatory chemicals. Trans fats are the worst, and the easiest to eradicate from your diet simply by staying away from processed foods whenever possible (or at least check labels for the word "hydrogenated" and avoid buying products that contain it).

Inflammation from food wouldn't be such a problem if we ate what our ancestors did—fresh foods high in fiber and vegetable matter. When they did eat meat, it was less likely to cause inflammation than today's meat. That's because their animals grazed on grass and other vegetable matter critical to the formation of omega-3 fatty acids, which counter inflammation. (These fatty acids make up the "good" fats in fish.) Today's cattle are fed on corn and are lower in omega-3s and higher in omega-6s, fatty acids that promote inflammation.

Even as late as the early 1900s the ratio of omega-6 to omega-3 fatty acids in the typical American diet was about 4:1—not bad. Today, however, with our increased consumption of processed foods, the ratio is closer to 25:1—way out of whack.

GETTING TESTED

The following tests can provide information on your level of inflammation. You can ask your doctor for the CRP or the "sed rate" tests, which are common; the others are more specialized tests your doctor might order to investigate the cause or degree of inflammation if inflammation is known to be present.

C-reactive protein (CRP). This simple blood test measures levels of CRP, a protein that serves as a marker for inflammation. Numerous studies find that the higher the level of CRP, the greater your risk of a heart attack. In fact, CRP may be even more predictive of heart problems than cholesterol. The evidence is so strong that the American Heart Association and other medical organizations recommend you have your CRP levels measured if you have any other risk factors for heart disease (such as being overweight, smoking, having diabetes, etc.). Eventually the CRP test could also be used to warn of illnesses such as colon cancer and dementia. With a few lifestyle changes like those noted here, your CRP levels could drop in as little as two to four weeks.

Erythrocyte sedimentation rate. Also called ESR or "sed rate," this test measures how fast red blood cells cling together, fall, and settle (like sediment) in the bottom of a glass tube during an hour. The higher the sed rate, the more inflammation. Although this is a good test to use for inflammatory diseases like inflammatory bowel disease or lupus, it is not as helpful as CRP for identifying the existence of an underlying inflammatory process that leads to an increased risk of heart disease or accompanies diabetes.

Omega-3 profile. This test, also called the "silent inflammation profile," measures the ratio of pro-inflammatory fatty acids (omega-6s) to anti-inflammatory fatty acids (omega-3s) in your blood. Remember, you should aim for a 4:1 ratio. You will probably have to find a specialized laboratory that does nutritional testing to get this test. Check with an integrative medicine provider, or even the nutrition department of an academic medical center.

Fasting insulin levels. High levels of insulin are a sign of insulin resistance and/or overproduction of insulin, either of which could be the result of inflammation. Both are risk factors for diabetes and heart disease.

Food and environmental allergy tests. It's possible to have allergies and not know it. Since allergies increase low-grade inflammation, it's worth getting an allergy test (blood or skin prick) to see where you stand.

Your diet also affects the inflammatory process in other ways. For instance, a diet high in animal products (at least those that are not organic) usually brings with it "toxins" like hormones and antibiotics that trigger an immune response and, you guessed it, inflammation. Red meat, especially if it's cooked over high heat, may also contain cancer-causing toxins, which again, trigger an immune response that causes inflammation. And if you're eating a lot of red meat, chances are you're not eating much fish or plant-based foods—so you're missing out on valuable omega-3 fatty acids and antioxidants, which help counter the effects of inflammation.

Lack of Sleep

When's the last time you had a good night's sleep? Probably on your last vacation (assuming your hotel room was far enough away from the

Best Remedies FOR CHRONIC INFLAMMATION

Diet

Eat fatty fish at least twice a week. It's high in omega-3 fatty acids, which counter inflammation. Good choices are salmon, tuna, sardines, mackerel, halibut, and anchovies. Purchase wild fish rather than farmed fish if possible; it's richer in omega-3s.

Use more olive oil, canola oil, and flaxseed oil. These are high in omega-3s. Olive oil contains an anti-inflammatory component so strong that researchers liken it to aspirin. It may be why people who follow the Mediterranean diet have such low rates of heart disease.

Cut back on regular margarine and most vegetable oils, including corn, cottonseed, peanut, safflower, sesame, soybean, and sunflower oil. All of these are high in pro-inflammatory omega-6 fatty acids. (Margarine that contains no trans fats or hydrogenated oil is okay.)

Weed out trans fats from your diet. These "partially hydrogenated oils" are rampant in packaged and fried foods. The FDA now requires that all food labels list trans fats.

Limit animal fat, especially red meat.

Sprinkle 1 tablespoon ground flaxseed (a fabulous source of omega-3 fatty acids) over salads, yogurt, and cereal at least once a day.

Snack on walnuts and pumpkin seeds (up to an ounce a day) and steamed soybeans (edamame).

Buy omega-3 enriched eggs.

Eat at least two servings of dark leafy greens a day (1/2 cup of spinach counts as one serving). They're high in folic acid and other B vitamins, which reduce levels of an inflammatory marker called homocysteine, and they're good sources of antioxidants, which reduce the oxidation that can cause inflammation (more on this in the next chapter).

elevator). Well, those restless nights are doing more than cause bags under your eyes. During sleep, physical as well as mental restoration occurs. This rest time allows your body to catch up with tasks like clearing toxins, for example, which, in turn, can reduce ongoing inflammation.

A growing body of evidence points to short-term sleep deprivation as a culprit in inflammation. Studies find increased levels of inflammatory chemicals in people deprived of sleep for several days. People with sleep apnea, a condition in which you stop breathing dozens or even hundreds of times in the night, never getting the kind of restorative sleep so critical to health, also have increased levels of inflammatory chemicals.

All of which could explain why people with painful conditions like osteoarthritis, chronic fatigue syndrome, fibromyalgia, and rheumatoid arthritis find their pain gets worse if they don't get enough sleep.

Include berries, red wine, and dark chocolate in your diet. All protect against inflammation.

Eat a variety of fruits and vegetables so you get a broad spectrum of antioxidants.

Drink several cups of black or green tea a day or take the equivalent amount in supplements for its anti-inflammatory effects.

Buy organic. Limit your exposure to pesticides and hormones that can trigger inflammation by buying organic produce (especially berries) and free-range poultry.

Lifestyle

Avoid allergens, particularly foods you may be allergic to.

Get 7 to 8 hours of sleep a night.

Lose weight if you're overweight.

Consider weekly acupuncture. Studies find that it can help reduce inflammation.

If you smoke, quit.

Exercise

Exercise at least 30 minutes a day. Studies find this much exercise can suppress low-level inflammation. Just don't overdo it—too much intense exercise could actually cause inflammation.

Medicine

Take a baby aspirin (81 milligrams) every day after you get your doctor's okay. Aspirin curbs inflammation.

Clear up existing infections, such as gum disease, ulcers, etc. If you have an ulcer caused by the *H. pylori* bacterium, your doctor should prescribe antibiotics.

Oxidative Stress

You'll hear a lot throughout *Best Remedies* about oxidation and free radicals. And we've made oxidative stress our second Super Threat. What in the world are we talking about?

Anytime any of your cells complete chemical reactions or make energy (which they have to do in order for you to live), they create by-products in the form of molecules called free radicals. These by-products are similar to the exhaust a car's engine creates when it uses gasoline for energy. Just as the exhaust pollutes the air, the free radicals pollute your body—even though, in a cruel twist of nature, you literally can't breathe without making them. This pollution stresses the body's capacity to keep itself healthy.

Free radicals do their harm by assaulting healthy cells. Their goal? Stealing an electron to replace one they're missing. (In case you don't remember your high school chemistry, an electron is a tiny, tiny particle with a negative charge). In the process, they create more free radicals. They also damage cells and, by extension, the surrounding tissue in a process called oxidation. This is the same process, by the way,

that rusts metal and turns the surface of a cut apple brown.

But in your body oxidation does much worse things. For instance, it can lead to heart disease. How? By turning otherwise relatively benign cholesterol particles floating in the bloodstream into dangerous enemies by making them more likely to stick to artery walls. Once they've made their

RELATED AILMENTS

- Allergies
- Alzheimer's disease
- Asthma
- Congestive heart failure
- Coronary artery disease
- Diabetes (type 2)
- Fibromyalgia
- Glaucoma
- High blood pressure
- High cholesterol
- Infertility, female
- Infertility, male
- Insulin resistance syndrome
- Macular degeneration
- Memory problems
- Menstrual cramps (dysmenorrhea)
- Muscle soreness
- Parkinson's disease
- Peripheral vascular disease
- PMS
- Rheumatoid arthritis

assault on the artery wall, the immune system has to go after them, setting in motion a process that brings on inflammation—which speeds the formation of plaque and paves the way for heart attacks and strokes.

Oxidation also eats away at the cartilage that cushions your joints. It can even damage a cell's DNA. Ideally, your immune system should recognize these damaged cells and head in for the kill, but sometimes it doesn't, and the cells keep dividing, creating more and more damaged cells that eventually become a cancer. The reason high levels of radiation sometimes lead to cancer is that radiation increases free radicals.

Oxidative damage can also contribute to Parkinson's disease. The hallmark of this disease is a lack of the neurotransmitter dopamine. Oxidation disrupts the function of a protein involved in the production of dopamine.

Free radicals are even culprits behind gum disease. That might not sound like a very big deal, but since gum disease is also linked with higher rates of heart disease, lung disease, and diabetes (all connected by Super Threat #1, inflammation), it really is. The immune response to the bacteria responsible for gum disease probably triggers increased free radicals.

Antioxidants to the Rescue

Fortunately, nature's not dumb. It has a defense for free radicals: antioxidants. These molecules have a chemical structure that allows them to absorb free radicals, rendering them harmless.

Your own body produces certain antioxidants. Others come from food. You probably recognize many of the names—especially vitamins E, C, and A. There's also beta-carotene, minerals like selenium, enzymes like glutathione and coenzyme Q_{10} (CoQ_{10}), and dozens or even hundreds of others (they haven't all been discovered yet).

> ## Highest-Antioxidant Foods
>
> Which foods have the strongest antioxidant powers? These 20 top the USDA's list.
>
> 1. Dried red beans
> 2. Wild blueberries
> 3. Dried red kidney beans
> 4. Pinto beans
> 5. Farmed blueberries
> 6. Cranberries
> 7. Artichokes
> 8. Blackberries
> 9. Prunes
> 10. Raspberries
> 11. Strawberries
> 12. Red Delicious apples*
> 13. Granny Smith apples*
> 14. Pecans
> 15. Sweet cherries
> 16. Black plums
> 17. Russet potatoes*
> 18. Dried black beans
> 19. Plums
> 20. Gala apples*
>
> *Eat the skin—that's where the bulk of the antioxidants are.

Unfortunately, as we age, our body produces fewer antioxidants. Stress also depletes our supply, as do certain medications like acetaminophen (Tylenol) and the cholesterol-lowering drugs known as statins. So do alcohol and cigarettes. In fact, smoking is a one of the strongest known destroyers of antioxidants. In a double whammy, cigarette smoke also contains toxins that increase the production of free radicals, requiring more antioxidants to neutralize them.

Finally, since most of the antioxidants in our diets come from fruits and vegetables—and since most of us don't eat enough of them—most of us get far fewer antioxidants from our food than we should.

No problem, you're thinking. I'll just take some antioxidant supplements. Not so fast! For some reason—and we're not sure why—getting antioxidants from supplements just doesn't provide the same benefits as eating antioxidant-rich foods. That doesn't mean you should forget about supplements; we still recommend them throughout the book, and we feel strongly that everyone should take a good multivitamin/mineral supplement every day. But if you want to prevent or reduce your risk of numerous chronic health conditions, including heart disease, stroke, cancer, and Alzheimer's disease, you should look to your diet first for help.

One likely reason that foods do what supplements can't is that antioxidants, as with most things in nature, work best together. Like players on a team, each has something a little different to contribute. And thanks to teamwork, teams can typically accomplish more together than any one player can accomplish alone. Only a diet rich in a variety of healthy foods can put the whole team to work for you.

The effects can be powerful. For instance, one study found that people who eat a lot of foods rich in vitamin E, like nuts, olive oil, egg yolks, and whole grains, had a 70 percent lower risk of developing Alzheimer's than people who don't. Another example: Numerous population studies have found that people who eat foods rich in beta-carotene have much lower rates of lung cancer than people who don't.

When scientists tried to duplicate this effect in cancer prevention studies using beta-carotene supplements, the results were, to say the least, disappointing. Researchers had to halt the trials early when they learned that beta-carotene

Best Remedies FOR OXIDATIVE STRESS

Diet

Cut out fried foods. The heat and saturated fat used to fry food creates pro-oxidant substances in the food.

Cut out trans fatty acids. These fats are very oxidative, not to mention really bad for your arteries.

Load up on fruits and vegetables (9 servings a day is ideal). This is where you'll get the majority of your antioxidants. Don't panic, we're not talking about truckloads of vegetables; one serving equals one piece of fruit, 1/2 cup of raw, cooked, canned or frozen fruits or vegetables, or one cup of raw, leafy vegetables like lettuce or spinach.

Drink green or black tea instead of coffee. They're full of powerful antioxidants called polyphenols. Coffee also contains antioxidants, but none as powerful.

Have a glass of red wine every day (if you have no alcohol-related problems or high blood pressure).

The polyphenols in red wine, grape juice, and pomegranate juice are powerful antioxidants, and the alcohol itself seems to reduce the risk of blood clots and inflammation. If you don't want to drink alcohol, consider drinking the same amount of dark Concord grape juice instead. A University of California-Davis study found drinking a glass a day for two weeks significantly increased the ability of LDL cholesterol to resist oxidation.

Drink 1 to 2 ounces of concentrated pomegranate juice a day. A study published in 2005 found the juice reduced the buildup of fatty plaque on coronary arteries in mice, and improved the health of human heart cells in the laboratory. Other fruit juices, including orange juice, also contain antioxidants. Stay away from juice with lots of sugar or corn syrup, though.

Follow a low-glycemic diet. We explain this in more detail in the chapter on insulin resistance (page 48), but basically this means loading up on

GETTING TESTED

How do you know if you're under oxidative stress? Well, if you're alive in the modern world, assume you are. Breathing, eating, and just about everything else result in free-radical production. The key is balancing those free radicals with enough antioxidants, from your own body's supply and from food.

Unfortunately, there aren't any commonly performed tests that measure levels of antioxidants in your blood; the tests that are available are used only in research settings. However, if you're suffering from any chronic disease or are under any physical or emotional stress, it's a safe bet that you need to increase your antioxidant intake.

---

supplements not only didn't prevent lung cancer in people at high risk for the disease, but appeared to *increase* rates of the disease, particularly among smokers. It turns out that by itself, without the benefit of other antioxidants found in fruits and vegetables, beta-carotene actually acts as an oxidant, *increasing* the production of free radicals.

So, while we do recommend a multivitamin, and we sometimes recommend antioxidant supplements in some of our Best Remedies, we'll say it again: Your diet is what's most important.

---

high-fiber foods including whole fruits and vegetables (with the skin included whenever possible). It also means avoiding processed foods, sweets, and "white" foods like white rice, white bread, and white pasta. These foods increase your blood sugar quickly, producing a corresponding increase in free radicals. Eventually you may develop insulin resistance, and this in turn increases oxidative stress.

Reduce calories. By eating less food you'll produce fewer free radicals. Of course, we don't want you to starve—but most of us could stand to eat a little less.

Use honey as a sweetener instead of sugar. Honey contains powerful antioxidants.

Exercise

Stay physically active. About 30 to 60 minutes of moderate exercise a day is ideal. This amount induces a mild oxidative stress that stimulates your body's production of antioxidants.

Supplements

Take a multivitamin/mineral every day to ensure you're getting adequate antioxidants and other nutrients. That's not just our opinion. That's the opinion of Harvard researchers writing in a landmark article published in the *Journal of the American Medical Association* in 2002. They noted that most people don't get the optimal amount of vitamins through their food. (As we've said already, this doesn't get your diet off the hook; you still need to eat lots of fruits and vegetables.) *Note:* If you're a man or you're a woman who's no longer menstruating, pick a multivitamin that does not contain iron.

Take a separate vitamin C/flavonoid supplement even if your multivitamin contains vitamin C. This is especially important if you're a smoker or you're under significant physical or emotional stress, which increases the body's usage of antioxidants. Take 500 milligrams once or twice a day.

Insulin Resistance

Picture a line of people waiting to get into a shelter to give hungry people food. Unfortunately, the doorknob on the front door is broken, so the people are left standing in the street. As more and more people arrive to help, the crowd grows, with nowhere to go. Their arms are full of food, but the people inside go hungry.

That's a little bit like what happens with insulin resistance. In this condition, the body's cells stop responding as quickly or completely as they should to the hormone insulin, produced by the pancreas. Insulin—the doorknob—is supposed to "open" cells so that blood sugar (glucose), the body's main source of fuel, can get in. In an attempt to solve the problem, the body produces more insulin, but that doesn't do much good. So both blood sugar and insulin build up in the bloodstream. Over time, the insulin-producing cells in the pancreas wear out from all the effort, and you develop full-blown type 2 diabetes.

What does all this have to do with aging? Quite a lot.

First, we tend to become more insulin resistant as we age. That's just a fact, and while we have lots of theories, we don't know exactly why.

Second, insulin resistance and high blood sugar both contribute to inflammation. That may be one reason why older people tend to have more inflammation than younger people do. It also contributes to oxidation (we *told* you, the Super Threats are hopelessly intertwined!). In fact, common complications of diabetes once thought to be the result of long-term damage from high blood sugar, including eye and nerve problems and heart and kidney disease, are now also thought to result from oxidative damage caused by high insulin levels.

Researchers are starting to explore other links between high insulin levels and chronic diseases. For instance, there's some evidence that insulin resistance may contribute to Alzheimer's disease. For one thing, unlike muscle tissue, the brain doesn't store glucose; it needs a steady, constant supply to function properly. With insulin resistance, that doesn't happen, and brain cells become damaged. Second, insulin helps regulate a protein indirectly associated with the development of protein clumps in the brain that are typical of Alzheimer's. Too much insulin means too much of the protein.

Another danger of insulin resistance: People who have it tend to be overweight, which causes its own set of problems involving many of the Super Threats. At the same time, in another cruel twist, insulin resistance makes it harder to lose weight because the excess blood sugar with nowhere to go eventually gets stored in—you guessed it—fat cells. Adding insult to injury, excess insulin may even stimulate your appetite.

All in all, insulin resistance is pretty darn bad for your health. Consider the results of this study from Stanford University. For six years the researchers followed 208 people who started out perfectly healthy, with normal blood sugar and insulin levels. At the end of the study, 70 percent of those who developed the greatest insulin resistance also developed chronic diseases such as high blood pressure, cancer, heart disease, stroke, and type 2 diabetes. None of those with normal insulin resistance had any sign of chronic disease.

Why We're Insulin Resistant

The causes of insulin resistance are many, but being overweight is a big one. Blame those fat cells. They are stuffed with fatty acids created from excess blood sugar. These fatty acids keep insulin from working normally in muscle, fat, and liver tissue.

As we've mentioned earlier, the worst type of fat—both a cause and an effect of insulin resistance—is the fat around your middle. It doesn't take much to improve the situation, though. Studies find losing as little as 10 pounds can significantly reduce insulin resistance.

To see if you need to lose belly fat, check your hip-to-waist ratio. While standing, measure your waist in inches at its smallest point. Don't pull in your stomach or hold your breath. Write the number down. Now measure your hips in inches at the widest point. Divide your waist measurement by your hip measurement to determine your hip-to-waist ratio. It should be about .80 for women, and .95 for men.

Other causes of insulin resistance include:

Lack of exercise. Too much sitting is one of the biggest risk factors for insulin resistance. Conversely, exercise, particularly strength training, is one of the best ways to prevent or treat it.

Here's how it works. When you start exercising, your muscles need extra fuel, so your body sends a signal to the liver to begin releasing stored glucose. That supply gets used up pretty quickly, though, so your body turns to other sources for energy—namely fat cells. Fat cells release glucose by breaking down fatty acids, the stuff they're filled with. Voilà! Less fat.

Exercise also forces your body to work harder in order to get blood sugar into cells, lowering your blood sugar level. It also lowers your blood sugar another way: If you exercise often enough, your body will actually grow new blood vessels to bring more oxygen and nutrients—and blood sugar—to muscles, leaving less blood sugar floating in the bloodstream.

Lack of sleep. Given that the average American gets less than seven hours of sleep a night (15 percent get less than six), it's safe to say we're a sleep-deprived nation. Some researchers think that may be the reason behind the growing epidemic of insulin resistance and its kissing cousin, metabolic syndrome.

The links between sleep and blood sugar first surfaced in the late 1990s, when researchers at the University of Chicago found that depriving healthy young men of a good night's sleep raised their blood sugar almost to diabetic levels. Later studies by the same group found that lack of sleep significantly increased insulin resistance in healthy adults, putting them at risk for diabetes and other health problems. Meanwhile, a Harvard Medical School study published in 2003 found that women who slept five or fewer hours a day were nearly a third more likely to develop diabetes.

No one knows why too little sleep affects blood sugar levels, but there are some theories.

GETTING TESTED

Several tests can measure blood sugar and insulin levels. Ask your doctor which ones, if any, are appropriate for you. If you have a history of diabetes in your family, and abnormal scores on any of these tests, take the results seriously. You're already at high risk for diabetes because of your genetic background; the fact that your levels are even a little abnormal may indicate you're on your way to a problem, even if they're not bad enough to suggest you already have insulin resistance or diabetes.

Fasting blood glucose levels. This blood test measures your blood sugar level after you fast overnight.

Fasting insulin. Your insulin level is measured after you've fasted overnight.

Insulin sensitivity test (IST). During this test, you receive an intravenous infusion of a glucose solution and insulin over three hours, along with a drug to prevent your body from releasing its own insulin. Blood samples are taken during the three hours to determine your insulin sensitivity.

Insulin tolerance test (ITT). This is a simplified version of the IST (above). It measures the decline in blood levels of glucose after a large, intravenous dose of insulin. Several insulin and glucose levels are taken over the next 15 minutes.

Oral glucose tolerance test (OGTT). In this test you drink a sugar solution and your glucose and insulin levels are measured at various intervals over the next two to four hours.

Postprandial testing. Your blood glucose levels are tested two hours after a meal.

One theory is that the quantity and quality of your sleep affects your body's ability to control the release of various hormones like insulin. Another theory is that lack of sleep increases two hormones that boost appetite, so you eat more. That may be one reason studies also find that chronically shortchanging your sleep puts on the pounds. Insulin resistance is also linked with sleep apnea and other sleep-related breathing disorders, although no one's sure which is the chicken and which is the egg.

Simple carbohydrates. We're not recommending the Atkins diet, but it's true that certain low-carb, high-protein diets tend to reduce insulin resistance. That's because unlike carbohydrates, protein and fat don't raise your blood sugar or insulin level.

Not all high-protein diets are created equal, though. Diets that focus on fatty foods like bacon, steak, and cheese are full of saturated fats—which *increase* insulin resistance. So make sure most of your protein comes instead from fish, beans, and lean poultry.

Bonus: Diets high in protein, fiber, and healthy monounsaturated fat (the kind of fat in olive oil, nuts, and avocados) also raise levels of "good" cholesterol and reduce blood fats called triglycerides, a risk factor for heart disease, in most people.

Notice we mentioned fiber. That's right, the rough stuff in whole grains, whole fruits, and vegetables—and yes, these are carbohydrate foods. The point isn't to avoid all carbs. Rather, be selective about which carbs you eat. Shun the simple carbs, those that come with little fiber, like fruit juices, white bread and pasta, doughnuts, chips, etc. These are the ones that tend to contribute most to insulin resistance.

Fruits and vegetables, on the other hand, help control or prevent it, in part by providing critical antioxidants. The antioxidant pigments found in yellow, orange, and red fruits and veggies have been found to reduce fasting insulin levels. In one study, people who consumed plenty of beta-carotene, one of these pigments, were less likely to develop insulin resistance.

Chronic stress. When we're under stress, our bodies release "stress" hormones that increase blood sugar. The system is designed to get fuel to muscles fast in case we need to fight or flee. In the short term it works just fine, but when stress stays high, so do blood sugar and insulin levels.

You can't eliminate all the stress in your life, but you can reduce its effects on your body. Using stress management techniques like deep breathing can significantly improve blood sugar and insulin levels by reducing stress hormones.

Mineral deficiencies. Low levels of certain minerals, particularly chromium, calcium, and vanadium, may increase the risk of insulin resistance or make existing insulin resistance worse. Supplementing with these minerals can help.

Smoking. Cigarettes and even nicotine products like the patch and nicotine gum have been linked with insulin resistance.

Low levels of vitamin D. A study in the *American Journal of Clinical Nutrition* found that the lower the level of vitamin D in apparently healthy young people, the higher their insulin resistance. See our advice under "Best Remedies for Insulin Resistance," below.

Best Remedies FOR INSULIN RESISTANCE

To reduce your risk of insulin resistance, or improve your cells' ability to use insulin if you already have it, follow these Best Remedies:

Exercise

Get at least 30 to 60 minutes of physical activity a day. At least two days a week, do some form of resistance exercise (such as weightlifting, Pilates, or calisthenics).

Diet

Eat six small meals a day rather than three large meals. This reduces blood sugar spikes (and can help you lose weight), especially if you include a protein and/or healthy fat source with each meal.

Minimize processed or "white" foods in your diet, including white bread and white pasta.

Add more "whole foods" to your diet, particularly orange, yellow, and red fruits and vegetables.

Aim to get at least 25 grams of fiber a day. This shouldn't be difficult if you're following the other recommendations here. Use a fiber supplement if for

some reason you really can't manage to get enough fiber into your diet.

Reduce the amount of saturated fat in your diet by favoring protein sources like fish and beans over red meat and full-fat dairy.

Increase the amount of "good" fat in your diet in the form of fish, olive oil, omega-enriched eggs, nuts, avocados, etc.

Lifestyle

If you smoke, quit.

Supplements

If you're at increased risk for insulin resistance, take 200 micrograms chromium picolinate, 1,500 milligrams calcium, and 100 milligrams vanadium daily (no more; higher levels could be dangerous).

Take at least 400 IU vitamin D as part of a daily multivitamin or calcium supplement, up to 800 IU. You need more of this vitamin as you age. If you're over 70, aim for 600 IU a day.

Super Threat #4
Immune Stress

You learned in the chapter on inflammation (Super Threat #1) that an immune response is, surprisingly, a double-edged sword, creating inflammation even as it repairs damaged tissue and rids the body of bacteria and viruses. But of course you can't live without an immune system. There would be no way to destroy mutated cells that could lead to cancer, no way to keep infections in check, no way, in fact, to even eat an apple without putting yourself in grave danger. Your immune system is your personal defense system, ready to deploy the "troops" when a threat arrives. If it's weak, you're in trouble.

Consider this: Autopsies find that the major cause of death in the elderly is not cancer or heart disease, but an increased susceptibility to infection. For instance, one study found that death rates from pneumonia, influenza, bronchitis, and gastroenteritis increased with age, whereas death rates from various cancers and stroke remained the same or decreased.

That's because our immune system, like many other parts of our body, weakens as we age. This is why older people generally don't respond as well

to vaccinations as younger people, and why the vaccines they get may not last as long. A weakened immune system explains why something like West Nile virus may feel like a mild case of the flu to a 30-year-old, but kill a 70-year-old.

Even if you're young, it's important to maintain a strong immune system. First, to have a strong starting point as you age. Second, to ward off

❦ Helpful Hint

Check Your Meds

Numerous medications can play havoc with your immune system. While some drugs like corticosteroids are *supposed* to suppress your immune system, others that might affect it include antibiotics, antipsychotics, antidepressants, anticonvulsants, blood pressure medications, and H_2 blockers. You'll be amazed to know that even anti-inflammatory painkillers (such as aspirin and ibuprofen) may suppress the immune system with chronic use and/or at high doses, at least in susceptible people.

RELATED AILMENTS

- Allergies
- Alzheimer's disease
- Asthma
- Athlete's foot
- Bronchitis
- Canker sores
- Chronic fatigue syndrome
- Colds
- Cold sores
- Conjunctivitis
- Coronary artery disease
- Ear infection
- Eczema
- Fatigue
- Fibromyalgia
- Flu
- Gum disease
- Hepatitis
- Herpes
- HIV/AIDS
- Inflammatory bowel disease
- Lyme disease
- Rheumatoid arthritis
- Shingles
- Sinusitis and sinus infection
- Ulcers
- Urinary tract infection
- Warts
- Yeast infection

infections that can increase inflammation and free-radical production—Super Threats that lead to chronic disease.

Take heart disease, for instance. We talked earlier about the role of inflammation in the buildup of plaque on artery walls. Researchers now think that chronic bacterial or viral infections may contribute to chronic inflammation by triggering an immune response (which, as you remember, involves inflammation). In fact, several large, population-based studies find a connection between certain viruses and bacteria and heart disease. Culprits include the bacterium *Chlamydia pneumoniae* (which causes bronchitis and pneumonia), the bacterium *H. pylori* (which causes gastric ulcers), cytomegalovirus (a type of herpes virus that usually causes no symptoms), herpes simplex virus (HSV), and bacteria that cause gum disease.

At least two bacteria also cause cancer: the human papilloma virus (HPV), which causes cervical cancer, and *H. pylori*, which can lead to stomach cancer.

Low-grade infections may even play a role in Alzheimer's disease. There's a link between the disease and *C. pneumoniae*, the herpes simplex virus, and, possibly, cytomegalovirus.

Again, we're not suggesting these organisms *cause* Alzheimer's. But they trigger inflammation that contributes to the disease's development, particularly in people who are already genetically predisposed to the disease.

The good news? Many of the same things we recommend to combat the other Super Threats—diet, exercise, stress reduction—can help you maintain a strong immune system.

Diet: Your First Line of Defense

Without the vitamins, minerals, and essential fatty acids contained in the food you eat, no cell functions properly, especially not immune system cells.

The worst problem? Malnutrition. Not the potbellied, spindly-armed kind of malnutrition you're used to seeing in images from third-world countries, but the more subtle malnutrition—deficits of important micronutrients—that is common in industrialized nations, particularly in the elderly.

Studies find about 10 to 25 percent of the elderly have some form of nutritional deficit, a figure that may be as high as 50 percent for older people hospitalized for any reason. Malnutrition and infection are a chicken-and-egg conundrum; while malnutrition increases the risk of infection, infection also increases the risk of malnutrition.

Older people are often deficient in iron, and this deficiency can affect the immune system enough to increase the risk of infection. Supplementing with iron and other trace minerals such as selenium can improve the immune system enough to reduce the number of respiratory and urinary tract infections in older people.

The key micronutrients for immune health seem to be zinc, selenium, B vitamins (particularly

B_6, B_{12}, folic acid, and riboflavin), iron, vitamin A, beta-carotene, and vitamin C.

That doesn't mean you should head out to the drugstore and stock up on supplements. Although we recommend a multivitamin/mineral (studies find it not only increases immune function in older people but reduces infections), we don't want you taking lots of individual nutrient supplements on a daily basis.

Nutrients are meant to work together. Too much zinc, for instance, can *hurt* immune response, while supplementing with iron if you're not deficient could interfere with your body's absorption of zinc. If you find you're getting sick a lot, ask your doctor to test your iron levels before you take a supplement.

Also consider your dieting habits. Yo-yo dieting—constantly going on and off a diet—can really do some damage to your immune system. Researchers have long known that intentionally losing weight makes natural killer cells, which normally attack cancer cells and viruses, less effective. But a study of 114 postmenopausal women ages 50 to 75 who were overweight or obese (but otherwise healthy) revealed that the more diets the women had been on in their lifetime, the weaker their natural killer cell activity.

That doesn't mean you should give up on losing weight. But if you keep losing and regaining the same 20 pounds, it might be time to consult a qualified nutritionist about an eating plan you can live with, not another quick-fix, drop-ten-pounds-in-two-weeks diet.

The Chronic Stress Connection

Like so many other things in life and in health, stress can be bad or good, depending on how much of it you have and how long it lasts.

Much of what we know about the effects of stress on the immune system come from studies

---

Your Defense Team

Like a sports team or construction crew, the immune system contains many different players that work together to get a job done. These players include:

Border protection. Your skin (which keeps out invaders), the mucous lining of your stomach and lungs (which traps invading bacteria), hairs that move mucus and bacteria out of the lungs, stomach acid (which kills bacteria), "good" bacteria in your gut that prevent bad bacteria from taking over, and urine, which flushes bacteria out of your bladder and urethra.

Ground troops. Cells that swoop in, destroy invaders or corrupt cells, gobble up the mess, and go on their way. They have names like neutrophils, granulocytes, monocytes, macrophages, and natural killer cells.

Special forces. These are cells that have had some training in attacking specific threats. This is the system behind vaccinations. You "train" cells called B lymphocytes to produce antibodies, chemicals designed to activate under a specific threat. Because B lymphocytes have good memories, they're able to produce the antibodies quickly next time they encounter the threat. The antibodies latch onto the invader, sending a chemical signal to other immune cells to come and destroy it.

---

of caregivers, who, you can imagine, are under unrelenting, ongoing stress. That's the type of stress that's most harmful to your immune system. Short-term stress (the kind you have when you're getting up to give a speech), on the other hand, actually *strengthens* the immune system.

Why? When you're confronted with an acute stressor like public speaking, your immune system revs up to meet the challenge. But if you're dealing with day-in, day-out stress, it eventually burns out like a motor that's been running non-stop. That's why the activity of natural killer cells deteriorates after divorce, why older people are more likely to be diagnosed with cancer when they're stressed and depressed after the death of a loved one, and why social isolation as well as marital discord can impair immune function.

How does the immune system burn out, exactly? Like most systems in the body, it has a feedback loop. After it finishes attacking foreign invaders with inflammatory chemicals, the brain sends out cortisol—yes, also the stress hormone—to shut down this inflammatory response. But if your body releases cortisol all the time, as it does under chronic stress, then your immune system is constantly suppressed.

If you get a cold when you finally go on vacation after a stressful work cycle, or you experience three herpes outbreaks in the year you're going through a divorce, it's your body's way of telling you the stress is too much.

The Exercise Answer

Although intense exercise (such as a two-hour run) can temporarily depress your immune system, getting no physical activity at all can be much more harmful over time. When researchers studied the blood of 56 people ages 62 and older who received flu shots, they found that those who got at least 20 minutes of exercise three or more times a week had the highest levels of antibodies to the flu viruses two weeks after the shot compared with those who exercised less—a sign of immune strength.

It doesn't take much physical activity to rev up your immune system. A review of more than 600 studies found that three or four brief sessions of strength training a week and moderate aerobic exercise (30 to 45 minutes) on most days are enough to increase the number of natural killer cells, reducing infections.

Other studies find that people who get moderate physical activity suffer fewer colds than couch potatoes, and that walking briskly for 45 minutes a day most days of the week can cut

GETTING TESTED

Various tests provide clues to the health of your immune system. Ask your doctor which, if any, you might need. These include:

Complete blood count (CBC). This includes measurements of white blood cells, which belong to the immune system.

Antibody tests. These measure the levels of various antibodies in your blood to evaluate your immune status against particular invaders, diagnose an autoimmune condition, or diagnose an allergy.

Iron test. This blood test measures the levels of iron in your blood.

Immunization challenge test. In this test you're immunized with a common vaccine, like a flu shot, to see if your body develops antibodies to it—a sign of a healthy immune system.

Skin response to known allergens. A tiny dose of something you've been exposed to before, like the mumps antibody, is placed under your skin. A reaction at the site of the injection proves that your immune system can respond to this kind of challenge. The traditional tuberculosis test is one example.

Food allergies. Testing your blood can sometimes reveal the existence of food allergies. You should eliminate or drastically reduce these foods in your diet to avoid chronically over-stimulating the immune system through repeated allergic responses.

your sick days in half over a 12- to 15-week period. Even gentle exercise programs like t'ai chi can increase immunity.

Exercise can help kids' immune systems too. In one Canadian study, children who participated in sports were less likely to get sick enough to miss school.

How does exercise help? It increases circulation, speeding immune cells' movement through the body so they destroy invaders before they get a foothold. It also lowers stress hormones and helps you eliminate toxins via breathing and sweating.

A word of warning: An intense workout of two hours or so can actually temporarily suppress your immune system, increasing your risk of common infections like colds and flu. So keep your workout intensity moderate—that means you can still talk to the person next to you—and limit workouts to no more than an hour. Also forgo most exercise when you're actually sick, even if it's just a cold.

Best Remedies FOR IMMUNE STRESS

To maintain a strong immune system, we recommend you do the following:

Diet

Eat brightly colored produce. It's high in beta-carotene and vitamin C, which support the immune system.

Eat a cup of live cultured yogurt every day. Researchers find it boosts immune cell activity, even when you're under chronic stress.

Get iron from leafy greens and shellfish. Leafy greens like spinach and kale, and shellfish, are also good sources of trace minerals like zinc.

Sprinkle wheat germ on salads, cereal, or yogurt. It provides iron as well as important B vitamins.

Use garlic for seasoning. Rich in antioxidants, especially selenium, garlic can increase production of natural killer cells.

Cut the fat from your diet. Studies find that people following diets with about 15 percent of calories from fat have stronger immune systems than those following diets containing 30 or more percent of fat.

Switch to tea. Researchers from Harvard University found greater immune activity in tea drinkers compared to coffee drinkers. They suspect that an amino acid in brewed tea called L-theanine may be involved in tea's immune benefits.

Eat more mushrooms. They're great immune stimulators. Although the dark-brown Chinese or shiitake mushrooms are best known for their health effects, even white button mushrooms can temporarily boost immune function.

Limit sugar. High amounts of sugar in your diet are linked to poor immune function. And don't forget that fruit juice is loaded with sugar.

Stick to one serving or less of alcohol a day. A toxin, alcohol suppresses the immune response.

Eat organic whenever possible. This reduces your intake of toxins like hormones and pesticides that stress your immune system.

Bake, broil, and roast—but don't fry. Frying transforms fats into toxic forms that stress your immune system.

Get adequate protein. Protein foods, with their high levels of zinc, iron, and B vitamins, are critical

The Sleep Solution

There's a reason all you want to do is sleep when you're sick. It's because your body does its best repair and restoration work while you're snoozing. This is also the reason that you're more likely to get sick when you're not getting enough shut-eye—that maintenance work gets put on hold, and things start to fall apart.

Many studies find that the more severe the lack of sleep or the worse the quality of sleep, the less natural killer cell activity. One reason alcoholics are thought to be more susceptible to a host of infectious diseases like tuberculosis, HIV, and hepatitis C may be the effects of alcohol-related sleep disturbances.

The connection between sleep and immune function is a two-way street—not only does lack of sleep affect production of important immune system chemicals and cells, but when production of those cells and chemicals is reduced, that, in turn, affects the quality of sleep.

---

for a healthy immune system. Most of us get enough; this is primarily an issue for vegetarians and the elderly.

Eliminate any foods to which you might be allergic. Repeated allergic responses can weaken the immune system.

Avoid foods that contain artificial colors and flavorings.

Supplements

Take a daily multivitamin/mineral supplement that contains at least 20 milligrams elemental zinc and 100 micrograms selenium, as well as 300 to 400 IU vitamin E.

Exercise

Get at least 30 minutes of moderate exercise (a brisk walk or bike ride with hills is ideal) at least three days a week.

Lifestyle

Practice deep breathing and mental imagery (described on page 60) at least three times a day for five minutes to reduce stress. A deep-breathing technique called the Nishino Breathing Method, which combines deep breathing, visualization, and gentle exercise such as relaxing and twisting, enhanced the natural killer cell activity of 17 of 21 subjects after just one 90-minute class, while reducing their average stress level.

Get at least eight hours of sleep in every 24-hour period. Rats deprived of sleep die, most likely because of an immune system breakdown that allows an influx of deadly bacteria.

Laugh often. In one study, after watching a funny video, men had higher levels of numerous immune system cells, and the effect lasted up to 12 hours. The former editor of *The Saturday Evening Post*, Norman Cousins, attributes his survival from a mysterious, life-threatening illness to humor. He started watching Marx Brothers movies every day and is certain the resulting laughter strengthened his immune system enough to fight off the illness.

Elevated Stress Hormones

The body's reaction to stress serves a very useful purpose. If there's a fire in your house, for instance, it will help you get out. How? At the first sign of trouble (the smell of smoke, perhaps), your system releases a cascade of "stress hormones" like adrenaline and cortisol, which send a volley of chemical signals to various parts of your body to gear up for action. The liver releases glucose to provide fast energy to muscles; the lungs expand to take in more oxygen; the heart beats faster to send more oxygen-rich blood throughout your body. Meanwhile, your bowel and intestinal muscles contract as blood is shunted from the digestive system to other parts of your body deemed more critical in the moment at hand.

But if this stress response happens constantly, say, because you're faced with tight deadlines at work or you're troubled by a difficult relationship or financial problems, then it doesn't do much good at all. In fact, it can lead to serious health problems, including high blood pressure, heart disease, heartburn, constipation, irritable bowel syndrome, and depression.

Ongoing stress can also make you fat in all the wrong places. That's because the stress hormone

cortisol is a powerful appetite trigger. Just as bad: Chronically elevated cortisol levels stimulate the growth of fat cells in the abdomen, resulting in belly fat, which is linked to inflammation and insulin resistance. (If it's starting to seem that just about everything that happens in the body is linked together, that's because it is!)

You also discovered in the last chapter that elevated levels of stress hormones suppress your immune system, increasing your risk of infection. Studies find people with high levels of stress hormones don't make as many antibodies when they get immunized as people with lower levels. Also, their wounds take longer to heal, and they're more likely to have flares of viral diseases like herpes, shingles, and chronic fatigue syndrome.

Stress also cranks up levels of free radicals, leading to greater oxidative stress (Super Threat #2), which damages cells and tissues. That damage can be particularly severe in the brain, even harming the hormonal system that regulates the stress response, leading to more intense and prolonged responses to stress. It's a vicious cycle.

Finally, chronic stress increases your risk of insulin resistance (Super Threat #3) and diabetes by constantly sending out chemical signals to your liver to release more glucose.

Unfortunately, as you age, your body is less able to take stress in stride. Studies find that older people tend to release more stress hormones in reaction to a stressor than younger people do.

So. Enough negative stuff about stress. What can you do about it? Plenty. While you can't necessarily get rid of all the stress in your life, you can practice techniques to damp down your body's reactions to it and protect your health.

The Power of Positive Thinking

The first thing we want you to do is teach yourself to view the negative in a more positive light. Think of the ability to do this as a personal shield against the harmful effects of stress. We don't mean you should adopt an "everything's rosy" Pollyanna attitude. That wouldn't work.

Positive thinking doesn't mean ignoring reality, but looking at it differently. Take the survivors of any major disaster. There's no way to downplay the horror of the situation for those who lost everything. But while some people really dwell on what they lost, others begin to focus almost immediately on the possibility of new opportunities and new experiences that might now be available. That kind of redirecting your thoughts, studies show, can help you physically and mentally recover quicker and more fully from stressful situations.

Even a more minor situation—like an impossible deadline at work—can be reframed in a more positive light. Instead of tearing your hair out in panic, take a step back and think of all the "impossible" deadlines you've met before, and remind yourself that you'll probably meet this one too.

Sometimes a situation is only as stressful as you view it. In one study, researchers asked women to place themselves on a picture of a ladder representing socioeconomic status—with those best off

RELATED AILMENTS

Chronic stress either causes or contributes to the following ailments:

- Acne
- Anxiety
- Back pain
- Canker sores
- Chronic fatigue syndrome
- Colds
- Cold sores
- Constipation
- Coronary artery disease
- Dandruff
- Depression
- Diabetes (type 2)
- Diarrhea
- Diverticulitis
- Dry mouth
- Eczema
- Erectile dysfunction
- Fatigue
- Fibromyalgia
- Flu
- Headache
- Heartburn and GERD
- Herpes
- High blood pressure
- High cholesterol
- Hives
- Infertility, female
- Infertility, male
- Insomnia
- Insulin resistance syndrome
- Irritable bowel syndrome (IBS)
- Memory problems
- Migraine
- Neck pain
- Nicotine addiction
- Obesity
- Psoriasis
- Rheumatoid arthritis
- Shingles
- Tinnitus
- TMJ
- Ulcers

at the top and those worst off at the bottom. Women who perceived themselves as lower on the ladder had higher stress hormone levels than women who perceived themselves as higher up. Yet all the women had similar incomes.

Start small. Stuck in traffic? Instead of steaming, pop in your favorite CD, or spend a few minutes doing deep breathing.

Learning to Relax

You can teach your body to relax, in essence, telling it to take it easy and not respond so much to stressors. These relaxation techniques help counter the physiological effects of stress, which is why they're effective in treating a variety of stress-related conditions, including chronic low back pain, coronary artery disease, headache, and insomnia. Best of all, you can use them on your own (although you'll need training for the biofeedback).

Deep breathing. You wouldn't think such a thing as deep breathing could make any real difference when it comes to stress hormones. But it does. Most adults are breath holders, using rapid, shallow breathing, especially when they're stressed. That's why the first advice you get when you're upset is to take a slow, deep breath. And that's what we want you to do. Count to four as you slowly breathe in through your nose, consciously pushing out your stomach by pushing down with your diaphragm. This is the active phase of breathing. Then count to four as you exhale through your mouth, pursing your lips like you're going to whistle and watching your stomach slowly fall. Repeat 5 to 10 times.

Meditation. Meditation involves focusing your mind on a particular word or thing (like your breathing) to the exclusion of everything else. It can change just about everything that relates to your stress level and state of mind, from your blood pressure to your stress hormones.

To practice a basic form of meditation, find a quiet place. Sit upright, your arms and hands relaxed in your lap, your eyes looking down but slightly open. (If you practice meditating in this posture, it's easy and unobtrusive to sit like this anytime during the day, scan your body for tension, then let go enough to trigger the remembered state of relaxation.) Breathe slowly through your nose, concentrating on each breath. If you like, think of a particular word as you exhale. Choose something simple like "peace."

Try to focus only on your word and your breathing. If thoughts intrude, let them float away. Meditate for 2 or 3 minutes. Practice daily until you can increase the time to 10 minutes.

GETTING TESTED

Although there aren't any commonly available tests to measure stress (the ones that exist are used only in research settings), we usually ask people to measure their blood pressure when they feel very relaxed, then measure it again just after an upsetting event. Usually your pressure increases as much as if you were running, evidence of the stress on your body. Other signs of stress in your body include tight muscles, tremors, trouble concentrating, fatigue worse than you'd expect given your activity level, acid stomach, diarrhea and other stomach problems, and headache.

Other ways to tell if you're feeling stressed is to put your hands to your face to see if they're warm or cold. Cool hands are a sign that your body is directing blood away from the periphery (arms and legs) to feed the core of your body as part of the stress response. Hand temperature, in fact, is how the mood rings of the '70s worked.

Mental imagery. This is really a form of meditation, only you focus on an image of a place or experience that relaxes you. But don't stop with the visual—you want to engage all your senses. So, for instance, if you're envisioning a beach scene, feel the sunlight on your back or the hot sand under your feet, smell the salty air, and hear the waves rolling in.

Biofeedback. With biofeedback you learn to consciously control something that's normally involuntary, like blood pressure, sweating, or muscle tension. Initially, you need special training with a trained biofeedback professional, who will use instruments that give you "feedback" on the thing you're trying to control. Eventually you can use the technique you learned on your own. Forms of biofeedback include:

- **Electromyogram (EMG),** which measures muscle tension and is often used for anxiety, constipation, and urinary problems.

- **Electroencephalogram (EEG),** which measures brain wave activity.

- **Thermal biofeedback,** which measures skin temperature and is often used to treat headaches and reduce blood pressure.

- **Electrodermal activity,** which measures changes in perspiration.

- **Finger pulse,** which is used to lower blood pressure, manage heartbeat problems, and reduce anxiety.

- **Breathing rate monitoring,** which is used for asthma and anxiety.

Progressive muscle relaxation. This simple technique has been shown to help people cope with anxiety and improve their ability to relax. Start at the tips of your toes and curl them tightly. Then relax them completely. Next, flex your feet up toward your face, then relax them completely. Continue with every major joint and muscle from the tips of your toes to your forehead, on both sides of your body. The goal is to show you how tightly you keep everything clenched, and give you a sense of what it feels like to have your muscles fully relaxed, a feeling that, with practice, you should be able to repeat without going muscle by muscle.

Best Remedies FOR ELEVATED STRESS HORMONES

Lifestyle

Attempt a "glass half-full" approach toward negative situations.

Treat yourself to a massage at least every two weeks if you can afford it.

Use essential oils, candles, and room sprays with relaxing scents like lavender, geranium, bergamot, chamomile, and rose essential oils. Scent is one of our strongest senses, directly linked to the most primitive portion of our brains.

Take up a hobby that includes repetitive activity, like knitting, needlepoint, or woodworking.

Practice deep breathing or meditation twice a day for 10 minutes at a time.

Soothe with music. Listening to music has been shown to help people with chronic pain hurt less, relax patients before surgery, reduce anxiety, and improve sleep. The idea is that part of your brain is "distracted" by the music.

Tend and befriend. Lack of social support and simple loneliness can increase cortisol levels. So make an effort to reach out to others and nurture your connections. Next time you come home from work with your shoulders tighter than a hangman's noose, talk to a friend. As the saying goes, a worry shared is a worry halved.

Exercise

Get at least 30 minutes of moderate physical activity a day.

Sign up for a yoga class. Yoga, with its mindfulness, deep breathing, and stretching components, calms the stress response system and stems the release of stress hormones, providing a sense of calm alertness that continues long after the final Downward Dog. Once you learn the poses, you can practice yoga at home.

Toxin Exposure

There's a saying in medicine: "There are no harmless substances, only harmless ways of using them." That's a good adage with which to begin this chapter, since anything—even water—can be toxic (drink too much water and you throw off your chemical and electrolyte balance, which, in the extreme case, can result in death).

So while you might think of things like cigarette smoke, pesticides, heavy metals, industrial chemicals, and alcohol as the primary toxins you need to beware of, they're only the tip of the toxic iceberg. Even the biochemical processes that keep cells working result in a tremendous amount of toxic by-products your body has to break down and dispose of. Heck, even "healthy" things like food and medicine have components your body needs to dispose of—and these components are technically toxins.

Obviously, you can't stop eating or drinking water or taking medicines you need. But you can limit your exposure to unnecessary toxins. You can also take steps to keep your body's detoxification system—primarily your liver—strong. If your detox system is impaired, your body could develop the physical equivalent of a toxic waste problem, leading to increased inflammation (Super Threat #1), oxidative stress (Super Threat #2), and a weakened immune system (Super Threat #4). By now you know what that means—an increased risk of numerous diseases of aging.

Consider the damage that toxins can cause:

Air pollution, particularly tiny particulates that lodge in the lungs, can thicken the blood and increase inflammation.

Lead exposure on the job can result in memory and learning ability declines nearly 20 years after the initial exposure. Additionally, it contributes to high blood pressure. Even small amounts of lead exposure for young children can lead to devastating neurological damage.

A high level of mercury from freshwater fish, dental fillings, or environmental exposure may increase your risk of heart attacks as well as death from all cardiovascular diseases. Researchers suspect mercury somehow encourages the oxidation of LDL cholesterol, which, you'll remember, makes these particles much more dangerous to arteries. High mercury levels are also thought to contribute to autoimmune diseases like multiple sclerosis and lupus by overactivating the immune system.

- Allergies
- Alzheimer's disease
- Asthma
- Bronchitis
- Chronic fatigue syndrome
- Coronary artery disease
- Diarrhea
- Diverticulitis
- Inflammatory bowel disease
- Irritable bowel syndrome
- Eczema
- Endometriosis
- Fatigue
- Fibromyalgia
- Hangover
- Headache
- Heavy menstrual bleeding
- Hepatitis
- High blood pressure
- High cholesterol
- Hives
- Infertility, female
- Infertility, male
- Memory problems
- Muscle soreness
- Parkinson's disease
- Psoriasis
- Rheumatoid arthritis
- Rosacea
- Scleroderma

Cigarette smoking dramatically increases inflammation, with the effects lasting years after you've stubbed out your last butt. That may be one reason smoking is linked with Parkinson's and Alzheimer's diseases, as well as cardiovascular diseases and cancer.

Numerous environmental toxins, including solvents, metals, and pesticides, are thought to contribute to neurological diseases like Alzheimer's and Parkinson's. Heavy metals like copper, iron, lead, manganese and zinc may act as catalysts that generate free radicals, resulting in the oxidative damage that is a hallmark of these diseases.

Your Detoxification System

Ever bought a bushel of clams in the summer? They're still alive when you get them, and to ensure good eating without sandy grittiness, you're supposed to put them in a bowl of water with cornmeal. The clams filter the water and cornmeal mixture through their muscle, removing any impurities, like sand, at the same time.

Your liver works something like that. At any one time, one-fourth of your entire blood supply is filtering through your liver, being detoxified.

Detoxification is a two-phase process that involves a chain of chemical reactions you only want to know about if you plan to become a doctor or biochemist. But here's the short version.

In the first phase, the liver uses certain enzymes to make toxic substances less toxic and easier to get out of your body. This process, however, creates lots of free radicals, which can damage the liver. Ideally, the antioxidants in the liver take care of those free radicals, but if your store of antioxidants is low or toxin levels are high, the free radicals win out, leading to oxidative stress and liver damage. This can start a vicious circle—the damaged liver can't handle the toxins and doesn't make enough antioxidants to manage the free radicals, leading to increased oxidative stress and increased liver damage.

Certain medications like Prozac (fluoxetine) or H_2 blockers like Tagamet (cimetidine) can make for a sluggish phase 1, allowing even relatively mild toxins to build up to a dangerous level.

During phase 2 of detoxification, the liver adds additional enzymes to make toxic molecules water soluble so your body can dispose of them through bile, urine, perspiration, or breathing. If this phase doesn't work properly, you expose yourself to dangerous inflammation that may be linked with conditions such as rheumatoid arthritis.

If either phase of detoxification comes up short, toxins build up in fatty tissue, particularly in the brain and endocrine system (think glands that produce hormones). That's why many researchers believe certain brain diseases, like Alzheimer's and Parkinson's, as well as some hormonally related conditions, like infertility, menstrual problems, and premature menopause, may be related to our exposure to fat-soluble toxins like heavy metals in today's environment.

Why is this? As toxins build up, free-radical production increases, and you know where that leads: increased inflammation, cellular damage, and increased risk of numerous chronic diseases, including cancer.

So how do you maintain a healthy detoxification system? We're so glad you asked.

Turn Down Your Toxin Exposure

As you might imagine, the more toxins you're exposed to, the harder your detox system has to work. And the harder anything works, the more likely it is to falter or break down. That's why heavy drinking, taking too much acetaminophen (Tylenol), or even eating a single poisonous mushroom can destroy your liver.

Reducing your exposure to toxins starts with the obvious: Stop smoking, drink alcohol only in moderation, and don't take drugs you don't need. But some toxins are less obvious. For instance, most foods contain additives, whether it's the coloring or preservatives in prepared foods, the hormones and antibiotics in animal foods, or pesticide residues on produce. This is one of the many reasons we recommend eating fresh foods and organic foods whenever possible.

Additionally, be sure that the cleaners you use and the carpets and other items you buy for your house are "green." Studies find that compounds called volatile organic compounds (VOCs) released from building materials, carpets, office machines, furniture—even cleaning products— can lead to illness, a sign they're overwhelming your body's ability to detoxify itself.

Even simple habits, like popping an aspirin for a headache, spritzing on hair spray every morning, or sweetening your tea with aspartame, increase your toxic load, which is why daily aspirin therapy is a bad idea if you have liver problems. We're not saying these things on their own make you sick, but the cumulative effects, particularly if your detox system isn't working at an ideal level to begin with, may bring you a step closer to disease.

Improve Detoxification With Diet

Beyond reducing the toxins you're exposed to, the next most important step to staying "detoxed" is eating well.

Important Nutrients

Certain nutrients are critical for an effective detox system, specifically: vitamins B_2 (riboflavin), B_3 (niacin) B_6, B_{12}, and folic acid, as well as certain flavonoids (antioxidant plant chemicals found in tea, dark chocolate, grape juice, and wine, among other foods) and fats.

You also need adequate antioxidant support during phase 1, meaning plenty of beta-carotene, vitamin C, vitamin E, coenzyme Q_{10}, and the antioxidant minerals selenium, zinc, copper, and manganese. Recall that these antioxidants protect the liver by neutralizing the free radicals released during the process of breaking down toxins.

Other important compounds for antioxidant support during phase 1 are thiol compounds, found in garlic, onion, and cruciferous vegetables like broccoli, cabbage, and cauliflower. These compounds are also critical for driving the chemical reactions of phase 2.

Friendly Bacteria

Strange as it sounds, food contains toxins your liver has to detoxify. But what if there were a kind of protective shield that prevented such toxins from ever leaving your gut, so your liver didn't have to deal with them?

There is. It's the "friendly" bacteria in your stomach and colon, also known as probiotics. These prevent the absorption of certain toxins. Probiotics also produce vitamins K and folic acid, as well as immune-enhancing compounds and natural antibiotics that help reduce levels of nasty bacteria that inhabit your gut.

We recommend probiotic supplements (such as acidophilus) quite a lot throughout *Best Remedies* for a variety of conditions, most related to the digestive or immune system. You can also get probiotics in yogurt that contains active cultures. You can even go a step further with prebiotics, organisms that help form probiotics. If you eat plenty of dietary fiber from fruits, vegetables, whole grains, and legumes, you should have plenty of prebiotics. Still, prebiotic supplements are often the best way to ensure a good supply if you're subject to gastrointestinal problems or have a weak detox system.

Best Remedies FOR TOXIN EXPOSURE

Diet

Limit alcoholic drinks to no more than one or two a day.

Get 8 to 10 servings of fruits and vegetables, including at least 2 servings of cruciferous vegetables, every day.

Drink at least 8 glasses of water a day.

Stick to organic produce and meats and poultry raised without hormones or antibiotics whenever possible.

Supplements

Take a B supplement vitamin daily.

Take a daily multivitamin that contains at least 100 micrograms selenium, 200 IU vitamin E, 500 milligrams vitamin C, and 2,500 to 5,000 milligrams beta-carotene.

Take two probiotic capsules at bedtime and make sure you get plenty of fiber every day from foods like vegetables, whole grains, and whole fruit with the skin.

Take milk thistle extract standardized to silymarin 175 milligrams two or three times a day to protect the liver if you know you're going to be exposed to a higher-than-usual load of toxins (traveling to a third-world country, for instance).

Lifestyle

Don't take medication you don't need.

Stop smoking and stay away from people who smoke and from smoky places.

Open the windows in your home to air out volatile compounds.

Buy "green" products for your home. Purchase furnishings, wall coverings, and floor coverings made of natural materials that don't emit toxic fumes or compounds. And use natural cleaning products.

The 7-Day Super Protection

PLAN

So how do you put all our advice from this chapter into action? You take it one step at a time. Combating all six Super Threats to slash your risk of age-related ailments may sound overwhelming—but it really isn't. That's because many of the measures that combat one Super Threat also combat others. To get you started, we've put together this 7-Day Super Protection Plan, designed to jump-start your efforts. By taking just a few small "anti-aging" steps every day, you'll soon be cutting your risk for the diseases that speed the aging process, and also reversing—or a least minimizing—damage from health conditions you may already have.

Day 1

8 a.m. In a small notebook, starting this morning, write down everything you eat and drink this week. Studies find that people who keep detailed food diaries are more likely to lose weight and keep it off than those who don't. Even if you don't need to lose weight, a one-week food diary will help you to see where your diet is lacking in terms of fruits and vegetables, healthy fats, fiber, and other good-for-you nutrients.

10 a.m. Sort through your kitchen cabinet and pantry and toss anything that has trans-fatty acids. (Hint: If you see the word "hydrogenated" in the list, it has 'em.) Also get rid of any corn, cotton-seed, peanut, safflower, sesame, soybean, and sunflower oil. If you don't have olive or canola oil, put them on your shopping list.

1 p.m. Go to your favorite health food store or pharmacy and stock up on a quality multivitamin, a B complex supplement, a C vitamin supplement, a calcium-magnesium-vitamin D supplement, and fish oil. When you get home, put them in a basket on your kitchen counter next to the coffee maker so you remember to take them daily.

4 p.m. Plan a meatless dinner tonight. Try a bean dish, a tofu dish, or whole grain pasta topped with soy crumbles, canned or fresh tomatoes, fresh herbs, onions, garlic, and grated carrots. Remember to eat a salad before you start dining—you'll eat less overall.

QUIZ: What Are You Drinking?

In a typical week, which of the following do you drink?

____ Tea (chock-full of antioxidants to reduce oxidative stress)

____ Soda (full of calories and sugar, contributing to all Super Threats)

____ Water (helps with detoxification; drink purified to reduce toxins from local water sources)

____ Fruit juice (okay as long as it's unsweetened and no more than 1 1/2 cups a day; also aim for full-pulp juice to increase fiber)

____ Wine (one glass a day is great for countering oxidative stress, relieving stress, and reducing inflammation; just make sure you don't exceed that amount)

Day 2

8 a.m. Make a fruit smoothie for breakfast with 1/2 cup blueberries, 1/2 cup strawberries, 1 banana, and 1 scoop of soy protein powder along with 1 cup skim milk or soy milk.

10 a.m. Pull out the yellow pages and find the closest yoga, Pilates, or t'ai chi center. Call and sign up for the first class that fits your schedule.

Noon. Go for a lunchtime walk around your neighborhood or your office complex for 20 to 30 minutes. If the weather is bad, find an indoor mall or walk the halls (and stairs) of your office building if it's large enough.

6 p.m. Dinner tonight is iron-rich shrimp sautéed in olive oil and garlic with sliced red, yellow, and orange peppers served over brown rice with a side salad. There, you've just added a layer of protection against nearly all six Super Threats. Substitute firm tofu or skinless chicken breast if you don't eat seafood.

QUIZ: How Sleep-Friendly Is Your Bedroom?

How many of the following steps have you taken to make your bedroom more sleep-friendly? Recall that a good night's sleep helps keep nearly all six Super Threats at bay.

____ Added room-darkening shades

____ Bought a white-noise machine

____ Removed the television and computer

____ Cleared out clutter, leaving a soothing environment

____ Painted the walls a soothing color (such as sage green)

____ Added a small night-light so I don't have to turn on the light if I get up to go to the bathroom

____ Bought new, good pillows

Day 3

8 a.m. Scramble up two omega-3 fatty acid-enriched eggs and serve atop a piece of whole grain toast with a side of cantaloupe for breakfast.

11 a.m. Do the grocery shopping for the week and choose organic produce (especially when buying strawberries, apples, grapes, and pears), free-range chicken, and naturally raised meats (no hormones or antibiotics). Also pick up two types of fish to fix for dinner. Put one package in the freezer and use the other for dinner tonight.

3 p.m. Pull out the bike that's been gathering dust in the garage and go for a ride through the neighborhood. If the weather's bad, clear the detritus off the stationary bike or treadmill and fire it up.

10 p.m. Turn off the television and computer, put the pile of work away, and sit quietly for 10 minutes to meditate as you begin unwinding for bed.

QUIZ: Did You Find the Fiber Today?

How many high-fiber foods did you eat today to get your 25 grams?

____ An apple (4 grams)

____ 1 cup bran cereal, such as Kellogg's Raisin Bran (8 grams)

____ 1 cup black beans with no added lard or other fat (19 grams)

____ 2 slices seven-grain bread (6.5 grams)

____ 1/2 cup raw broccoli (4 grams)

____ 1/2 cup canned chickpeas (6 grams)

____ 3 dried figs (10.5 grams)

____ 1/2 cup fresh peas (9 grams)

____ Other

Day 4

8 a.m. Have a cup of tea this morning instead of coffee (caffeinated is fine), and use honey to sweeten it to get a good dose of antioxidants to start your day.

9 a.m. Call your doctor and schedule a physical. It will include blood work to measure your glucose/insulin levels, liver and kidney function, etc.

3 p.m. Have an afternoon snack. Remember, you're trying to eat six times (small portions) a day to reduce blood sugar swings. A good option: a bowl of cut-up fruit and a handful of walnuts (antioxidants, fiber, protein, and healthy fats all rolled up into one).

7 p.m. Go see a comic movie with your partner or friend. Laugh heartily to reduce stress and strengthen your immune system.

QUIZ: Are You Getting Your Antioxidants?

Which of the following high-antioxidant fruits (preferably organic) have you eaten this week?

___ Blueberries

___ Raspberries

___ Strawberries

___ Cherries

___ Plums

___ Apples

Day 5

9 a.m. Make an appointment for a dental cleaning and examination to make sure you don't have the beginnings of gum disease.

10 a.m. Drink a glass of pomegranate juice with your morning snack for a huge dose of antioxidants.

3 p.m. Have a cup of yogurt with live cultures for your afternoon snack with a tablespoon of ground flaxseeds sprinkled on top. The probiotics in the yogurt enhance your immune system and reduce toxin absorption. The flaxseeds provide blood sugar-reducing fiber and omega-3 fatty acids that quell inflammation.

6 p.m. Stop at the store on your way home and pick up a filter for your kitchen faucet. The filter clears out most toxins in your water supply, helping you reduce oxidative stress and inflammation, as well as giving your liver a break.

QUIZ: Are You Controlling Your Stress?

How many of these stress-reducing tools did you use this week?

___ Deep breathing

___ Positive thinking to reframe a negative situation

___ Meditation

___ A relaxing hobby like needlepoint, knitting, painting, or woodworking

___ A walk, bike ride, swim, or other aerobic activity

___ Aromatherapy

___ A massage

___ Yoga or t'ai chi

___ A warm bath with aromatherapy oils

Day 6

All day: Serve yourself a little less food than you would normally (unless, of course, you're trying to gain weight). This is one of the best ways to lose weight, and losing weight is one of the best ways to address nearly all six Super Threats.

5 p.m. Go to your local wine store and ask the salesclerk to recommend a good cabernet or merlot for dinner tonight (stick with one glass, though).

7 p.m. Sauté a mix of chopped enoki, chanterelle, portobello, shiitake, and oyster mushrooms (or any two from the list) with a clove of minced garlic in olive oil. Serve over whole wheat pasta and get the benefits of the mushrooms' immune-enhancing effects.

10 p.m. Take two probiotic capsules before you go to bed to strengthen your detoxification system.

QUIZ: Are You Allergic?

Food and airborne allergies can increase inflammation and stress your detoxification system. But many people don't even know they have allergies. Ask yourself the following questions. If you answer yes to one or more questions, you may want to see an allergist for testing.

1. Do I have a runny nose, itchy eyes, and sneezing only during certain times of the year?
2. Do I get itchy red rashes on my skin?
3. Do I often have wheezing and congestion?
4. Is my skin very dry?
5. Do I find I start sneezing and my nose starts running after eating certain foods?
6. Do I ever feel short of breath after eating certain foods?

Day 7

7 a.m. Take a buffered baby aspirin with your breakfast to reduce inflammation (if your doctor says it's okay).

10 a.m. Peruse gardening catalogs or online sites and make a plan for your own garden. Even if you live in a small apartment, container gardening can still provide stress relief. If that's not practical, make a plan to walk regularly in a public garden both for the exercise and the stress relief.

3 p.m. Make an appointment with a massage therapist for your first session. Check the yellow pages or ask a friend or your doctor for a referral, and find out if your insurance will cover it. Massage is a wonderful stress reliever and a good way to clear out toxins that accumulate in your muscles.

6 p.m. Make a super salad for dinner tonight and get nearly all your daily servings of fruits and vegetables at once. Our favorite combines a base of raw spinach with sliced mushrooms, a diced apple, a can of drained mandarin oranges, a diced red pepper, and a sprinkling of canned chickpeas. Add some drained, canned tuna (albacore to reduce the risk of mercury exposure) or a piece of grilled, wild salmon for some healthy omega-3s and immune-enhancing protein, and mix with a light olive oil and balsamic vinegar dressing to counteract every Super Threat on the list.

PART 3

The Best Remedies

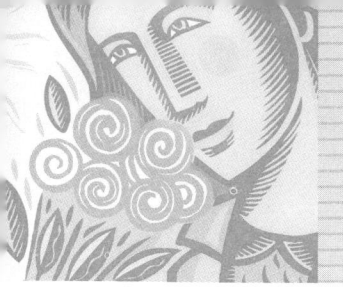

Allergies

The sneezing, sniffling, and itchy eyes of allergic rhinitis are plenty annoying. They can lead to poor sleep, fatigue, and an overall sense of feeling just plain lousy. Allergies can even trigger sinusitis or an asthma attack. And chronic allergies cause inflammation in the body, which, as you read in Part 2, is simply bad for your health.

What does inflammation have to do with allergies? Practically everything. When an allergen such as pollen or mold enters the body, the immune system launches an all-out attack. Immunoglobulin E (IgE) antibodies trigger mast cells in your nose, eyes, lungs, and elsewhere to release inflammatory chemicals, such as histamine and leukotrienes. It's these chemicals that cause the inflammation—and the congestion, itching, and other symptoms of an allergy attack—that most allergy remedies (including the herbal remedies here) target. Supplements that discourage the release of these chemicals can even help you have fewer allergy attacks if you take them regularly.

Do This Now

Follow this sequence of actions at the first sign of an allergy attack. If you have frequent attacks, keep reading for ways to keep seasonal or chronic allergies under control.

1. Take a Claritin once every 12 hours.

2. Also take 2 to 3 freeze-dried nettle capsules immediately. Repeat with 1 to 3 capsules three to four times a day over the next 24 to 48 hours.

3. Spray an over-the-counter saline solution such as Ocean, Ayr Mist, or Simply Saline Rinse into your nose to get rid of allergens and thin the mucus. Or mix your own solution using 4 ounces of water and 1/8 teaspoon salt. To get it into your nose, use an ear bulb syringe (like the kind used to clean out a baby's nose), a neti pot, available in health food stores, or a waterpick. To use the waterpick, you'll need a special adapter called a Grossan nasal adapter, available in most drug and health food stores. Run the waterpick on its lowest setting.

4. If your sinuses are still clogged, boil a pot of water, remove from heat, place on a heat-safe surface, and add 10 drops of eucalyptus oil. If you don't have any eucalyptus oil, use peppermint oil. Then lean over the pot with a towel over your head to keep in the steam. Breathe deeply through your nose (if you can) until the water cools.

Why It Works

Antihistamines do what their name implies: They neutralize histamines. Newer antihistamines such as Claritin last longer and are less likely to cause drowsiness than older drugs such as Benadryl. A word about antihistamines: Don't use them if you have glaucoma, problems urinating, or benign prostatic hyperplasia (BPH). If the regular over-the-counter dose is too much for you, or the side effects bother you, consider using children's allergy medicine.

The leaves of nettle, or "stinging nettle," contain histamine, making them a common component in homeopathic allergy remedies. (Recall from Part 1 that homeopathy uses minuscule doses of the chemical causing the illness to resolve the condition.) Nettle leaves also contain acetylcholine, a chemical often released at nerve endings during stress. It dilates blood vessels, which can help relieve stuffiness. Additionally, nettle leaves contain quercetin, one of the antioxidant plant chemicals called polyphenols. Studies find that quercetin can prevent the release of inflammatory chemicals from mast cells—which is one step better than blocking them once they're released.

As for the fragrant steam treatment, eucalyptus and peppermint oil contain menthol (the same stuff you find in Vicks VapoRub). When inhaled through steam, it helps open the nasal passages and bronchial tubes, improving breathing and relieving congestion.

Other Medicines
Herbs and Supplements

Butterbur. This herb has been used for centuries to treat allergy symptoms. Now clinical trials find it really does work. One trial comparing butterbur to a placebo found it was just as effective as Allegra in improving nasal symptoms in people with year-round allergies. Choose a standardized extract with 8 milligrams of petasine per dose and make sure the extract is free of toxic constituents called pyrrolizidine alkaloids. The usual dose is 50 to 100 milligrams twice a day. Take it every day during allergy season, and otherwise just when you're having symptoms.

Quercetin. As we mentioned earlier, this powerful antioxidant helps prevent the release of histamines. Take two to four 500-milligram capsules every four to six hours when you have allergy symptoms; otherwise, take one to two capsules three times a day to help prevent future allergy attacks.

Zinc. An mineral important to the immune system, zinc also helps prevent the release of histamine. Take 15 milligrams a day to prevent allergy symptoms, and up to 30 milligrams a day for up to a week when your allergies are flaring.

Over-the-Counter Drugs

Oral decongestants. If your nose is so stuffy that you have trouble breathing at night or you're snoring, add an over-the-counter decongestant like Sudafed (or generic pseudoephedrine

GETTING TESTED

If you don't already know what you're allergic to, allergy testing can tell you. The gold standard is skin tests, called immediate-type hypersensitivity skin tests. They're typically used to test for allergies to airborne allergens, insect stings, and penicillin by identifying the presence of IgE antibodies to a particular allergen. And yes, they involve a lot of shots. But the needles are very thin and they honestly don't hurt much.

Your doctor may also suggest blood tests. There are several types, including the radioallergosorbent test, or RAST. They're not nearly as good as skin testing, however, and should only be used when skin testing isn't an option; for instance, if you have a skin disease that makes it hard to read the results.

Blood tests are also sometimes used to help identify food allergies, but they are not foolproof. The most reliable way to diagnose a food allergy is an elimination diet, in which suspect foods are cut from the diet and gradually reintroduced.

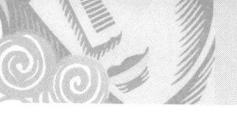

tablets). Take it during the day, however; these drugs may keep you awake at night.

Nasal spray decongestants. If you need something at night, try a nasal spray decongestant like Afrin. One or two squirts in each nostril will relieve congestion for up to 12 hours. Nasal sprays won't keep you awake like oral decongestants, but don't use them for more than three days. If overused they can have a "rebound" effect, resulting in increased swelling when you stop using them.

Eye drops. Plain "natural tears" drops rinse allergens from the eye, while astringent or decongestant drops like Visine or Allergan Relief shrink blood vessels to take the red out. Antihistamine eye drops, like Visine-A, also reduce the itching and swelling caused by the release of histamine (your eyes have a *lot* of mast cells).

Prescription Drugs

If over-the-counter remedies don't do the trick for you, see your doctor. There is an entire arsenal of prescription medications that not only relieve allergy symptoms but also prevent allergy attacks.

Nasal steroid sprays such as Flonase and Rhinocort AQ work by reducing inflammation. They can take a few days to begin working, and you have to use them every day during allergy season for them to be effective.

✤ Helpful Hint

Timing Is Everything

Try taking your allergy medication at night, about an hour before you hit the sack. Nasal congestion from allergies tends to be worse at night and early in the morning, often interfering with sleep. Some studies suggest that antihistamines taken in the evening are more effective than those taken in the morning.

Mast cell stabilizers such as Intal work by preventing the release of inflammatory chemicals like histamines and leukotrienes from mast cells. Because they stop allergies earlier in the process, they are one step better than antihistamines, which prevent the action of histamine *after* it's released.

Long-acting antihistamines such as Clarinex and Zyrtec contain the same active ingredients as their over-the-counter cousins, but they last longer with a single dose.

Leukotriene modifiers were initially developed to treat asthma, but because they work by stemming production of leukotrienes, they can also help with severe allergy symptoms. One leukotriene modifier, Singulair, is approved for use in allergic rhinitis.

Other Approaches

Acupuncture. There's some evidence that acupuncture can damp down allergic reactions. Several studies comparing acupuncture to a sham technique in adults and children showed good results in easing symptoms of seasonal allergies.

Homeopathy. In one well-designed study of 51 patients, a homeopathic remedy chosen based on the patient's specific allergy reduced symptoms 28 percent compared to a 3 percent reduction in the placebo group. But for the best results you'll need to see a naturopath, who will prescribe the remedy that's right for you. If you don't want to visit a naturopath, you can look for an over-the-counter homeopathic allergy medicine such as Boiron Sabadil, available in health food and drug stores.

Massage therapy. When you inhale pollen or something else that you're allergic to, huge numbers of immune cells are released in response to the allergen. The process eventually leaves a collection of dead cells and cellular debris in its wake. This "garbage" needs to be cleared through the body's lymph system. Lymphatic drainage

massage is said to help to drain the lymph system by boosting the flow of lymph (an almost-clear liquid) through the body.

Postural drainage. With this technique, you use warm, moist heat to drain your sinuses. Wet a washcloth under hot water, squeeze out the excess water, then lie flat on your back with the washcloth over your sinus areas for 10 to 15 minutes.

Black tea bags. To soothe swollen, itchy eyes, moisten two black tea bags with cool or cold water. Squeeze out the excess water, close your eyes, and place a tea bag over each eye. Lie quietly for a few minutes and allow the astringent tannins in the tea and the cool water to work.

Prevention

The best way to cope with allergies is to prevent attacks before they start. The prescription drugs mentioned above can help, as can butterbur, quercetin, and zinc. Here are three other approaches to prevention.

Take fish oil every day. Fish oil reduces inflammation in the body. It also helps your heart and the rest of the body—not just your allergies. Take 1,500 milligrams a day.

Even before allergy season begins, start taking bee propolis. Made by bees, this substance contains various flavonoids, including quercetin, and is thought to inhibit inflammation related to allergies. Start taking 500 milligrams two to three times a day four to six weeks before allergy season begins (assuming you have seasonal allergies) or take daily if you have perennial allergies. Don't take if you're allergic to bees.

Consider allergy shots. Also called desensitization shots or immunotherapy, they work by gradually desensitizing your immune system to the substance to which you're allergic. They take several weeks (and often dozens of shots) to do the job, and don't work for everyone, but if your allergies are really making you miserable, they're worth a try.

Limit your exposure to allergens. Closing the windows and running the AC, using a vacuum with a HEPA filter, replacing carpeting with hard flooring, and changing bed linens (especially pillowcases) often help limit your pollen, dust mite, and mold exposure. Running a dehumidifier can also keep mold growth in check. Ask your doctor for more ways to reduce your allergen exposure.

Asthma

If you've had asthma since you were a child, then you know how treatment of this disease has changed over the past two decades. We used to treat asthma as an acute illness, one in which you took medication only when you couldn't breathe. Today we know that it's a chronic condition, one that involves inflammation of the airways—even when you think you are breathing clearly.

Asthma is a perfect condition for an integrative medicine approach. Modern asthma drugs—like corticosteroids and leukotriene modifiers—do an amazing job of controlling the inflammation when taken on a daily basis. Meanwhile, alternative remedies and lifestyle changes, including something as simple as eating more fatty fish and Brazil nuts, can decrease your dependence on medication.

One warning: Asthma is a serious disease. It needs to be treated with conventional medication during attacks, not herbs alone. Also, if you haven't done so already, talk with your doctor about an asthma management plan. As part of this plan, you'll learn how to use a peak flow meter and determine which medications you need on a daily basis and which rescue medication you'll use during attacks. Remember, you are the most important element when it comes to the daily management of your asthma.

Do This Now

Follow this sequence of actions at the first sign of an asthma attack. If you have frequent attacks, keep reading for ways to keep chronic asthma under better control.

1. Use your peak flow meter. If you are in the red range, go immediately to the emergency room. If you are in the yellow range, keep reading.

2. Use your rescue medication. This is usually a bronchodilator such as Proventil (albuterol). If you don't feel relief within 15 minutes, use it up to twice more, 15 minutes apart. Once you feel relief, continue using it every four to six hours during the next 24 hours to make sure you don't have another asthma flare.

3. If you've been prescribed a steroid inhaler, take an extra dose about 5 to 10 minutes after using the bronchodilator.

4. If significant allergy exposure triggered your allergy attack, take 25 milligrams of Benadryl.

5. Take 1 to 2 grams of quercetin every 4 to 6 hours as symptoms persist.

6. Drink one or two cups of strong caffeinated coffee or tea (as long as you are not also taking theophylline).

7. Take in as deep a breath as possible, then exhale through pursed lips (as if you were going to whistle, only don't make the sound). Repeat this for several minutes.

8. Recheck your peak flow meter after an hour. If you haven't significantly improved, call your doctor.

Why It Works

Bronchodilators, or rescue medications, open and keep open the large and small airways in your lungs. But they don't do much for inflammation, so they shouldn't be the only medication you're using. If you find you're using your rescue medication several times a week, your asthma is not well controlled and it's time for a talk with your doctor.

Quercetin is a powerful flavonoid, an antioxidant plant chemical that helps prevent the formation of histamines and reduces inflammation.

As for the caffeinated drink, we recommend it because caffeine contains compounds, similar to the asthma medication theophylline, which have an airway-opening effect. Theophylline is rarely prescribed any longer, but the active ingredient in it, methylxanthine, is found in coffee. Plus, the warmth of the liquid helps to relax constricted airways.

The breathing technique, called pursed lip breathing, puts more pressure on your airways, holding them open so they don't collapse during exhalation. Don't wait until an asthma attack to try this for the first time; it works best if you've been practicing it regularly.

Other Medicines
Herbs and Supplements

The use of natural remedies to treat asthma dates back thousands of years. In fact, several prescription medications began as herbal remedies. While there are literally dozens of herbs you could take to treat asthma symptoms and help prevent attacks, we recommend the following.

Vitamin C with flavonoids. Take 500 milligrams three or four times a day when your symptoms are flaring, or 250 milligrams three or four times a day when your lung function is in the green range. Several studies find that vitamin C not only reduces asthma symptoms but may also help prevent them. Some people with asthma have lower levels of vitamin C in their blood and sputum (mucus). The vitamin is considered a natural antihistamine. An added bonus: Large doses (1 to 2 grams) may prevent exercise-induced asthma. (They may also cause diarrhea, however, so cut back if you have this problem.) It's always better to get vitamins through your diet; most fruits and vegetables are high in vitamin C, especially red bell peppers, kiwifruit, broccoli, strawberries, cantaloupe, and oranges.

Quercetin. This flavonoid works both to treat and prevent attacks. Take one to two 500-milligram capsules three times a day and consume more foods rich in quercetin, such as apples (with the skins) and onions.

Other Approaches

Acupuncture. Several studies support the use of acupuncture to help prevent and even treat asthma attacks. Overall, studies find that acupuncture during asthma attacks can improve airflow about half as much as an inhaled beta2-agonist, such as Ventolin or Proventil.

Steam inhalation. To ease your breathing, use either the steam treatment described on page 72 in the allergy section or a cool mist humidifier if the heat from the steam bothers you.

Prevention

In most instances, asthma is just an extreme reaction to an allergen, or trigger. So identifying your asthma triggers and controlling your exposure to them is very important.

Beyond that, there are plenty of approaches that can help prevent asthma flares.

Take a preventive prescription drug if you need one. See "Preventive Asthma Drugs," page 78. What you take and when you take it will depend on the severity of your asthma and whether it is classified as mild intermittent (no medication necessary), mild persistent, moderate persistent, or severe persistent. Ask your doctor where you fall on the continuum. Although daily anti-inflammatory medication is usually recommended for mild persistent asthma, a study published in the *New England Journal of Medicine* in 2005 found that it may not be necessary. We suggest you talk to your doctor about this.

Try butterbur. We talked about the use of this herb to treat allergies on page 73. It's also effective for asthma. In one study, 80 adults and children with asthma took between 50 and 150 milligrams a day (depending on age) of a butterbur extract called Petadolex for two months. The number, duration, and severity of their asthma attacks, as well as measures of asthma severity including peak flow and forced expiratory volume, all dropped while they were taking the supplement. Plus, after two months on Petadolex, more than 40 percent of those using asthma medications were able to reduce the amount of medicine they needed.

Block histamine with pycnogenol. This supplement, derived from the bark of pine trees that grow near the sea in France, helps relieve asthma by combating inflammation and preventing the release of histamine. It also relieves swelling, helping you breathe easier. Take 50 to 100 milligrams twice a day.

Get more essential fatty acids. Take 3 grams of either fish oil or evening primrose oil daily to reduce inflammation. You can also get essential fatty acids through your diet, ideally deepwater fish like mackerel and tuna (eat three times a week) or ground flaxseed (sprinkle on yogurt and cereal and aim for one or two tablespoons a day).

Preventive Asthma Drugs

Unlike rescue medications, which abort attacks in progress, these drugs help with long-term asthma management.

Inhaled corticosteroids

These drugs (such as Pulmicort) may take up to a month of daily doses before you notice an effect. Studies show that people with mild asthma taking inhaled steroids can reduce their dose without compromising the drug's effectiveness, so ask your doctor if you're taking the lowest possible dose.

Mast cell stabilizers

Your doctor may prescribe these drugs (Nasalcrom, Intal, or Tilade) if allergies trigger your asthma attacks. They prevent the release of inflammatory chemicals like histamine from mast cells. Be patient, though; it may take up to three weeks before you experience the full benefit. Also, these drugs don't work in everyone and some require use up to four times a day.

Leukotriene modifiers

Leukotrienes are among the molecules that mast cells and other immune system cells release when they encounter allergy triggers. Leukotriene modifiers such as Singulair stem the tide of leukotrienes, come in pill form, and have minimal side effects. They are particularly useful in preventing exercise-induced asthma and asthma triggered by allergens.

Inhaled beta2-agonists

These drugs, which include Serevent and Foradil, are long-acting bronchodilators that work for 12 hours, so you might want to take them at night. However, they don't treat inflammation, so if you're prescribed one, make sure your doctor also treats you with a corticosteroid or other anti-inflammatory drug. You can get both in one with Advair. *Warning:* Don't try to use Serevent as a rescue medication; it works slowly and isn't meant to be used during an attack.

Oral steroids

These drugs are prescribed only if you have very severe asthma, and then only for a short period of time until your symptoms come under control.

Supplement with magnesium. This mineral, often given intravenously during an asthma attack, relaxes the smooth muscles that line your airways, minimizing the spasms that are characteristic of an asthma attack. People with asthma often have low levels of magnesium in their blood, so we recommend supplementing with 250 milligrams twice a day. You should also increase the magnesium in your diet. Good sources include halibut, almonds, cashews, soybeans, spinach, and whole grain cereal.

Supplement with selenium. This trace mineral is a valuable antioxidant, yet people with asthma typically have very low levels in their blood. Supplementing with 200 micrograms daily can significantly improve asthma symptoms. Your best dietary source is Brazil nuts, with 544 micrograms per ounce.

Make it better with bee pollen. Bee pollen, or bee propolis, seems to prevent the release of leukotrienes and other inflammatory chemicals. Intrigued by this information, researchers from Cairo, Egypt, tested the supplement in 22 people with asthma, comparing them with another 24 who received a placebo. Those taking the supplement had far fewer and much less severe nighttime asthma attacks, as well as significant improvements in their lung function. Start with one capsule per day, gradually increasing up to three a day as long as you have no side effects. Don't take if you're allergic to bee stings.

Take up yoga. We know stress plays a role in asthma flares, so it's important to make changes in your life to help reduce it. One approach that has shown good results in numerous studies is yoga. Yoga encompasses relaxation and meditation as well as regulated breathing exercises through the pranayama part of the work. In one study of 17 adults with asthma, those who learned yoga and meditation and practiced it three times a week for four months not only reported they were more relaxed but were able to reduce the amount of beta2-agonist they used. Other studies find improved peak flow meter readings in yoga practitioners.

Keep a journal. The simple act of writing about stressful experiences can significantly improve your asthma symptoms. At least, that's what researchers at the State University of New York at Stony Brook School of Medicine found when they asked 58 asthma patients to write about either the most stressful events of their life or about nonstressful events. After four months, lung function in the stressful-event-writing group improved significantly, while the others showed no change. Whenever you're feeling stressed, take 10 minutes to sit in a quiet place, open a notebook, and let the voice in your head come out on the page.

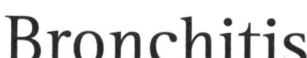

Bronchitis

When you have a deep rattling cough that just won't quit, you probably have bronchitis—inflammation of the bronchial tubes that results in a chest full of phlegm. Contrary to popular belief, bronchitis is not usually a bacterial infection requiring antibiotics. It's most often a complication of a viral infection (such as a cold), and can usually be treated with home remedies. Having said that, if you're coughing up dark yellow or green mucus, chances are you're dealing with a bacterial infection, and you should see a doctor.

Acute bronchitis is gone for good once it clears up, but with chronic bronchitis, the cough comes back again and again. It's usually caused by irritation to the lungs from gases or particles—especially cigarette smoke. Our advice? Stop smoking.

Do This Now

Follow this sequence of actions when you're suffering from an acute bout of bronchitis.

1. Take as deep a breath as possible, then exhale through pursed lips (as if you were whistling, but don't whistle).

2. Boil a pot of water, remove it from the heat, and place it on a heat-safe surface. Add 10 to 15 drops of eucalyptus oil. If you don't have any eucalyptus oil, use peppermint. (Don't use any essential oils if you're wheezing.) Lean over the pot with a towel over your head to keep in the steam. Breathe deeply until the water cools.

3. Make a chest rub by mixing 30 drops of massage or carrier oil like almond, jojoba, or avocado (neutral oils that are well absorbed by the skin) with 5 to 10 drops of eucalyptus or wintergreen oil. Rub the mixture onto your chest, then apply a hot-water bottle to help your skin absorb it, or cover your chest with a thin cotton towel or piece of flannel, then put a heating pad on top. Now snuggle under the blankets.

4. If your cough is productive—that is, you're coughing up phlegm—you don't need any cough medicine during the day. (Better to cough up the phlegm than leave it in the chest.) If not, take 1 to 2 teaspoons every 6 hours of an expectorant cough medicine that contains guaifenesin to help thin the mucus in your lungs. If your cough keeps you up at night or is dry and comes in waves that you can't stop, try 1 to 2 teaspoons every 12 hours of a cough suppressant that contains dextromethorphan, such as Delsym.

Why It Works

The pursed lips breathing technique puts pressure on your airways, holding them open so they don't collapse during exhalation and enabling you to breathe easier.

Studies find that inhaling oils that contain menthol, or rubbing them on your chest, can reduce spasms in smooth muscle surrounding the breathing tubes. The oils also thin mucus so it's easier to cough it up. This is also how expectorant cough medicines work. Cough suppressants that contain dextromethorphan, on the other hand, work on the brain to elevate the threshold for coughing. They are meant to halt dry, hacking coughs. It's best not to suppress a wet cough.

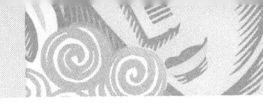

Other Medicines
Herbs and Supplements

Fenugreek. Take two capsules of fenugreek (capsules are typically between 350 and 500 milligrams) three to four times a day to thin mucus.

Bronchipret. If you're coughing but not bringing up much mucus, try this multi-herbal formula that makes your cough more productive. Take 3 to 4 tablets a day, either swallowing them or letting them dissolve on your tongue. You can also try Sinupret, a German herbal remedy often used for sinusitis that helps thin mucus. See Resources, page 365, for buying information.

Esberitox. If you think your bronchitis is heading toward a bacterial infection, start with this combination herbal formula before asking for an antibiotic. Clinical trials find it's effective in treating respiratory infections like bronchitis. See Resources, page 365, for buying information.

Prescription Drugs

If you have chronic bronchitis, your doctor will likely treat you with several prescription medications, including a bronchodilator like albuterol (Ventolin or Proventil), anti-inflammatory medications such as prednisone to reduce airway swelling, and Atrovent, which helps block the production of mucus.

Other Approaches

Garlic. Although the thought of eating four to five raw cloves of garlic a day might turn you off, we urge you to try it. Garlic is a traditional herbal remedy for respiratory infections. To safely eat raw garlic (it can burn the mouth), peel and crush fresh cloves, then mix with a small amount of rice, mashed potatoes, or pasta. While the smell of garlic in your breath isn't great for romance, it shows that the active compound in the garlic has gotten into your lungs. Don't eat a lot of garlic if you're taking a blood-thinning medication like Coumadin or are scheduled for surgery in the next two weeks.

Massage. Regular massage may help prevent, as well as treat, respiratory infections. Not any massage will do, however. A technique called percussive massage, in which the therapist uses a slapping or cupping motion on your back, helps loosen mucus.

A humidifier. Constant coughing and a good night's sleep don't mix. Run a cool humidifier in your bedroom to help you sleep.

Prevention

Stop smoking. We've already said it, but we'll say it again: If you are prone to bronchitis, stop smoking. Cigarette smoke suppresses the body's ability to clear mucus from the lungs (and of course it damages the lungs). Also limit exposure to harsh chemicals and odors. Even using bleach or a strong cleaner like Ajax in a poorly ventilated space can trigger coughing.

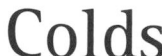

Colds

We can clone mammals, send a spacecraft to Mars, and invent fat-free cheesecake, but we can't cure the common cold. And we probably won't ever be able to. After all, there are more than 200 viruses that cause colds. But while we can't cure colds, we are getting better at making them shorter and less severe. Using integrative remedies, you can reduce the duration of your cold from the typical ten to twelve days to five to eight. You can also help prevent a cold by addressing two Super Threats: a weak immune system and chronic stress.

Do This Now

Follow this sequence of actions at the very first sign of a cold.

1. Suck on a zinc lozenge containing at least 6 to 13 milligrams of zinc gluconate every two waking hours (don't chew or swallow whole). Don't suck on more than 10 in one 24-hour period or you may get nauseated.

2. Every time you pop a zinc lozenge in your mouth, also spray Zicam, a zinc nasal gel formulation, in each nostril.

3. Additionally, take an herb called *Andrographis paniculata* unless you're pregnant or trying to become pregnant. Good brands include TriMune, made by Nature Made (it also contains vitamin C, zinc, and echinacea), and Kold Kare. Follow the dosage instructions on the label.

4. Prepare (or have someone else prepare) a pot of chicken soup and eat a steaming bowlful.

Load it up with garlic, and add a teaspoon of hot red pepper flakes for added effect.

5. If you're very congested, take two 30-milligram pseudoephedrine tablets every four to six hours, or 120 milligrams in a 12-hour formulation. Try to avoid taking it near bedtime, as it may interfere with your sleep.

6. If you're sneezing a lot, take an antihistamine such as Chlor-Trimeton or Claritin according to package directions.

7. If your throat is sore, gargle with warm salt water.

Why It Works

Zinc is an important mineral for the immune system. Numerous studies find that sucking on zinc lozenges at the first symptoms of a cold can reduce their severity and help you feel better faster. Zicam, available in drugstores, is a homeopathic remedy containing zinc. A study conducted at the Cleveland Clinic Foundation found that people who used Zicam nasal gel recovered from their cold three times faster than those taking a placebo, even when participants began taking Zicam the second day of their cold symptoms. You can get Zicam five different ways: the nasal gel pump, nasal gel swabs, chewable tablets, melt-in-your-mouth tablets, and mouth spray. For best effects, continue using for 48 hours after your cold symptoms end.

The herb andrographis has been used for centuries to treat colds and fevers. There's quite a bit of research on it, with several studies finding that it not only reduces the duration of cold symptoms but also reduces the number of colds if taken on a regular basis. Although echinacea is more popular, we think andrographis works better. It has many different effects on the body, but the one that's probably most related to its effects on colds is its ability to reduce inflammation, the culprit behind most cold symptoms. The herb also stimulates the immune system and can help the body produce certain antibodies, chemicals generated in reaction to foreign invaders like cold viruses.

Grandma recommended chicken soup for a cold, and so do we. It isn't just unfounded folk medicine. Scientists have actually studied chicken soup and, at least in the lab, it proved to have real healing effects. The soup inhibited the movement of white blood cells called neutrophils. These cells are designed to gobble up bacteria and other microorganisms; they are released in huge numbers when you have a cold. Neutrophils rushing to infected sites are a major cause of the inflammation and other symptoms associated with a cold. Chicken soup has other benefits too. The steam helps open up clogged nasal passages, the broth provides liquid for hydration, the spiciness of the hot pepper opens your sinuses and gets mucus flowing, and the garlic has immune-boosting benefits. Plus, not to be minimized, you can't eat steaming hot chicken soup while on the go—you have to take time out. Getting rest is a critical "ingredient" in your recovery.

ℰ Helpful Hint

Blow the Right Way

You probably go through a box of tissues every few days when you have a cold. Make sure you're using them properly. Don't just blow no-holds-barred; that can send germ-filled mucus into your ears. Instead, hold one nostril closed with a finger, then gently blow.

Finally, gargling with salt water soothes a sore throat in two ways: The warmth increases blood flow to the throat, which helps fight the infection, and the salt clears away dead white blood cells and other "garbage," making room for healthy new tissue. You can boost your gargle with a squeeze of lemon; the acidity helps kill off bacteria and viruses.

Other Medicines
Herbs and Supplements

Echinacea. This popular herb is another option for fighting colds. We think it's definitely second to andrographis, but it's easier to find. Not all echinacea is created equal, however. The most effective form is a tincture, or water alcohol extract, of *Echinacea purpurea* and/or *Echinacea angustifolia*. Mix 1/4 to 1/2 teaspoon of the tincture in 1 to 2 ounces of hot water and drink every four to six hours.

Slippery elm. If you're coughing, look for an herbal cough formula, lozenge, or tea that contains slippery elm, a natural throat-coating mucilage. A good tea that's been clinically tested is called Throat Coat, which contains slippery elm, licorice root, and other herbs. Marshmallow root (not to be confused with the marshmallows you eat) is another herb that coats a sore throat.

Honey and lemon. Drinking hot water with honey and lemon is a simple yet effective way to soothe a sore throat. The honey coats the throat, while the lemon acts as an astringent, shrinking swollen throat tissue. Honey is also a humectant (a substance that draws moisture) and is naturally antiseptic.

Fenugreek. An herb used to make curry, it can also thin mucus and relieve a cough. Take two 300- to 400-milligram capsules three or four times a day. It will make your urine smell like barbecue sauce, but don't worry; it's not harmful.

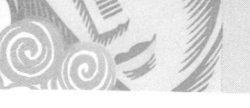
Over-the-Counter Drugs

Oral decongestants. If your nose is so stuffy that you have trouble breathing at night or you're snoring, use a decongestant like Sudafed (or generic pseudoephedrine tablets). But these drugs dry you out and can keep you up at night, so try other remedies first.

Nasal sprays. If you need something at night, try a nasal spray decongestant like Afrin. One or two squirts in each nostril will relieve congestion for up to 12 hours. Nasal sprays won't keep you awake, but don't use them for more than three days. If overused, they can have a "rebound" effect, resulting in increased swelling when you stop using them.

Cough suppressants. If your cough is really driving you crazy and herbal cough syrups and other remedies don't do the trick, try a cough syrup containing the cough suppressant dextromethorphan. For nighttime coughs, choose a product like Delsym, a slow-release version that lasts for 12 hours. Avoid products with extra ingredients like decongestants or aspirin if you don't need them.

Lozenges. To numb the pain, look for a lozenge that contains benzocaine, an anesthetic.

Other Approaches

Steam inhalation. Try the steam treatment described on page 72 (in the allergy chapter) or use a cool-mist humidifier with mentholated essential oils such as pine, eucalyptus, or peppermint added to unclog stuffy sinuses without medication.

Chest rub. Make a chest rub by mixing 30 drops of massage or carrier oil like almond, jojoba or avocado (neutral oils well absorbed by the skin) with 5 to 10 drops of eucalyptus or wintergreen essential oil. After rubbing the mixture onto your chest, apply a hot-water bottle to help your skin better absorb it, or cover your chest with a cotton towel or piece of flannel, then put a heating pad on top. Snuggle under the blankets. A simpler option is to rub some Vicks VapoRub or other chest rub containing eucalyptus and/or menthol on your chest, then cover with a warm flannel shirt (try tossing it into the dryer for five minutes). Throw a heating pad on top for extra effect.

Plenty of liquids. When you're sick, your metabolism speeds up and you burn more calories and use more water. Add to that fact your increased mouth breathing and possibly a fever, and you can see why you need to drink more liquids. Hot liquids provide a triple whammy: They replenish fluids, soothe the throat, and prevent viruses in the throat from replicating.

Prevention

By addressing two Super Threats—decreasing the stress in your life and strengthening your immune system—you can significantly cut down on the number of colds you suffer every year, and maybe even get through the year cold free! So check back in Part 2 for our recommendations on battling these two Super Threats, especially if you're experiencing recurrent colds.

Now, if everyone around you has a cold, do the following.

Wash your hands at least once every two hours for at least a minute, and generally avoid touching your eyes, nose, and mouth.

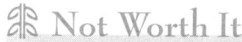 Not Worth It

Goldenseal

Although many echinacea formulations are packaged with the herb goldenseal, there's no evidence that goldenseal can prevent or even decrease cold symptoms. Additionally, the plant is an endangered species.

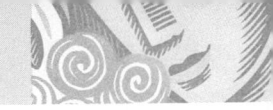

Head for the health club and sit in the sauna for 15 minutes twice a week. Some health clubs will even give you a day pass. Studies find that regular sauna use can reduce the incidence of colds.

Hit the sack early. When cold season is upon you, it's time to get an extra hour of sleep a night to support your immune system.

Clean phones and doorknobs every day with an antiseptic preparation like Lysol or rubbing alcohol. You can also try a dilute solution of antiseptic essential oils such as eucalyptus, thyme, and tea tree. Mix 10 drops of each in 3 ounces of an equal mix of rubbing alcohol and water.

Take andrographis or Esberitox. Andrographis, described on page 82, is one of the few herbal therapies with good research suggesting it prevents as well as treats colds. Take 2 pills three times a day for 10 days with a standardized preparation of 30 milligrams of andrographolides per tablet. Another one to try, either instead of or in addition to andrographis, is the German herbal preparation Esberitox. Available in most health food stores, it contains two types of echinacea as well as white cedar and wild indigo extracts. Numerous studies testing its use in patients with weak immune systems as well as in healthy patients find it increases immune response. Take 3 pills, three times a day.

Cut back on alcohol, which suppresses the immune system.

Keep a humidifier running in your home to keep your mucous membranes moist so they're better able to ward off viruses.

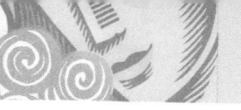

Flu

Unlike the common cold, which is annoying but ultimately harmless, the flu can be dangerous—even deadly. Your best bet? Focusing on the twin Super Threats of chronic stress and immune weakness. With a strong immune system, you're much more likely to fight off this potential killer.

If you do get the flu, act fast. Prescription antiviral medications can help you get better faster, and numerous studies find that natural remedies can also significantly reduce the amount of time you suffer—but you need to take them at the very first sign of symptoms, or as a precaution during flu season.

Do This Now

Follow these six steps at the first sign of the flu.

1. Call your doctor and ask for an antiviral medication such as amantadine, rimantadine, zanamivir, or oseltamivir.

2. At the same time, start taking 1 tablespoon of the liquid elderberry extract Sambucol four times a day for three to five days.

3. Also start taking the homeopathic remedy *Anas Barbariae Hepatis et cordis extractum 200c*, more commonly known as Oscillococcinum or Flu Remedy. Follow the dosage instructions on the package.

4. To relieve headache and achiness, take 500 to 1,000 milligrams of enteric-coated aspirin, 200 milligrams of ibuprofen, or 500 to 1,000 milligrams of acetaminophen every four to six hours, or 275 milligrams of naproxen twice a day. Don't take acetaminophen if you have

liver disease. Don't give aspirin, ibuprofen, or naproxen to children or adolescents (use acetaminophen instead).

5. Now that you're medicated, work on bringing your fever down to make yourself more comfortable. Start with cool compresses on the pulse points at the neck, throat, and wrists.

6. If your fever is still high and you're still achy, add a cup of Epsom or sea salt to a warm tub, soak for 20 minutes, then wrap up warmly and lie under blankets to induce a sweat. Adding 10 to 15 drops of eucalyptus or peppermint oil to the bath will help with congestion, cough, and muscle aches.

Why It Works

Antiviral drugs can decrease the severity and length of your infection if you take them within the first day or two of symptoms. They're particularly helpful if you got the flu even though you were vaccinated, because chances are you're dealing with a different strain from the ones in the vaccine.

Sambucol also fights the flu directly. One well-designed study of 60 patients, all of whom had the flu, found that those who received the supplement were nearly recovered by the third or fourth day of treatment, whereas it took seven to eight days for the people in the placebo group to feel better. Researchers think that compounds called anthocyanins in elderberry may be responsible; they boost the immune system and also seem to prevent the flu virus from sticking to cells.

The other treatments are all about making you more comfortable and relieving aches and pains. The warm bath has an added effect: it causes a

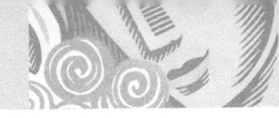

slight increase in body temperature, which makes bacteria-killing enzymes more effective, potentially helping to prevent a secondary bacterial infection when your defenses are down.

Other Medicines

Herbs and Supplements

Fenugreek. If you're coughing, take 2 capsules three or four times a day. This herb helps thin mucus and also soothes a dry cough. (Note that it makes your urine smell sweet.)

Over-the-Counter Drugs

Cough suppressants. If you want to use a cough suppressant, choose one that contains dextromethorphan. At night, try Delsym, which lasts for 12 hours.

Other Approaches

Sports creams. For body aches, massage a pain-relief rub or sports cream like Ben-Gay or Tiger Balm onto the achy areas.

Fluids. Drink lots and lots of fluids, both hot and cold. Avoid caffeinated and overly sweet drinks like sodas and undiluted fruit juices.

Prevention

Consider a flu shot. Although a flu shot is often considered the best bet for preventing the flu and should definitely be a part of any flu prevention program for the elderly, young children, and anyone with a compromised immune system, there is some evidence that healthy people with a strong immune system may do just as well with approaches like the ones described here.

Start taking American ginseng extract or the Chinese ginseng extract Ginsana once flu season begins. Several clinical trials find that taking

---

Is It the Flu?

Use this chart to help you determine if you have a cold or the flu.

	Cold	Flu
Fever	Rarely	Yes, usually high, with a sudden onset
Headache	Rarely	Severe
Aches and pains	Slight	Significant
Fatigue, weakness	Some	Severe
Stuffy nose	Yes	Occasionally
Sneezing	Yes	Maybe
Sore throat	Yes	Occasionally
Chest discomfort	None or mild	Yes
Cough	Hacking	Severe (sometimes)

---

either one significantly reduces your likelihood of getting the flu. Take 100 milligrams of Ginsana twice a day for up to two weeks when flu exposure risk is highest, or 200 milligrams twice a day of Cold-fX, an American ginseng extract (see Resources, page 365, for buying information).

Add "green drinks" rich in chlorella, a type of algae, to your diet. Available at health food stores, these drinks, such as wheat and barley grass, are very high in antioxidants and chlorophyll (the stuff that makes plants green), which stimulates the immune system. In one study on 124 healthy adults, those 55 and older who received a chlorella-derived supplement once a day for four weeks had a much greater immune response against certain strains of the flu than those who got a placebo.

Wash your hands frequently with soap and hot water.

Get enough sleep. Lack of shut-eye lowers your immune defenses.

Take a daily multivitamin/mineral supplement that contains antioxidants, including at least 200 IU of vitamin E.

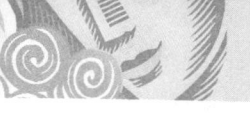

Sinusitis

Is it a cold, the flu, allergies or sinusitis? Given the overlapping symptoms like congestion, fever, and headache, it can be hard to tell. Plus, one often leads to the other. Congestion from colds or allergies provides a breeding ground for viruses and bacteria, which can lead to sinusitis.

The dead giveaway that you're dealing with sinusitis, however, is a heavy feeling of pressure in your face. You can also blame sinusitis for a pounding headache that gets worse when you lean over, a toothache, and green or gray nasal drainage and postnasal drip.

Many of our remedies mimic those we recommend for allergies and colds, since you're trying to attack many of the same issues, especially thick mucus and inflammation.

Do This Now

If you think you have sinusitis, follow these steps to clear your sinuses for fast relief.

1. Start with nasal irrigation. Add 1/4 teaspoon salt to 1 cup warm water. To get it into your nose, use an ear bulb syringe (like the kind used to clean out a baby's nose), a neti pot, available in health food stores, or a waterpick. To use the waterpick, you'll need a Grossan nasal adapter, available in drug and health food stores. Run the waterpick on its lowest setting. Flush your nasal passages two to three times a day.

2. Next, bring a pot of water to a boil. Remove it from the heat. Add 10 to 15 drops of eucalyptus oil, then place a towel over your head and shoulders and inhale the steam for 10 to 15 minutes. Do this at least twice a day.

3. Practice postural drainage. Wet a washcloth under hot water, squeeze out the excess water, assume the proper position depending on where you're most congested, then apply the cloth for 10 to 15 minutes per sinus. To drain the frontal sinuses (behind the forehead), sit upright. To drain the maxillary sinuses (behind the cheekbones), lie on the opposite side (i.e., if your left sinus is clogged, lie on your right side). To drain the ethmoid sinuses (behind the bridge of the nose), lie on your back.

4. If your sinuses are still clogged, mix 1 teaspoon horseradish with 1/2 teaspoon olive oil and 1 tablespoon lemon juice. Eat 1/4 teaspoon at a time until you feel your sinuses start to drain. Eat it mixed with rice or mashed potatoes if necessary to protect your mouth and stomach from burning.

5. If you are still congested and in pain, turn to an over-the-counter decongestant like Sudafed.

Why It Works

Studies find that using nasal irrigation before you turn to antibiotics and decongestants helps these medications penetrate the nasal cavities better. The salt water also decreases swelling, which improves drainage. Nasal irrigation may also help flush out bacteria.

The warm, moist heat of postural drainage, coupled with gravity, helps clear congested sinuses.

The heat of the horseradish helps thin mucus, encouraging drainage.

Decongestants do what their name implies. But don't use them for more than a few days. They

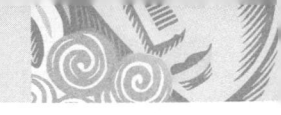

dry up mucus, leaving it hard and sticky and blocking the small openings of the sinuses.

Other Medicines
Herbs and Supplements

Ginger compress. Grate a large gingerroot into 1 pint boiling water and simmer for 15 minutes. Strain. Soak a washcloth in the tea, then apply to your face as part of your postural drainage.

Sinupret. This German product contains a handful of herbs with mucus-thinning, anti-inflammatory, and antiviral properties. Studies have found it protects people with chronic sinusitis from infection and aids recovery in those with acute sinusitis when taken with antibiotics and decongestants. Follow the package directions.

Pycnogenol/grape seed extract. This antioxidant helps reduce inflammation associated with sinus allergy and irritation. Take 50 milligrams three times a day.

Fenugreek and thyme. To thin mucus, take two fenugreek capsules with one thyme capsule two to three times a day.

Prescription Drugs

If you have acute sinusitis, your doctor may decide to prescribe an antibiotic if self-care measures fail. If you have chronic sinusitis, defined as sinus infections lasting 8 to 12 weeks, your doctor may prescribe nasal corticosteroids such as Flonase or corticosteroid tablets, and/or medications that thin the mucus, such as guaifenesin.

Other Approaches

Acupressure. Press hard on the outer edge of your nostrils at the base of your nose with your index fingers. Then put your thumbs on either side of your nose and firmly press on the cartilage (the part that moves back and forth), holding for 30 seconds, then releasing. Now press the areas next to your inner eyes with your left thumb and index finger as you use your fingers and the heel of your other hand to grab the muscles on both sides of your spine at the back of your neck, pressing on all four points for about a minute.

Prevention

Treat your allergies. If you're prone to sinus infections, have your doctor check you for allergies, and reduce your exposure to allergens.

Eat sinus-friendly foods. Eat more spicy foods, which promote mucus drainage, and limit sugar and alcohol, which interferes with the immune response. Alcohol also swells nasal and sinus membranes. Eliminate foods that leave you congested. For many people, this includes ice cream or milk, possibly signifying an allergy to dairy.

Consume more antioxidants. Studies suggest that people who are prone to sinus infections have low blood levels of antioxidants. So eat more fruits and vegetables, and consider these supplements: 250 milligrams vitamin C, 100 to 200 IU vitamin E, 5,000 IU beta-carotene, 200 micrograms selenium, and 25 milligrams zinc.

TIME TO WORRY

Call your doctor if your condition doesn't improve after two days of home treatment and your symptoms include:

- Persistent pain and pressure in the central part of your face

- Headache around your eyes that doesn't respond to Tylenol or aspirin

- Fever of 101°F or higher, especially if accompanied by facial pain

- Nasal discharge that is thick, discolored, foul tasting, or foul smelling

Snoring

The butt of late-night-comedian jokes, snoring is no laughing matter. In fact, one of the major causes of snoring—sleep apnea, a condition in which breathing may be interrupted up to 300 times a night—is associated with heart disease, heart attack, and premature death.

Nearly half of us snore at any one time, and one quarter of us every night. Why do we snore? Many reasons, ranging from a stuffed nose to sleeping position. The primary cause of a snore, however, is the vibration of the soft palate (the soft, fleshy part of the roof of your mouth) and the uvula, that fleshy tip that hangs down the back of your throat, as air passes through. If you're overweight or you've had too much to drink, these tissues are more likely to sag and obstruct the flow of air—and you're more likely to snore.

Even if your snoring doesn't bother you, it probably bothers the person you share your bed with. Since good sleep is important to good health, if you love your partner, you'll address your snoring.

Do This Now

Follow this sequence of actions for fast relief of short-term snoring. For chronic snoring, read on for more advice.

1. Go to the drugstore for some nasal strips to wear at night.

2. Before you go to bed, elevate the head of the bed by placing a couple of bricks or boards under the legs. If you can't raise the head of the bed, add a couple of pillows so your head and neck rest much higher than the rest of your body.

3. Get used to sleeping in a non-snoring position, generally *not* on your back. An old trick: Sew a pocket to the back of your pajamas and put a tennis ball into the pocket.

4. Before you turn out your light, spritz an aromatherapy spray called Helps Stop Snoring in each nostril.

5. If you're congested, take an oral or nasal decongestant spray before bed to relieve congestion (don't do this more than three nights in a row, however).

6. Run a humidifier in your bedroom at night.

Why It Works

Nasal strips work by lifting and opening nasal passages so you can breathe through your nose, not your mouth (mouth breathing is a major reason for snoring). In one study, 35 people with a history of heavy snoring wore nasal strips for two weeks. Both the participants and their partners evaluated their sleep and snoring. Overall, 52 percent of the participants' partners reported less snoring, while 66 percent of the snorers reported less daytime sleepiness.

By raising the head of your bed, you keep your head and neck elevated. This helps reduce snoring in two ways: it drains a stuffy nose or sinuses and opens up the throat so the uvula has more room to hang freely.

The nasal spray contains a variety of essential oils, including mint, lemon, close, fennel, thyme, and lavender, and is said to tighten, or tone, soft tissue, preventing it from obstructing airflow and vibrating. A study of 120 serious snorers found

that the partners of 82 percent of those who received a dose of the oil said their partners' snoring improved. That compared to 44 percent of partners of those who tried a placebo. The spray is available in drugstores in the United Kingdom and online at helpsstopsnoring.co.uk. Other snoring sprays are available in the United States but lack clinical evidence behind them. There's no harm in trying them, though.

By sending water vapor into the air, a humidifier prevents your nasal passages and throat from drying out, which contributes to snoring.

Other Approaches

Mouth splint. An orthodontic appliance called a mouth splint, or mandibular advancement splint, keeps your lower jawbone from falling back during sleep, which contributes to snoring.

Neck brace. If you tend to snore when your head is tilted forward, talk to your doctor about a soft neck brace to wear while you sleep.

CPAP. If you are diagnosed with sleep apnea (and if you're a serious snorer, you should be evaluated), the first thing your doctor should try is a treatment called CPAP: continuous positive airway pressure. A mask that fits over your nose and mouth while you sleep drives air through your nose, forcing your airways open. This approach works in up to 90 percent of people with sleep apnea and can be used as long as you need it.

Surgery. For severe snoring, your doctor may want you to consider surgery. Several surgeries can help reduce or eliminate snoring, including nasal surgery, in which polyps or nasal irregularities are corrected; soft palate surgery, also called uvulopalatopharyngoplasty (UPPP), in which the surgeon expands air passages and tightens flabby tissues in the throat and palate; and thermal ablation palatoplasty (TAP), an umbrella term for a host of procedures designed to shrink excess tissue in the palate, uvula, tongue, and nasal passages.

Prevention

Lose weight. One major cause of snoring is overweight or obesity, so losing weight is critical. Losing just 10 percent of your body weight can make a big difference.

Finish dinner (and drinks) at least three hours before you go to bed. Eating a heavy meal or drinking alcohol before you go to sleep makes the tissue at the back of your throat more relaxed, increasing your snoring.

Get some exercise. Exercise can tighten loose muscle that may lead to posture problems that result in snoring.

Control your allergies. Your bed—with its bedcovers, pillows, and mattress—is a prime source of allergens, particularly dust mites and pet dander, and people who are fine during the day may find they get congested at night. For more on specific allergies and allergy testing, see pages 72-75.

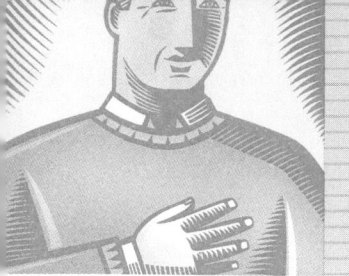

Constipation

An occasional bout of constipation isn't anything to worry about. But if you are constipated several times a month, you may have an underlying condition that requires medical attention. For instance, constipation can be a sign of irritable bowel syndrome (see page 116), colon cancer, bowel obstruction, or appendicitis. It can also be a side effect of medications, including certain calcium channel blockers, narcotics, aluminum antacids, and antidepressants.

You might also have a condition called anismus, or pelvic floor dyssynergia, in which you're unable to have a bowel movement because you contract instead of relax the muscles of the pelvic floor. Researchers suspect it may account for up to half of all cases of chronic constipation. Jump down to the prevention section; we've addressed it there.

There is no "rule" on how often you should have a bowel movement. Some people go every day (maybe even two or three times), others once every couple of days. Medically, you're considered constipated if you haven't had a bowel movement in three days.

Do This Now

When you just can't go, try these gentle remedies before trying anything else.

1. Drink two cups of coffee, warm water with lemon, chamomile tea, or warm prune juice.

2. Now take 1 to 2 teaspoons of psyllium seed and/or husk (also called ispaghula or *Plantago ovata*). If you don't have a bowel movement within 12 hours, take another 2 teaspoons.

3. At the same time you take the psyllium seed, take 300 to 600 milligrams of magnesium.

4. If you have still not had a bowel movement after 24 hours, take a stool softener such as Colace or Surfak, following the package instructions.

Why It Works

The warm liquids trigger the urge to have a bowel movement after a meal. Coffee works well because the caffeine and other chemicals act as mild irritants; that's why many people have a bowel movement after their morning coffee. Chamomile helps relax the muscles around the bowel. Prunes are high in fiber and plant chemicals that help move stool through the colon.

Psyllium is a "bulking agent," the gentlest of all laxative forms, and should be the first laxative option when you're constipated. Don't expect immediate results; it acts relatively slowly (within about 24 hours). Magnesium also acts as a laxative. In fact, one side effect of too much magnesium is diarrhea.

Stool softeners work by helping liquids mix with your stool, so they're softer and easier to pass.

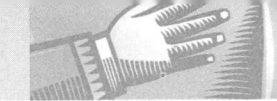

They're so gentle that many doctors recommend them after childbirth or abdominal surgery. Like psyllium, they may take a day or two to work.

Other Medicines
Over-the-Counter Drugs

Lubricant laxatives. These laxatives, including mineral oil, coat the stool, making it easier to expel. Don't take them at the same time as any medicine, though, because they can interfere with the body's absorption of drugs.

Saline or osmotic laxatives. These laxatives, including milk of magnesia, contain magnesium, sulfate, phosphate or citrate ions, which stay in the colon and attract water to the colon to soften the stool. Don't use if you have kidney damage or congestive heart failure.

Stimulant laxatives. These laxatives, including castor oil, Ex-Lax or Senokot, and aloe, should not be your first choice. They force the bowel muscles to contract. Use only if your doctor recommends.

Prescription Drugs

Hyperosmolar laxatives. These drugs, including Kristalose (lactulose), sorbitol, and MiraLax (polyethylene glycol), hold water in the stool, increasing the softness and bulk. One warning: When the bacteria in your colon breaks them down, the result is gas and bloating.

❧ Helpful Hint

Go When You Have the Urge

By sitting on the toilet whenever you feel the urge, or even at regularly scheduled times (such as after breakfast), you can strengthen that mind/gut connection and "train" yourself to have regular bowel movements.

Zelnorm. This drug is sometimes prescribed for chronic—not acute—constipation. It can have severe side effects, so consider it a last resort.

Other Approaches

Homeopathy. One of the most common patent remedies recommended for occasional acute constipation is nux vomica. Look for it as a single remedy or as part of a combination product to treat constipation.

Massage therapy. Massage your abdomen in a clockwise direction with 5 drops of ginger, peppermint, or orange essential oils mixed into 20 drops of a massage or carrier oil (like almond or castor oil). These oils provide warmth, promote increased blood flow, and relax the muscles and tissues of the abdomen. You can also use the oils in a warm bath for a similar effect.

Prevention

Eat more fiber. We can't stress enough the importance of fiber in preventing constipation. Aim to get between 25 and 30 grams a day from whole fruits, vegetables, beans, and whole grains. One way to get your daily fiber is with a morning bowl of oatmeal with fresh fruit or prunes. It one study it worked much better than laxatives—and the oatmeal cost 93 percent less.

Supplement with Metamucil. If you can't get enough fiber from your diet, add a fiber supplement like Metamucil once a day.

Get your fill of fluids. Getting enough fluids is critical to making stool pass easily.

Try biofeedback. If you have (or suspect you have) the condition described above called anismus, biofeedback might be the answer. Several studies find that it helps not only in the short term but also 6 to 12 months after completing the training. Ask your doctor where you can go in your area to receive biofeedback training.

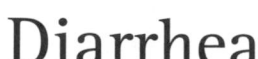

Diarrhea

Like constipation, diarrhea is a symptom, not a disease, one with numerous possible causes. You could have the classic traveler's diarrhea, an intestinal virus, a reaction to medication, or a chronic digestive condition like irritable bowel syndrome or inflammatory bowel disease (see those entries). Even a severe response to stress or something as simple as suddenly cutting out caffeine could lead to diarrhea.

These steps help you get through a bout of short-lived diarrhea. Cases lasting more than 48 to 72 hours require a doctor's attention due to the dangers of dehydration.

Do This Now

1. Stop eating solid food and begin drinking clear liquids, including electrolyte replacement drinks (like Rehydralyte, an adult version of Pedialyte), clear broth, water, and tea. If this slows the diarrhea, remain on the clear liquid diet for 24 hours.

2. After 24 hours on the clear liquid diet, add foods back slowly, starting with simple starches (rice, bread, dry crackers) and bananas. If you can handle these foods without a return of the diarrhea, add simple proteins such as grilled chicken. Do not eat cow's milk products or fatty food for 48 to 72 hours after a bout of diarrhea.

3. If the liquid diet didn't slow your diarrhea within several hours, try stool-thickening agents such as Kaopectate or Diasorb. Take 1 tablespoon with each loose bowel movement. Don't take more than five doses a day.

4. If the stool-thickening agents don't help, move on to the antimotility drug Imodium AD, available in drugstores, or Lomotil, which requires a prescription.

Why It Works

Most diarrhea is related to something you ate. Cutting out solid foods gives your digestive system a rest. Clear liquids reduce the risk of dehydration. Also, broth and electrolyte replacement drinks contain sodium and other important minerals lost through the diarrhea. When it's time to eat again, we recommend bananas because they're high in magnesium and potassium. These minerals help tighten the smooth muscle surrounding the colon, important because one reason for diarrhea is overactivity of those muscles. Bananas are also binding.

Kaopectate and other stool-thickening agents slow the movement of stool through the bowel by either absorbing water in the intestine or thickening the stool, making it less watery. Imodium and Lomotil relax the smooth muscles surrounding the bowel, slowing the movement of the intestinal contents so your colon has more time to absorb liquid.

Other Medicines
Herbs and Supplements

Carob powder. This natural stool-thickening option, available in health food stores, has been used to treat diarrhea in Turkey since ancient times. A study on 80 children conducted there found it significantly improved symptoms when combined with an oral rehydrating solution

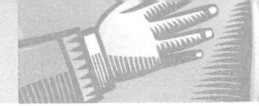

(Pedialyte) compared to the solution alone. Take 1 tablespoon of carob powder moistened with water or diluted soy milk—*not* cow's milk—every time you have a loose stool. Don't take more than five doses a day.

Black walnut husks or hulls. The husks and hulls are astringent, or drying, agents, so they remove water from the stool. Take 1 to 2 capsules of ground husks three or four times a day. You can find them in health food stores.

Probiotics. Probiotics replace friendly bacteria in your gut that can not only stop traveler's diarrhea and diarrhea associated with antibiotics, but also help prevent it in the first place. Take 1 to 2 capsules with each loose bowel movement, up to six a day.

Over-the-Counter Drugs

Pepto-Bismol. The "pink stuff" contains a small amount of aspirin and bismuth subsalicylate, a salt derived from the natural metal bismuth. Although we don't know exactly why it works, it's likely that it decreases inflammation and/or combats the bacteria that may be causing diarrhea. Take 1 tablespoon with every bout of diarrhea, but don't take more than five doses a day. Don't give this to children who have a fever, because it contains aspirin. Pepto-Bismol will temporarily turn your stool black.

Prescription Drugs

Xifaxan (rifaximin). This is an antibiotic that has been widely used for years in Europe for the treatment of traveler's diarrhea and was recently approved for use in the United States. Unlike other antibiotics that can *cause* diarrhea, Xifaxan isn't absorbed into the bloodstream; it stays in your gut to do its job before it is eliminated through the feces. If your doctor wants to put you on an antibiotic for your diarrhea, ask about this one.

Prevention

Avoid dairy. Many adults, particularly Asians, are lactose intolerant, meaning their body doesn't make enough of an enzyme required to digest a sugar called lactose found in dairy products. A major symptom is diarrhea. If you're prone to diarrhea, cut all dairy except active-culture yogurt and see what happens. Another option is to take an over-the-counter lactase enzyme (such as Lactaid) about 30 minutes before eating dairy.

Add psyllium. This high-fiber supplement can help prevent chronic diarrhea. Try sprinkling 1 to 2 tablespoons a day on yogurt to help with chronic diarrhea by adding bulk to the stool.

Take Pepto-Bismol. You can help prevent traveler's diarrhea by taking 1 tablespoon of Pepto-Bismol several times a day while traveling in third-world countries.

Drug and Supplement Culprits

If you take lots of dietary supplements and have loose stools, stop all supplements (check with your health-care practitioner first). Prioritize the products you are taking, then slowly resume taking the most important ones, adding one new product every three to five days until you identify what might be causing the diarrhea. Magnesium-containing supplements (including antacids) are a key culprit.

Also, several prescriptions and over-the-counter drugs can cause diarrhea, including antibiotics, laxatives, colchicine (used to treat gout), quinidine (used to treat abnormal heart rhythms), selective serotonin reuptake inhibitor (SSRI) antidepressants like Prozac, and ACE inhibitors. If you think your medications might be to blame, talk to your doctor about adjusting the dosage or switching to a different drug.

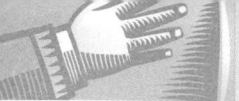

Diverticulitis

Diverticulosis and its cousin, diverticulitis, are diseases of the 20th century and our high-fat, low-fiber Western diet. By age 60, one in ten people are thought to have diverticulosis, or small pouches in their large intestine. It is only when those pouches become inflamed or infected, however, that you have a real problem. Now you have diverticulitis, which affects up to one in four people with diverticulosis and can occur on a regular basis.

If your condition is serious, expect to be hospitalized for intravenous antibiotics and, possibly, surgery. Diverticulitis is nothing to mess around with—it can lead to a perforated colon, abscesses in your colon, or fistulas, in which two areas of the digestive system become connected.

But for "uncomplicated" diverticulitis, try the remedies recommended here. Also, see the Constipation entry on page 92; chronic constipation is a key contributor to diverticulosis and can trigger a diverticulitis attack.

Do This Now

If you're experiencing lower abdominal pain, a slight fever, and/or changes in your bowel movements, see your doctor, and follow these steps for immediate relief.

1. Do not suppress the urge to have a bowel movement even if you think it will hurt.

2. Take Tylenol or aspirin (500 to 1,000 milligrams) or ibuprofen (200 to 400 milligrams).

3. Get into bed and apply a heating pad to your abdomen. Even better, spread castor oil mixed with 10 drops of ginger oil over your abdomen, then cover with a cotton or wool cloth before putting the heating pad on top.

4. Pull up the covers and rest.

5. While you're attacking the pain, also switch to a liquid diet. You should see a major improvement in 24 to 48 hours. If not, move on to the next step.

6. Take an antibiotic.

Why It Works

The liquid diet gives your bowel time to rest and may help a low-grade infection heal. We recommend aspirin or ibuprofen because they attack the underlying cause of the abdominal pain: inflammation of the intestinal wall. Tylenol doesn't affect inflammation, but it will help with pain and is your best option if you have any bleeding or stomach pain.

The warmth of the heating pad relaxes muscles and increases blood flow to the abdomen. Castor oil fights inflammation and is also an excellent carrier oil for the ginger oil, which creates soothing warmth and dilates the blood vessels under the skin, helping the castor oil penetrate more deeply.

Finally, we want you to rest because your body needs to conserve its resources in order to heal.

WARNING

Don't use an enema during a diverticulitis attack, even if you feel like you need one. It could cause a leak in the colon.

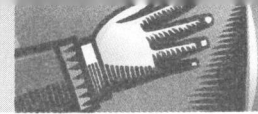

If you don't feel better after a day or two on the liquid diet, you probably need an antibiotic. Talk to your doctor about taking rifaximin, which studies suggest is the most effective antibiotic. It isn't absorbed by the stomach, but gets to the intestine, where it works its healing.

Other Medicines
Herbs and Supplements

Probiotics. A main cause of diverticulitis is the abnormal accumulation of fecal bacteria within the colon, which plays havoc with the normal balance of bacteria and other flora in the gut. Adding "good" bacteria via probiotics is an excellent way to restore that balance. Take 2 capsules with every meal and at bedtime for at least one to two months. If your symptoms respond, gradually decrease the dose until you only need one dose a day. We particularly recommend probiotics if you're taking an antibiotic, both to treat the underlying diverticulitis and to prevent the antibiotics from further altering the flora in your gut.

Over-the-Counter Drugs

Stool softeners such as Colace or Surfak, also known as emollients, are so gentle that many doctors recommend them after childbirth or abdominal surgery. They work by helping liquids mix with your stool, so they're softer and easier to pass. They may take a day or two to begin working.

Prescription Drugs

Asacol or Pentasa (mesalamine). This drug works within the large intestine to reduce inflammation as well as provide antioxidants to protect against further free-radical damage. (For a refresher on free-radical damage, see page 44 in Part 2.) For best results, talk to your doctor about taking the antibiotic rifaximin (Xifaxan) in addition to mesalamine; one large Italian study found that diverticulitis patients treated with both drugs had less severe symptoms and fewer bouts of recurrence in the 12 months after treatment than a group treated with the antibiotic alone.

Other Approaches

Acupuncture. Although there are no published studies on its use in diverticulitis, there is significant evidence showing that acupuncture can reduce inflammation. Particularly helpful are acupuncture points LI 11 (in a depression on the top of the arm, one inch in from the elbow joint) and LI 5 (on top of the wrist in the tiny depression at the base of the thumb). You can try acupressure at these points yourself, holding firmly for 30 seconds to a minute once or twice a day.

Prevention

Eat less meat, more fiber. These are the most important things you can do to prevent diverticulitis, particularly if you have diverticulosis. Aim for 25 to 30 grams of fiber a day. The best fiber source? Bran. Studies in patients getting a little less than an ounce a day (24 grams) of wheat bran for at least six months found significant improvement in nearly all diverticulitis symptoms. Vegetables, beans, and berries are also good sources of fiber. When you eat more fiber, drink plenty of fluids—at least six 8-ounce glasses a day. One caveat about certain fiber sources: If you've had a previous episode of diverticulitis, avoid nuts, seeds, and foods (such as strawberries) that have tiny seeds that could lodge in the diverticulosis pockets.

Get regular exercise. Physical activity is known to help keep your bowels regular, and there is some evidence that it may help prevent diverticulosis as well as diverticulitis. Aim for 30 minutes of mild to moderate exercise most days.

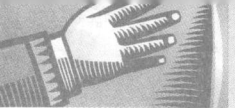

Flatulence

Flatulence is embarrassing and uncomfortable, but the problem usually "passes" quickly. If it recurs often, however, it could be a sign of irritable bowel syndrome, described on page 116. Or you may have a problem with bacterial overgrowth in your large intestine caused by undigested material entering the colon, where it is fermented by various forms of bacteria (hence the odor). You may also have a parasite, picked up during travel.

Be patient with our remedies. Nothing will make your gas go away immediately. It's produced in your colon, so anything you take via mouth requires several hours to get there.

Do This Now

1. Take 125 to 250 milligrams of an over-the-counter brand of simethicone, such as Mylicon or Phazyme, along with a dose of activated charcoal, available in drugstores. Don't exceed 500 milligrams of simethicone in one 24-hour period.

2. Sit on the floor and cross your right leg over your left leg so your right knee is aligned over your left knee. Then lean over as far as you comfortably can. You can also try lying on your back and pulling your knees up to your chest one at a time.

3. Take a walk around the block.

Why It Works

Simethicone is actually a detergent that transforms all the little bubbles in your intestine into larger bubbles so they pass more readily. (Find a private room to spend some time in because you'll still have gas, but at least it will be over with faster.) Meanwhile, the charcoal helps absorb odor by binding to odor-producing sulfur molecules.

Exercise and stretching—especially the stretches mentioned here—help you expel the gas. If you're walking outside, no one need be the wiser.

Other Medicines
Herbs and Supplements

Herbal tea. Mix 1 teaspoon chamomile, 1/2 teaspoon peppermint, 1 teaspoon catnip, 1 teaspoon basil, 2 crushed fennel seeds, and 1/2 teaspoon marjoram. If you don't have catnip or marjoram, just increase the amount of any of the other ingredients to make up for the missing herbs. Steep in 6 to 8 ounces of boiling water for 10 minutes. Strain and drink three or more cups a day. This mixture contains carminative herbs that aid digestion and antispasmodic herbs that decrease colon spasms.

Triphala. This Ayurvedic formula, available in natural food stores, is a digestive tonic consisting of three herbs: Amla (*Phyllanthus emblica* or *Emblica officinalis*), Hara (*Terminalia chebula*), and Bahera (*Terminalia belerica*). The dose depends on the brand, but the usual range is one to two tablets three times a day with meals.

Prescription Drugs

Xifaxan (rifaximin). This antibiotic is approved to treat traveler's diarrhea caused by *Escherichia coli* bacteria. But some patients have had good success using it for flatulence caused by an overgrowth of bacteria in the gut.

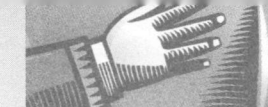

Other Approaches

Activated charcoal pads or underpants. If you have a serious problem with flatulence, these can absorb the odor and save you embarrassment. You can find them at medical supply stores or online. They are washable.

Prevention

Cut down on gas-producing foods such as onions, beans, broccoli, cauliflower, cabbage, and bran. When you do eat them (they are good for you, after all), take Beano at the start of the meal. Beano contains an enzyme that helps break down the types of carbohydrate in these foods that tend to cause gas. Rinse canned beans well before eating; soak dried beans overnight, then discard the water. Cook the beans in fresh water.

Find out if you're lactose intolerant. People who are lactose intolerant have trouble digesting the lactose in dairy products (except yogurt). Gas is often the result. Try cutting out dairy products for a few days and see if it helps. If it does, you're probably lactose intolerant. Take Lactaid (which contains the enzyme that breaks down lactose) before eating dairy products, and look for reduced-lactose milk.

Look to essential oils. Place a drop of peppermint, caraway, or fennel essential oil on a charcoal tablet and take one with every meal to help absorb gas.

Improve your digestion with probiotics. These supplements, such as *Lactobacillus acidophilus,* contain "good" bacteria that don't produce large amounts of gas as they break down nutrients. They also help prevent the overgrowth of other bacteria that linger in the digestive tract, feeding off partially digested carbohydrates and causing gas. Follow the package dosage instructions. Yogurt that contains active cultures is another source of probiotics.

Feed your "good bacteria" with prebiotics. Think of these nondigestible nutrients as fertilizer for the beneficial bacteria in your gut. They also help the bacteria attach more firmly to the wall of the gut, reducing gas. The most common prebiotics are fructo-oligosaccharides and inulin. Follow the package dosage instructions.

Erase gas with enzymes. Digestive enzyme products contain papain (from papaya) or bromelain (from pineapple) and/or the animal-based enzymes trypsin and pepsin. They aid digestion so that less poorly digested material gets to the large intestine. Follow the package directions.

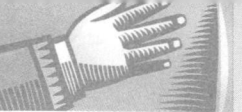

Gallstones

Gallstones, collections of crystals (from the size of a grain of sand to the size of a golf ball) often result from high levels of cholesterol in the bile, the fluid that breaks down high-fat, high-cholesterol foods and is stored in the gallbladder. Gallstones cause problems only when they block something. That "something" is most likely to be the bile duct, the small passageway between the gallbladder and the small intestine, through which bile passes.

If that duct becomes blocked, the pain can be excruciating. The blockage can also lead to infection in the duct and even abscesses in the liver, which is why surgery is often the first and only treatment discussed for gallstones.

Although heredity and a high-fat, high-cholesterol diet contribute to gallstones, one of the most common causes is, ironically, rapid weight loss, which raises levels of triglycerides (blood fats) and increases the amount of calcium in the bile—both key ingredients for stones.

Do This Now

During a gallbladder attack, take these steps.

1. Give your digestive system a rest. Consume only clear liquids for several hours.

2. Make a castor oil pack. Spread castor oil mixed with 10 drops ginger oil, 10 drops peppermint oil, and 10 drops chamomile oil over your abdomen, cover with cotton or wool flannel, then apply a heating pad over the spot where it hurts the most.

3. If you are still in pain after four hours of taking only clear liquids, take 1,000 milligrams of

Tylenol or aspirin, or 400 to 600 milligrams of ibuprofen, or 220 milligrams of naproxen.

Why It Works

If a gallstone is blocking a duct, your intestines won't work right. Eating increases the pain as food backs up in the stomach or sits in the intestine.

The main issue you're dealing with during an attack is pain. That's why we recommend using the castor oil pack with essential oils. The oils relax spasms in the bile duct. The ginger also dilates blood vessels in the skin so the other oils can be absorbed more rapidly. The pain relievers are, of course, for pain relief.

Other Medicines

Herbs and Supplements

Enteric-coated peppermint oil capsules. The menthol in peppermint contains compounds called terpenes, which prevent cholesterol crystals from forming in bile. Take 1 to 2 capsules three times a day between meals.

Choleretic herbs. These herbs, which include milk thistle (*Silybum marianum*), artichoke (*Cynara scolymus*), and dandelion (*Taraxacum officinale*), stimulate the flow of bile. They can help with intermittent gallbladder discomfort. Follow the dosage instructions on the package. Take along with the peppermint oil capsules.

Prescription Drugs

Bile salts. These work by slowly dissolving gallstones. Actigall (ursodiol) is the most commonly prescribed bile salt medication. Don't be

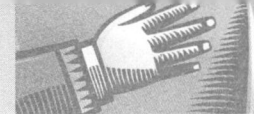

TIME TO WORRY

See your doctor or go the emergency room if:

- You have fever, nausea, and vomiting along with the pain in the upper right part of your abdomen.
- Your skin and/or the whites of your eyes have turned yellow.
- The color of your urine has changed drastically and become very dark, like Coke.
- The color of your stool has changed drastically and become very light, like gray clay.

surprised if your doctor doesn't mention this option, however; many gastroenterologists don't suggest it, because it takes a while to work (up to a year in some cases). Plus, the gallstones are likely to recur. But if you have small stones and an otherwise healthy gallbladder, along with mild symptoms, you're probably a good candidate.

Other Approaches

Surgery. Most conventional doctors will want to operate if you have gallstones. The procedure is called a cholecystectomy, and 90 percent are now done laparoscopically, meaning that the gallbladder is removed through a small incision in the abdomen rather than through a large opening. If the gallstones are in the bile or pancreatic ducts, they're removed through a different procedure using an endoscope, a tube with a camera on the end, that is passed through your mouth, down the esophagus, into the stomach and the small intestine. Although gallbladder surgery is generally safe, 20 percent or more of people who have their gallbladder removed still experience the pain they had before the surgery. Doctors don't know why, but suspect it may have to do with some underlying liver or gastrointestinal problem that led to the gallstones in the first place.

Lithotripsy. Gallstones can also be broken up through lithotripsy, or sound waves. One drawback: The stones tend to recur, which is why this procedure is rarely performed.

Acupuncture. Along with other forms of pain, acupuncture seems to help with the pain of gallbladder disease. It may also help "unstick" a gallstone. One published article on the use of electroacupuncture on 1,291 patients with gallstones reported that 91 percent expelled a stone. Of the 78 cases treated without acupuncture, none did..

Prevention

Take daily fish oil supplements. Take at least 3 grams a day. The omega-3 and omega-6 fatty acids in fish oil appear to reduce the amount of cholesterol in the bile.

Eat a low-fat, high-fiber diet. A diet low in saturated fat, cholesterol, and simple carbohydrates (like sugar and white flour), and high in fiber, can prevent gallstones in high-risk people. Also munch on a handful of nuts a day. One study found that an ounce of nuts every day seemed to reduce the risk of gallbladder disease.

Increase your coffee intake. Try drinking two or three cups a day. One study found it decreased the risk of gallstones in men by 40 percent. It doesn't appear to be an effect of the caffeine; high doses of tea actually seem to *increase* the risk of gallstones. However, if you already have gallstones, coffee or other caffeinated beverages may cause the gallbladder to contract, resulting in pain and/or causing a stone to lodge in the bile ducts.

Shake a leg. A brisk, half-hour walk a day can cut your risk of gallstones by about 20 percent.

Supplement with vitamin C. This vitamin is involved in breaking down cholesterol into bile acids. Get too little, and the amount of cholesterol in your bile rises. If you're at high risk of gallstones, take 2,000 milligrams a day of vitamin C in two or three doses throughout the day.

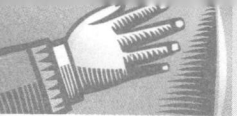

Heartburn and Gastroesophageal Reflux Disease

As you read through our remedies for heartburn and gastroesophageal reflux disease (GERD), it's important that you understand the difference between the two. GERD is a chronic digestive problem whose primary hallmarks are heartburn and acid reflux, the splashing up of stomach acid into the esophagus. Acid reflux occurs because a ring of muscle tissue called the lower esophageal sphincter, at the junction of the esophagus and the stomach, doesn't close tightly enough. GERD is a serious disease; left untreated, it can result in Barrett's esophagus, a precancerous condition in which cells from the intestine grow into the esophagus.

Heartburn is a symptom of GERD, but it may also occur on its own. It's that overly full, burning feeling you get when you've overdone it with heavy, rich foods, or gone to bed too soon after eating. The way you tell the difference between the two is that heartburn is primarily felt behind the breastbone (hence the name), whereas the primary symptom of GERD is a burning in the back of the throat and/or a chronic cough. Sometimes, however, you can also feel the pain of heartburn in your neck, throat, and even face.

Chronic heartburn can also be a sign of a peptic ulcer (see page 124) or irritable bowel syndrome (see page 116).

Do This Now

To soothe a bout of heartburn, follow these steps.

1. Drink a small glass of water (4 to 6 ounces).

2. Take a one-ounce dose of a liquid antacid, either Mylanta or AlternaGEL. You may repeat this every half hour or so for two or three doses.

3. Next, drink a cup of chamomile or slippery elm tea.

4. If you're still feeling the burning pain, take an over-the-counter H_2 blocker like Pepcid AC or Tagamet.

5. Finally, don't lie down; go for a walk instead.

Why It Works

The water dilutes stomach acid, washes any refluxed acid back down the esophagus, and may relieve some burning. Make sure you drink the water *first,* before taking the antacid, so it doesn't dilute the antacid.

The antacid is designed to absorb and neutralize stomach acid. The liquid is more effective than chewable antacids, if somewhat less convenient to carry around.

Chamomile is a carminative herb, meaning it aids digestion, while slippery elm is a demulcent, meaning it soothes and coats the stomach.

The H_2 blockers, or histamine-2 blockers, work by directly reducing the amount of acid your stomach produces. Zantac works fastest and all provide more long-term relief than antacids. H_2 blockers are also good heartburn preventives if taken before you eat.

Finally, walking takes advantage of gravity to help keep stomach acid where it belongs—in your stomach.

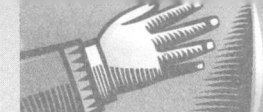

Other Medicines
Herbs and Supplements

Red pepper capsules. It might sound counterintuitive, but patients have had good results using ground red pepper capsules to relieve heartburn without reflux. One study on 30 people (without GERD or IBS) found red pepper capsules to be more effective than a placebo at decreasing the intensity of heartburn symptoms, probably by reducing the sensitivity of nerve fibers in the digestive system that send signals of pain to the brain. Take one 500-milligram capsule before breakfast, two before lunch, and two before dinner every day. If you have any burning during bowel movements, decrease the dose and work your way up. You'll need to take it for several days before you feel relief. Don't take it if you have acid reflux; the hot pepper in the backwash that comes up your esophagus can increase the pain. Also, if you're very sensitive to hot, spicy foods, skip this remedy.

Iberogast. This is a combination product containing the herbs *Iberis amara,* peppermint, and chamomile. Multiple studies show it's more effective in treating routine heartburn than a placebo and just as effective as the prescription drug Propulsid, typically prescribed for patients with GERD who have severe nighttime heartburn. Iberogast is available online and in health food stores.

Artichoke leaf extract. Clinical studies show good evidence that this herbal preparation (available in many health food stores) can relieve the symptoms of indigestion, including heartburn.

Peppermint. Peppermint is an age-old remedy for indigestion. You can skip the peppermint candy, however: Enteric-coated peppermint oil capsules, which are coated with a special substance so they travel to your small intestine without dissolving in your stomach, are the way to go. If you can find them, buy capsules made with caraway oil in addition to the peppermint for a more effective remedy. Take 1 capsule at the first sign of heartburn. *Caution:* Don't drink peppermint tea or take regular (nonenteric-coated) peppermint capsules; they reduce the tone, or tightness, of the esophageal sphincter, promoting acid reflux.

TIME TO WORRY

See your doctor if you have:

- Heartburn associated with shortness of breath, sweating, or pain in your jaw or left shoulder, hand or arm. This could be a sign of a heart attack. Call 911 and/or go to the nearest emergency room.

- You're vomiting blood or have severe difficulty swallowing.

- You have black, tarry, or maroon-colored stools along with the heartburn.

- Your heartburn hasn't responded to self-care for two weeks.

Over-the-Counter Drugs

Simethicone. Although they're marketed for gas and bloating, products that contain simethicone (such as Gas-X, Mylanta Gas Relief, and Phazyme) can help relieve that overly full feeling of heartburn. Take two chewable tablets or capsules, or a liquid dose (follow instructions on box) with meals or when you have symptoms. Don't take more than 500 milligrams in one 24-hour period.

Prescription Drugs

Proton pump inhibitors. Proton pump inhibitors like Prilosec, Prevacid, Reglan, Protonix, and Aciphex limit the amount of acid in

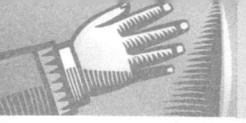

your stomach. They're usually prescribed for people with severe GERD symptoms and damage to the esophagus. They work best if you take them about 30 to 60 minutes before eating. You should only take them for the shortest time necessary to control your symptoms because they completely suppress acid production and you need some acid to digest your food. Plus, you shouldn't take them without also making some of the lifestyle changes we discuss in the prevention section.

Other Approaches

Traditional Chinese Medicine. Talk to a naturopath or herbalist about Kampo medicine formula TJ-43, a standard, prepackaged herbal formula. Studies find this remedy quite effective at relieving the burning and discomfort of indigestion.

Homeopathy. Dissolve a homeopathic heartburn preparation such as *Arsenicum album*, nux vomica, *Carbo vegetabilis*, *Kali carbonicum*, or *Lycopodium* under your tongue. If you don't have access to a homeopathic or naturopathic provider to guide you to the best treatment for you, look for a combination remedy at your health food store or drugstore designed for indigestion, heartburn, or GERD.

Prevention

Dramatically decrease the fat in your diet for several days, then follow a low-fat diet. Fat stimulates acid production in the stomach, as do alcohol and coffee. One study found that the more fat in your daily diet, the greater your risk of GERD symptoms and damage to the esophagus. High fiber intake reduced the risk of symptoms.

Lose weight. Excess fat around your abdomen puts more pressure on your stomach (one reason women suffer from heartburn late in pregnancy). You're far more likely to have heartburn or GERD if you're overweight.

Eat slowly and eat several small meals throughout the day rather than just a few large ones. This relieves the pressure on the stomach.

Stop eating three hours before you go to bed, and don't lie down, whether on the bed or couch, for three hours after eating.

✌ What About...

Surgery?

If your GERD continues despite prescription medications and other therapies, you may want to consider laparoscopic antireflux surgery. In this minimally invasive procedure, the surgeon creates a stronger sphincter at the bottom of the esophagus to prevent stomach contents from refluxing into the esophagus. The procedure has a 5 percent failure rate.

There are other options. The U.S. Food and Drug Administration has approved medical devices for several new procedures that fall somewhere between surgery and medical treatment for the treatment of chronic GERD. However, there are no long-term studies on the effectiveness of these treatments. They are:

- **Stretta procedure.** This procedure delivers radiofrequency energy to the area where the stomach and esophagus meet. This energy forms scar tissue in the area to tighten the sphincter and prevent reflux.

- **EndoCinch procedure.** A thin, flexible tube with a tiny camera is inserted down your throat. At the end of it is a small device that works like a miniature sewing machine. It places stitches in two different locations near the lower esophageal sphincter. The stitches are then tied together like a drawstring purse to tighten the sphincter.

- **Enteryx.** This procedure involves injecting a liquid into the wall of the lower esophagus that then solidifies into a spongy material to prevent reflux.

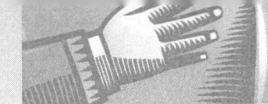

Quit smoking. Smoking not only weakens the lower esophageal sphincter, but it also seems to make stomach acid stronger by impeding the movement of bile salts (which aid digestion) from the intestine to the stomach. Plus, smoking damages the esophagus, making it harder for it to heal from reflux.

Sit up for 10 minutes after every meal. Sit with your eyes closed and focus on a mental picture of a peaceful scene to reduce stress and help you (and your digestive system) relax. Even if it doesn't improve the reflux, it can help you perceive the discomfort as less bothersome.

Try biofeedback. You'll learn how to consciously relax the muscles that govern the digestive system.

Take 1 to 2 chewable tablets of deglycyrrhizinated licorice (DGL) before each meal up to three times a day. It soothes and coats the stomach, preventing that burning feeling.

GETTING TESTED

If you've been diagnosed with GERD, your doctor may want to perform an esophageal endoscopy to check for damage to your esophagus. With this procedure, the doctor inserts a thin, flexible tube down your throat. It has a tiny camera on one end, which allows the doctor to see the condition of the esophagus and, if necessary, take a tissue sample to examine for any infection or other diseases, like Barrett's esophagus.

Take an H_2 blocker before you eat.

After meals, use carminative spices to aid digestion. You see these at Indian restaurants—a little dish of fennel seeds or cardamom. Caraway seeds are also carminative. Mix together 1/2 teaspoon seeds and chew after meals. Or drink a cup of chai tea after dinner; it includes many spices that aid digestion.

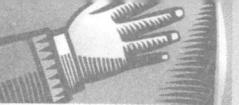
Hepatitis

The word *hepatitis* means inflammation of the liver. It's the type of hepatitis you have that determines your treatment options and prognosis. Most forms are viral, caused by the A, B, or C hepatitis viruses (and, more rarely, D). All are contagious, but in most instances your body fights off the virus after a few weeks. You may just think you had a bout of the flu.

Up to 75 percent of the time with hepatitis C (less frequently with the other viruses), however, the virus becomes chronic. Over time, it can lead to serious liver damage, specifically cirrhosis, in which fibrous scar tissue replaces normal liver tissue. Chronic hepatitis is also a leading cause of liver cancer, one reason for the high rates of liver cancer in Asia.

The second major type of hepatitis is called NASH (nonalcoholic steatohepatitis). This is a complication of obesity and is a common problem in obese children. It's also a complication of hepatitis C, so anything we suggest for hepatitis C can also be used for NASH.

Finally, there is toxic hepatitis, usually the result of excessive alcohol consumption or toxins such as poisonous mushrooms.

Our focus here is on chronic hepatitis, and our goal is to help you minimize liver damage and decrease your risk of cancer. If your condition is serious, you'll likely be treated with drug therapy (interferon and ribavirin). But studies find it's only effective in about 40 percent of cases and has numerous side effects. That's why an integrative approach is ideal for this complex condition. Complementary therapies can also help minimize the side effects of conventional therapy.

Our Best Advice

To help your body heal itself, follow these steps.

1. Start taking 140 to 200 milligrams of milk thistle standardized to 70% to 80% silymarin three times a day. We recommend the product Thistylin, by Nature's Way.

2. Get vaccinated for hepatitis A and B if you've been diagnosed with hepatitis C.

3. Stay away from acetaminophen (Tylenol) for pain. Use nonsteroidal anti-inflammatory drugs such as aspirin or ibuprofen instead.

4. Follow a low-iron diet if you already have severe hepatitis or cirrhosis. This means avoiding foods such as red meat and seafood.

5. Avoid alcohol.

6. Maintain a healthy weight.

Why It Works

Milk thistle is the best-researched herbal remedy for liver disease. It works as an antioxidant to prevent liver scarring. It also protects liver cells from toxins, enhances the liver's detoxification ability, and protects against the depletion of glutathione, one of the most important antioxidants in the liver.

You need the vaccinations because another infection on top of hepatitis C could really devastate your liver. Acetaminophen is a no-no because it can be hard on the liver. As for the low-iron diet, excess iron is a toxin that's stored in the liver. That's why phlebotomy, in which excess

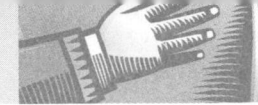

iron is removed from the blood, and a low-iron diet are common treatments for hepatitis C. Try to keep your iron intake at or below 8 milligrams a day. Alcohol is another toxin to avoid.

Hepatitis, especially hepatitis C, contributes to insulin resistance syndrome (see page 48). It can lead to weight gain and eventually to type 2 diabetes. Follow our recommendations on page 51 for preventing insulin resistance and on page 291 for maintaining a healthy weight.

Other Medicines
Herbs and Supplements

While herbal therapies won't eliminate the virus, studies find they help decrease inflammation while reducing levels of liver enzymes. Liver enzymes are released as liver cells die; fewer enzymes in the blood imply less cellular damage. Some herbs also have direct antiviral effects, decreasing the number of virus cells. The ones we recommend in addition to milk thistle are:

Licorice root. This herb has strong antiviral and anti-inflammatory effects. Studies find it can enhance the liver's detoxification ability and boost the body's ability to fight the virus. Take 250 to 500 milligrams two or three times a day. Have your doctor keep a close check for fluid retention, a blood pressure increase, or a decrease in potassium, which can occur with licorice. If you have heart disease, don't take it without a specific recommendation from your doctor.

S-adenosyl-L-methionine, or SAMe. This amino acid, also used for depression, plays an important role in various processes in the body, particularly the liver. Studies find levels of SAMe are low in people with alcoholic hepatitis. The U.S. government is sponsoring studies into the use of SAMe for other forms of liver disease. Start with 400 milligrams a day and increase the dosage to at least 400 milligrams twice a day.

Most clinical trials used 1,200 milligrams a day, which you could get in two doses of 600 milligrams, taken morning and evening.

Essential fatty acids. Children and adults with hepatitis have low levels of these antioxidants. We recommend at least 3 grams a day (up to 5 grams) of fish oil, flaxseed oil, or evening primrose oil (or a combination of the three).

Flavonoids. These antioxidants are present in many foods, particularly red or purple berries, teas, and other fruits and vegetables. Take 50 to 100 milligrams of resveratrol, grapeseed extract, or pycnogenol a day.

NAC (N-acetyl-cysteine). This amino acid contributes to the production of glutathione, used by the liver to break down toxins. Glutathione has a direct effect on how active the hepatitis B and C viruses are: The more glutathione, the less viral activity. One study found that adding NAC to interferon treatment for chronic hepatitis C significantly delayed the amount of time before patients' symptoms returned, compared to treating with interferon alone. Take 100 to 200 milligrams three times a day.

Vitamin K. In one small but significant study of 40 women with cirrhosis caused by viral pneumonia, those who took 45 milligrams of vitamin K a day to strengthen their bones were 80 percent less likely to develop liver cancer than those who didn't take the supplement. We recommend the same dose. You can also get vitamin K in dark leafy green vegetables.

L-carnitine. Studies find that high levels of this amino acid in the liver lead to less cirrhosis, while low levels are associated with greater inflammation and scarring. L-carnitine also helps reduce the fatigue associated with interferon therapy. Take 2 grams a day in two divided doses.

Traditional Chinese Medicine (TCM). Many herbal TCM formulas have been evaluated for use in hepatitis, in part because viral hepatitis is

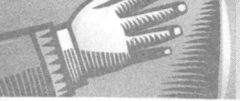

endemic in China. Many are used in combination with conventional therapy. Formulas include:

- **Bing Gan Tang.** When used with interferon treatment, this remedy reduced the amount of hepatitis C virus and improved liver function tests.

- **Yi Er Gan Tang.** Can improve liver function tests.

- **TJ-48.** This is used in Japan to counter anemia that often results from ribavirin therapy.

- **Mao-to.** This formula, given in conjunction with conventional ribavirin/interferon therapy, helped prevent treatment-related depression.

Prescription Drugs

Interferon alpha 2B and ribavirin. These two antiviral drugs are the standard medical treatment for chronic hepatitis C. Interferon is the chemical your immune system produces in response to a viral infection, so the drug makes you feel like you have the flu. That's why many people go off it or refuse to take it. Ask your doctor to use pegylated interferon, which stays in the body longer and has double the efficacy (it still has the side effects, however). Ribavirin works by interfering with the virus's ability to replicate. It may cause anemia as well as vomiting, diarrhea, constipation, and heartburn.

Other Approaches

Lycopene. If you're being treated with interferon and ribavirin, add more sources of lycopene, like tomato juice and tomato sauce, to your diet. In a study of 92 patients with chronic hepatitis C who were treated with the standard therapy, a lycopene supplement improved patients' ability to tolerate the full dose of ribavirin and reduced the anemia that's a common side effect with this treatment.

Green tea. Green tea is high in polyphenols, antioxidants that numerous studies find have a protective effect on the liver. Green tea also enhances the liver's detoxification ability. Choose any decaffeinated brand high in catechins and try to drink six cups a day.

Prevention

Get vaccinated for hepatitis A and B. No vaccine is available for hepatitis C.

Get a gamma globulin shot if you've been exposed to hepatitis A or B and haven't had a vaccine (which can take several months to begin working). It contains antibodies to the viruses.

Wash your hands thoroughly before you handle food.

Avoid risky behavior, like unprotected sex (always use a condom) and sharing needles. Blood transfusions, of course, should be used only when absolutely necessary.

Skip tattoos and piercings. If you can't resist, make sure the equipment is properly sterilized.

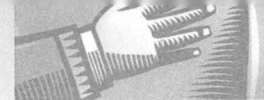

Hiccups

Hiccups are a strange phenomenon. There are nearly 100 causes, including everything from swallowing too much air or drinking too much alcohol to stress, fear, and irritating foods. Once in a while, hiccups can even be a sign of a serious medical condition, including pancreatitis (inflammation of the pancreas), heart attack, appendicitis, or pneumonia. Usually hiccups are short-lived, but in rare instances they can last for months or even years, causing severe health problems, even death.

Most cases of hiccups are harmless, though, and usually the tried-and-true folk remedies described below do the trick.

Do This Now

Hiccups usually stop on their own, but you can stop them sooner with these steps.

1. Swallow a tablespoonful of sugar or cocoa mix dry.

2. If that doesn't stop the hiccups, wrap a washcloth around your tongue and pull.

3. If you're still hiccuping, hold your breath as long as you can or breathe for several minutes into a paper bag.

4. If none of these remedies work, have someone apply a gentle version of the Heimlich maneuver. He should stand behind you, reach around your chest with both hands, clasp his hands and cross his thumbs, placing the thumbs just under the breastbone in the center of the ribs, then push in three or four times.

Why It Works

It isn't easy to swallow sugar or cocoa powder dry, and that's the point. The process of getting the crystals down your throat should interrupt the hiccup reflex.

Pulling on your tongue (you can also stick your finger down your throat) induces a gag reflex that may disrupt the hiccup reflex. It also stimulates the vagus nerve, which runs from the brain to the stomach. Stimulating this nerve also appears to interrupt the hiccup cycle.

Holding your breath or breathing into a paper bag increases levels of carbon dioxide in your blood, which is also thought to disrupt the hiccup cycle (people with severe hiccups may be given carbon dioxide to breathe).

The Heimlich maneuver seems to halt the contractions of the diaphragm that are the hallmark of hiccups. There's no need to push as hard as you would if someone were choking on food, though.

Other Medicines
Prescription Drugs

If your hiccups last for more than 48 hours, your doctor may prescribe one of several drugs, including the muscle relaxer baclofen, the antipsychotic Thorazine, or the anticonvulsant Depakote.

Other Approaches

Acupressure. With the tips of the fingers of both hands, press down along the center of your abdomen from the top of the abdomen to the pubic bone until the hiccups stop. Also try this: Use your thumbs to massage in a downward direction the shin of each leg, from your knee to your ankle.

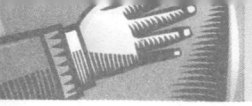

Incontinence, Urinary

This condition, just as common in women as in men, is one that simply isn't talked about. Yet it can significantly affect your quality of life, and is often one of the main reasons older people are put into nursing homes. Fortunately, it is relatively treatable.

There are different types of incontinence, with urge and stress incontinence (or a combination of both) being the most common. Urge incontinence involves an involuntary loss of urine associated with a strong sense that you have to go to the bathroom. This usually occurs when you're on the way to the bathroom. With stress incontinence, there's urine loss during coughing, sneezing, laughing or other physical activities, usually because of weak pelvic floor muscles. Much less common is overflow incontinence: The bladder overextends, usually due to a dropping of the reproductive and urinary tract organs (in women) or prostate problems (in men). This usually requires surgery to correct.

Our focus is on urge and stress incontinence. One caveat: The only thing that will work quickly is medication; complementary approaches take longer. To get a prescription, however, you have to tell your doctor about your problem, something fewer than half of those with urinary incontinence do.

Do This Now

These three steps should help solve your problem.

1. Begin performing Kegel exercises at least 10 times a day. To do them, pull in or "squeeze" your pelvic muscles as if you were trying to stop the flow of urine or keep from passing gas. Count to 10 as you hold the contraction. Relax, then repeat 10 times. You can do this as you sit at your desk or watch TV. No one will be the wiser.

2. Go to the bathroom whenever you feel the slightest urge. Gradually increase the amount of time between bathroom visits until your urine leakage stops.

3. While you're waiting for results from steps 1 and 2, minimize leakage and embarrassment by curbing the amount of liquid you drink before leaving the house and wearing protective padding. Add a drop of peppermint or grapefruit essential oil to the pad to help control odor.

Why It Works

Of all the behavioral changes you can make to improve urinary incontinence, study after study points to the benefits of pelvic floor exercises like Kegels. Strengthening the muscle that controls the urinary sphincter, which keeps urine in the bladder, will keep urine from leaking out—it's that simple.

Studies also find that going to the bathroom very frequently, then gradually lengthening the time between bathroom visits, a technique called bladder retraining, is very helpful for alleviating urge incontinence. You're training the bladder to get stronger and hold the urine longer, just like you'd train a muscle.

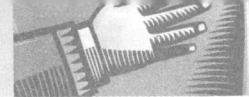

Other Medicines
Herbs and Supplements

St. John's wort. Although there aren't any studies using this herb in humans with incontinence, studies on rats found it slowed the transmission of signals in the rat bladder that led to urination. It also decreased bladder irritability (an irritable bladder is a leaky bladder). Given that other antidepressants seem to work for incontinence (St. John's wort is often used for depression), we recommend taking 300 milligrams three times a day.

Prescription Drugs

Tricyclic antidepressants such as Elavil, Tofranil, and Pamelor are often prescribed for urge incontinence. Like St. John's wort, they probably work by decreasing the irritability of the bladder. Also, a side effect of some antidepressants is urinary retention.

Anticholinergic drugs such as Ditropan (oxybutynin) or Detrol (tolterodine) reduce contractions of the bladder muscles and are approved for the treatment of urinary incontinence. They are best used for urge incontinence.

Other Approaches

Biofeedback. Through biofeedback, you can learn to better control the muscles that keep urine from leaking out of your body. One study of 35 women with urinary stress incontinence that compared biofeedback training to pelvic floor exercises found that nearly 70 percent of those who learned biofeedback avoided surgery compared to 52 percent of those in the pelvic floor exercise groups. Our advice: Try both suggestions. See page 60 in Part 2 for more on biofeedback.

Acupuncture. Acupuncture for urinary incontinence focuses on toning the bladder and kidney systems. In one study of 15 elderly women treated with 12 acupuncture sessions, all measures of incontinence (including urine leakage) significantly improved and remained improved three months later.

Magnet therapy. Perineal magnetic stimulation uses an FDA-approved machine to generate a pulsed magnetic field. You sit fully clothed on a chair that sends magnetic stimulation to your pelvic area. The magnetic field causes an electrical response in the nerves that control the bladder. Studies on this procedure are mixed, with most showing some benefits but not significantly more than other treatments. However, the procedure is painless and there are no side effects. If your health insurance covers it, we recommend trying it along with pelvic floor exercises.

Prevention

Lose weight. If you're a woman, the heavier you are, the more likely you are to have this problem, probably because the tube leading from the bladder to the vaginal opening (the urethra) is floppy.

Skip the tea. There's some evidence that heavy tea drinkers (but not coffee drinkers) are more likely to experience incontinence.

Stop smoking. Smokers are more likely to have incontinence than nonsmokers. We don't know why.

Get regular exercise. Any exercise that strengthens the core of your body will help prevent urinary incontinence. We recommend Pilates, a form of resistance training that strengthens your abdomen, back, and other core muscles. Look for a class with a certified instructor.

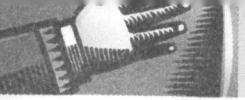

Inflammatory Bowel Disease

Inflammatory bowel disease (IBD) is really two diseases—Crohn's disease, which can affect any part of the digestive tract, and ulcerative colitis, which primarily affects the large intestine. Inflammation is the main underlying problem of both. Hence, most treatments—traditional and complementary—seek to stem the inflammation.

IBD requires significant interaction with your gastroenterologist; you're going to need prescription medication. However, one large study of 118 people with ulcerative colitis found that treatment with an integrative method of Chinese and Western medicine had far better results than treatment with medication alone.

Also keep in mind that if you have IBD, you also have an increased risk for other serious medical conditions, particularly colon cancer and osteoporosis. And you're at risk for becoming malnourished because your body doesn't get the nutrients it needs through food, so we recommend supplemental nutrients. If you have ulcerative colitis, you have a greater risk of blood clots, which is one reason we recommend you supplement with fish oil.

Do This Now

During a flare, take these steps for relief. To help prevent future flares, follow the advice in the rest of this entry.

1. Stop eating solid food. Instead, use a liquid diet product (called "enteral nutrition" or "medical food") such as UltraInflamX and follow the package directions. Even after you reintroduce solid foods, keep fiber low until you're in remission.

2. For a really serious flare, begin taking a corticosteroid such as prednisone by mouth, or a steroid enema, as prescribed by your doctor.

3. Next (or if your flare is not so serious), take an anti-inflammatory prescription drug such as Azulfidine (sulfasalazine) or mesalamine, as prescribed by your doctor.

4. Take one to three 300-milligram capsules of slippery elm, marshmallow, chamomile, or a combination product.

5. Also take 1/2 teaspoon valerian tincture (a liquid) and 1/2 teaspoon cramp bark tincture diluted in a small amount of warm water every one to two hours.

Why It Works

Enteral nutrition gives your bowel a rest, restores lost nutrients, and reduces the inflammation that whole proteins in food can trigger. In fact, some studies find that these diets can be as effective in the short term as corticosteroids in relieving symptoms. Enteric nutrition is also a good option if you have trouble eating enough to keep your weight up. The products can also be used as a vehicle for liquid supplements of fish oil, vitamins, and calcium, recommended below.

We want you to cut back on fiber as you reintroduce solid foods because it can irritate an already overly sensitive colon, making symptoms worse. As soon as the flare fades, however, resume eating plenty of fiber, which is actually critical to preventing flares.

Corticosteroids reduce inflammation by subduing the immune system. They're "heavy guns" and should be used for as short a time as possible

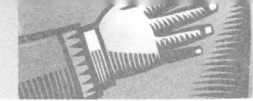
because they can cause serious side effects, from weight gain to mood disturbances to osteoporosis and high blood pressure. You can take them as a pill or an enema. Note that corticosteroids deplete a number of nutrients, so you must take a multi-vitamin/mineral at the same time, preferably in liquid from for easy absorption.

The anti-inflammatory drugs sulfasalazine and mesalamine (sold under many different brand names), as well as other, similar drugs work by reducing inflammation, particularly in the bowel and large intestine. They'll turn your urine and/or skin yellowish orange, but don't worry about it. They interfere with folic acid absorption, so also take a folic acid or B complex supplement while you're taking them.

Slippery elm, marshmallow, and chamomile are soothing herbs. Chamomile also aids digestion. The tinctures help with the abdominal cramps and pain. They relieve pain by relaxing the muscles around the bowel. They also have anti-inflammatory properties.

Other Medicines
Herbs and Supplements

Calm Colon. This Traditional Chinese Medicine formula, available in health food stores, is primarily composed of herbs that decrease inflammation. Ulcerative colitis patients have had excellent results when they use it just as they're entering the remission stage of the disease.

Herbal tea. Combine 1/2 teaspoon dandelion leaf and root, 1 teaspoon of lemon balm, and 1/4 teaspoon crushed fennel seeds. Mix with 6 ounces of boiling water and steep for 10 minutes. Strain and drink along with 300 milligrams of a standardized extract of St. John's wort three times a day. A study using a commercial product containing these herbs found that 23 of 24 patients with ulcerative colitis who took the product during a flare were pain-free by day 15 of the study.

Wheatgrass juice. One well-designed study in which 21 patients with ulcerative colitis drank 3 ounces of fresh wheatgrass juice (available in health food stores) a day or a placebo found that symptoms significantly improved in people who drank the juice. They also had far less rectal bleeding. Researchers suspect the antioxidative properties of wheatgrass juice are responsible for the positive effect. Stick with it for four weeks; it may take that long to see a benefit. If it works for you, continue taking 1 to 3 ounces a day.

Licorice (*Glycyrrhiza glabra* or *Glycyrrhiza uralensis*). Take 1 to 2 capsules three times a day at the end of a flare as you begin tapering off steroids. Licorice enhances the effects of steroids, so you may be able to reduce your steroidal dose sooner. Don't take for more than 5 to 7 days and make sure your doctor knows you're taking it.

Prescription Drugs

Immunomodulators. These drugs, which include Imuran (azathioprine), methotrexate, cyclosporine, and 6-MP (mercaptopurine), are serious drugs often used for cancer treatment. They suppress the immune system and work well—for about two to four months. Then they usually stop working. Potential serious side effects include inflammation of the pancreas and folic acid deficiency.

Remicade (infliximab). This drug works by blocking the immune system's overproduction of the protein TNF-alpha, an underlying cause of Crohn's disease. It's typically prescribed if your condition hasn't improved with other treatments. You receive it through an IV in a doctor's office on a regular basis, whether or not you're having symptoms. Its benefits are also relatively brief, so even if you're on this drug, you'll likely need others.

Antibiotics. Your doctor may prescribe antibiotics to reduce the amount of abnormal bacteria in the gut.

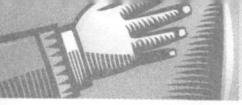

Nicotine. Studies suggest that nicotine replacement products like nicotine gum or patches can significantly improve ulcerative colitis symptoms. Ask your doctor if you should consider them.

Other Approaches

Surgery. You may need surgery to relieve strictures (narrowed passageways) in parts of your digestive system, and to decrease the risk of colon cancer by removing precancerous polyps and, in severe cases, the colon.

Acupuncture. Several well-designed studies find acupuncture can significantly improve symptoms in both types of IBD, probably because of anti-inflammatory effects. You will probably need 6 to 10 sessions to control a flare, followed by less frequent ongoing therapy. Studies find acupuncture works best when combined with Chinese herbal therapy and dietary changes.

Prevention

Check for food allergens. The most common offenders are dairy, wheat, eggs, and citrus. Ask your doctor to test your blood for IgG (immunoglobulin G, or gamma globulin) antibodies, a sign of food allergies. Eliminate these four foods for at least five days to see if there's any improvement, then slowly add back one at a time to identify which you're allergic to.

Eat more fish and cut back on vegetable oils. The omega-3 fats in fish and olive oil help counter inflammation, while most vegetable oils promote it.

Bump up your fiber intake. Get at least 25 to 30 grams from whole grains, vegetables, and fruit. If you want to supplement with a fiber supplement, choose 2 tablespoons a day of flaxseed, which is high in omega-3 fatty acids; oat bran (not wheat), 1 to 3 tablespoons a day; psyllium, 4 to 10 grams a day; or pectin (Citrucel), a soluble fiber that increases the amount of butyrate, an important digestive enzyme often low in people with IBD.

Avoid carrageenan, a seaweed-derived stabilizing agent used in many prepared foods such as ice cream, flavored milk products, and cottage cheese. It causes colitis in lab animals.

Avoid sulfites and additives, which are also irritating.

Cut down on sugar. It's been associated with a higher rate of ulcerative colitis.

Pick a stress reduction technique and practice it regularly. Stress plays a major role in triggering IBD flares. One study of 80 people with IBD found that those who received training in stress management showed significant improvement in their physical and psychological health, while those without the training showed no change. See Part 2, page 59, for more on stress reduction techniques.

Protect yourself with prebiotics and probiotics. These supplements help maintain a healthy bacterial environment in your gut, which can reduce inflammation. Some prebiotics may also help maintain your ability to produce the digestive enzyme butyrate. The most common prebiotics are fructo-oligosaccharides (which occur naturally in onions, asparagus, chicory, banana, and artichokes), and inulin (derived from chicory). There is a wide variety of probiotics. Take 1 to 2 capsules of prebiotics with each dose of probiotics. Take up to 1 billion organisms of probiotics a day divided into even doses with meals and at bedtime. Note that fiber contains prebiotic constituents, so if you are taking a full dose of fiber, you may not need the extra prebiotic.

Reduce inflammation with fish oil. This is an excellent source of anti-inflammatory omega-3 fatty acids. Take at least 3 to 5 grams a day, preferably as a liquid (available in some health food

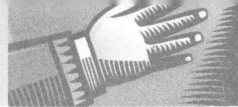

stores and online). This is a high dose, but you'll need this much to see benefits. Look for a liquid that's been treated so it's not very fishy tasting (the label will say something like "no fishy aftertaste"). If you're on a liquid food drink, add the fish oil directly to the drink.

Improve digestion with digestive enzymes. These supplements help break down food and complete digestion, as well as counter inflammation. Start with bromelain, which has been used in ulcerative colitis patients to good effect. Take 1 to 2 capsules with each meal.

Supplement with folate. This B vitamin can help reduce your risk of colon cancer and lower levels of homocysteine, an amino acid that can damage blood vessels and increase your risk of Alzheimer's disease. Levels are often high in people with Crohn's disease. Take 400 to 800 IU a day.

Take your calcium. Take at least 600 milligrams twice a day for a total of 1,200 milligrams. Studies find high levels of calcium can reduce the risk of colon cancer, and it will also help preserve bone density, a concern in people with IBD.

Ask your doctor if you need an iron supplement. If you're having any rectal bleeding or blood in your feces, you might. Take 326 milligrams of ferrous sulfate a day; if you have problems tolerating this form (i.e., constipation or nausea), switch to ferrous gluconate. When you take your iron supplement, wash it down with orange juice or take it with a vitamin C supplement to improve absorption.

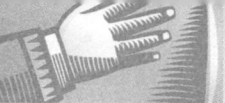

Irritable Bowel Syndrome

For years, doctors believed irritable bowel syndrome (IBS) was a psychological syndrome because they couldn't find any physical reasons for the bloating, gas, diarrhea, constipation, and abdominal pain that are its hallmarks. Today we know that IBS is a functional disorder, one diagnosed not through a specific test, but through a constellation of symptoms. That makes IBS, like many chronic conditions, ideal for an integrative therapy approach.

Keep in mind that IBS symptoms vary among individuals, and even within an individual over time. Some people have the diarrhea-dominant form, while others have the constipation-dominant form. Which remedies you follow depends on the form you have. Also, we didn't list specific remedies for diarrhea or constipation here; see those entries.

You may also note a dearth of "conventional" medical treatments for IBS; the reality is that there aren't very many. The U.S. Food and Drug Administration has approved only two drugs to treat IBS, one of which has significant side effects. While medications such as antidepressants may help some people, there's no clear consensus on how to medically treat IBS.

Finally, we urge you not to self-diagnose IBS. See your doctor. The symptoms are also the symptoms of a variety of other health conditions, ranging from simple constipation to the more serious inflammatory bowel disease (IBD) and even colon or ovarian cancer. Your doctor should be able to provide a diagnosis using the established standard for an IBS diagnosis called the Rome II criteria. If your case is mild, your doctor will probably recommend you start with self-care measures.

Do This Now

For fast relief of cramps and abdominal pain, take these steps. For longer-term solutions to IBS, follow the advice in the rest of this entry.

1. Take 1/2 teaspoon valerian tincture (a liquid) and 1/2 teaspoon cramp bark tincture (both available in natural food stores) every one to two hours.

2. Swallow an enteric-coated peppermint essential oil capsule.

3. While you're waiting for the herbs to work, apply heat to your abdomen with a heating pad or a castor oil pack. For the latter, spread castor oil mixed with 10 drops ginger oil over your abdomen, cover with cotton or wool flannel, then apply a heating pad.

4. If the pain persists, draw yourself a warm bath and soak until the water cools.

Why It Works

Patients have had excellent results using valerian and cramp bark to relieve abdominal cramps. Both are muscle relaxants. In the case of IBS, they relieve pain by relaxing the muscles around the bowel.

Studies on peppermint oil for IBS are numerous. The oil soothes pain, relieves nausea, and relaxes smooth muscles (like those that control digestion). It also helps you pass gas, thus relieving bloating. In one study, 110 people with IBS symptoms took either a peppermint oil capsule called Colpermin or a sugar pill three to four times a day, 15 to 30 minutes before eating, for one month. Seventy-nine percent of those taking

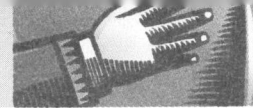

the peppermint oil said they had less abdominal pain, 83 percent had less bloating and fewer bowel movements, and nearly 80 percent had less gas and stomach rumbling. Less than half of those taking the placebo reported improvements in these areas. Use an enteric-coated brand of peppermint oil capsules so the oil gets to your small intestine without being digested first.

Heat relaxes, and castor oil has anti-inflammatory effects. It's also an excellent carrier oil for the ginger oil, which soothes and relaxes and also dilates the blood vessels under the skin, helping the castor oil penetrate more deeply.

The warm bath is relaxing both mentally and physically. Given that IBS is strongly related to stress, anything that soothes and relaxes will also help you unclench your stomach and other digestive muscles.

Other Medicines
Herbs and Supplements

Probiotics. Take one to two doses of probiotics with every meal, at least 1 billion live organisms a day (the number of live organisms in each dose should be noted on the label of the brand you're taking). The studies on probiotics are mixed, depending on the type used. One of the most recent and most interesting involved 77 people with IBS who received either *Lactobacillus salivarius*, *Bifidobacterium infantis*, or a placebo for 10 weeks. Those taking *B. infantis* had less abdominal pain, bloating, constipation or diarrhea than those taking *L. salivarius* or the placebo. Researchers also discovered that participants with IBS had much lower levels of anti-inflammatory immune system chemicals called interleukine-10 and much higher levels of pro-inflammatory immune system chemicals called interleukine-12 than those without IBS. The ratio between the two chemicals evened out in those receiving the *B. infantis* probiotic.

Iberogast. This is a combination product containing the herbs *Iberis amara*, peppermint, and chamomile. (See Resources, page 365, for buying information.) One well-designed clinical trial found that patients taking Iberogast for four weeks had much less pain and other IBS symptoms than those taking a placebo. Take 20 drops in warm water three times a day. This herb is particularly helpful if you also have indigestion.

Triphala. This Ayurvedic formula is considered both an astringent (something that dries and contracts) and a laxative, so it's beneficial for the diarrhea-dominant and constipation-dominant forms of IBS. It consists of three herbs: Amla (*Phyllanthus emblica* or *Emblica officinalis*), Hara (*Terminalia chebula*), and Bahera (*Terminalia belerica*). The dose depends on the brand, but the usual range is one to two tablets three times a day.

Digestive bitters. These herbs, including gentian and dandelion, have a bitter taste that stimulates the digestive process, beginning in the mouth. One half hour before meals, mix 10 to 20 drops of an elixir of either or both of these herbs in up to 20 ounces of warm water. Sip slowly over five or 10 minutes. You need to do this for several months.

Demulcents (soothing herbs). These herbs include marshmallow, slippery elm, and aloe juice. Don't use aloe if you have diarrhea-dominant IBS, however, because it acts as a laxative. The other two can be used regardless of which type of IBS you have. You can find these herbs in capsule forms. Take one to three 300-milligram capsules with meals to help relieve post-meal IBS symptoms.

Prescription Drugs

Serotonin (5-HT4) agonists. Low levels of serotonin (a neurotransmitter) in the gut may play a role in IBS, according to some researchers.

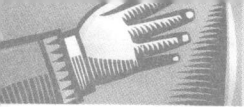

These drugs increase the amount of serotonin. Two are available:

- **Lotronex.** Lotronex is approved only for use in women with diarrhea-dominant IBS. Because it carries the risk of very serious side effects, including ischemic colitis, or inflammation of the colon, it is prescribed as a last resort. You and your doctor will have to sign several consent forms before receiving the drug.

- **Zelnorm.** Like Lotronex, Zelnorm is also approved only for women, in this case for women with constipation-dominant IBS. It doesn't carry the same risk of side effects as Lotronex, so no special forms are required. It is generally prescribed only for short-term treatment, however, usually four to six weeks.

Antidepressants. Tricyclic antidepressants (amitriptyline, nortriptyline, desipramine, etc.) are often prescribed for IBS, at doses much lower than those recommended for depression. Studies find these drugs improve the balance of serotonin and dopamine (another neurotransmitter found in the gut). Paxil, which belongs to the selective serotonin reuptake inhibitor (SSRI) class of antidepressants, is also effective for IBS. Antidepressants seem to work best for people with the diarrhea-dominant form of the disease.

Smooth muscle relaxants. For the painful spasms of IBS, muscle relaxants such as Levsin and Pamine, and the sedative Donnatal, can provide fairly quick relief.

Other Approaches

Acupuncture. In the only clinical trial of acupuncture for IBS, in which researchers used a real or fake acupuncture treatment (placebo) on patients with IBS, those who received the real thing said their pain and other symptoms improved significantly. However, when researchers completed the analysis of the study, they didn't find any statistically significant differences. We still think it's worth trying. Your acupuncture therapist should focus on points in the liver, large intestine, spleen, stomach, and gallbladder channels.

Prevention

Weed out your food triggers. One large study found IBS symptoms were related to meals in 63 percent of participants. Specific problems came from foods rich in carbohydrates, as well as fatty food, coffee, alcohol, and hot spices. To identify your food-related triggers, keep a food diary for two weeks. Write down everything you eat along with all IBS-related symptoms and look for any correlations. If you notice a certain food seems to trigger symptoms, eliminate that food for three days and see if you notice any improvement. Common trigger foods include dairy, beans, and gas-producing foods like onions, cabbage, and broccoli.

After you've identified food triggers, gradually move your diet to a low-fat, plant-based diet with few refined foods. That means avoiding white breads, pasta and white rice, packaged foods, and sweets. You don't have to switch all at once; start gradually by eliminating red meat, dark poultry, and dairy from one meal a day and adding one serving of fruits or vegetables a day. Changing your diet too abruptly can trigger an IBS flare.

Eliminate sweeteners such as fructose, sorbitol, mannitol, or large amounts of simple sugars.

Avoid very cold drinks and/or foods, especially just after eating. Many traditional healing systems such as Ayurveda and Chinese Traditional Medicine believe cold liquids and foods (like ice cream) extinguish the digestive fire, which, translated into Western-speak, means they

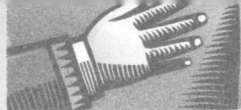

reduce your body's ability to adequately digest your food.

Limit caffeine and alcohol, which irritate the digestive system.

Add fermented foods such as yogurt that contains active cultures and sauerkraut to your diet to improve the ratio of good-to-bad bacteria in your gut.

Manage stress. This is critical in preventing IBS flares. While all forms of stress management therapy discussed in Part 2 are useful, a growing body of evidence points to the benefits of hypnotherapy. In one well-designed study, 204 people with IBS underwent 12 weekly hypnotherapy sessions. Seventy percent of participants said their symptoms initially improved, and of those, 80 percent still felt better at least five years after the therapy ended. Plus, participants receiving hypnotherapy visited their doctors less, and used less medication.

Other mind-body therapies with good scientific evidence behind them include yoga (particularly for diarrhea-dependent IBS), relaxation/stress management training (this could involve everything from meditation to relaxation visualization), cognitive-behavioral therapy (in which you learn techniques to better manage your reaction to stress), and biofeedback. We don't expect you to try all of these! Pick the one that works best for you given your own personality and schedule.

Exercise and stretch, particularly if you have constipation-dominant IBS because movement stimulates bowel activity.

Improve digestion with carminative spices. You see these at Indian restaurants—a little dish of fennel seeds or cardamom to aid digestion. Other carminative spices include cinnamon, caraway, cloves, anise, fenugreek, and ginger. You can chew a few seeds after eating to help with digestion, or grind several into a powder and sprinkle over your food or beverage. You can also take your carminatives as a tea (chai contains many carminative herbs). Read labels carefully, however; if you have diarrhea-dominant IBS, make sure you're not taking a tea meant as a laxative.

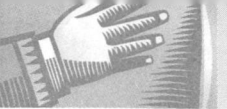

Kidney Stones

Kidney stones can form anywhere along the urinary tract, generally for two reasons: because your urine becomes too saturated with salts (primarily calcium salts) that result in stones, or because your kidneys don't make enough of substances like citrate that prevent stones. Citrate normally attaches to calcium, escorting the calcium out of your body through your urine. About 80 percent of stones are composed of calcium; the remainder are composed of uric acid, cystine, or, rarely, struvite (a compound made of magnesium, ammonium, and phosphate that forms in the presence of infection).

Do This Now

These five steps will help with the pain of a kidney stone.

1. Take 1,000 milligrams of Tylenol and 220 milligrams of naproxen (Aleve).

2. Drink 1 quart of water as quickly as you can. Drink another quart over the next 12 hours.

3. Take 1/2 teaspoon valerian tincture (a liquid) and 1/2 teaspoon cramp bark tincture (both available in natural food stores) in a small amount of warm water every one to two hours.

4. Apply a heating pad or hot compress to the sore area. For even better results, spread castor oil mixed with 10 drops of ginger, peppermint, or juniper oil where it hurts, cover with cotton or wool flannel, then apply a heating pad. You can also soak in a very warm bath to which you've added 1 cup Epsom salt and up to 10 drops of ginger, juniper, or peppermint oil.

5. If you still have pain, take any other pain medication your doctor has given you. It may also be time to head to the hospital for intravenous fluids and injected pain medication.

Why It Works

The pain relievers should take the edge off the pain. The point of drinking lots of large volumes of liquid is to increase your urine output, which will hopefully wash small stones out of the kidney. The valerian and cramp bark tinctures help ease cramps and abdominal pain, as do the heating pad and the oils.

Other Medicines
Herbs and Supplements

You may be able to find prepared tea bags of these herbs in natural food stores. Skip these if you're pregnant.

Gravel root (*Eupatorium purpureum*) is traditionally used to relax the muscles around the ureter and ease the passage of stones. Put 1 gram

✿ Helpful Hint

Save Your Stone

If you've never had a stone before, urinate into a container and strain the urine, keeping an eye out for the stone. Do this until you pass the stone. Save the stone in a clean glass container and take it to your doctor for analysis. Its makeup helps determine what, if any, therapy your doctor prescribes to prevent other stones.

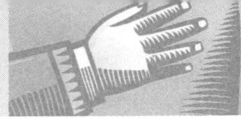

chopped root in 8 ounces boiling water. Simmer for 10 to 15 minutes. Strain and drink one cup several times a day during an acute attack.

Parsley leaf and root tea. Parsley helps increase urine output. It also increases blood flow to the kidney and the rate at which the kidney filters substances, leaving fewer substances around that can turn into stones. Steep 2 grams finely chopped dried parsley root in 5 ounces boiling water for 10 minutes. Strain and drink up to one cup three times a day.

Prescription Drugs

Potassium citrate (Urocit-K, Polycitra-K). Taking potassium citrate for four to six months makes your urine more acidic, which can dissolve small stones and help prevent others. Take 20 to 30 milliequivalents, or mEq, a day. You can either buy this at the health food store as a potassium-magnesium citrate supplement, or your doctor can prescribe it. Don't take if you are also taking potassium-sparing diuretics.

Other Approaches

Lithotripsy. This sound wave therapy is often used to break up stones into sandlike granules so they're easier to pass.

Surgery. Sometimes the doctor will use forceps to pull a stone through a small incision in the skin, or remove stones in the ureter via a flexible scope inserted through the urethra.

Prevention

Drink more fluids. You need to drink at least 1 1/2 to 2 quarts of fluid a day to dilute your urine to discourage stone formation. If your tap water has a high mineral content (i.e., you have hard water), drink bottled water or filter the tap water. Some of the liquid can be in the form of diluted juices, especially cranberry juice, lemonade, orange juice, or weak tea, all of which help make your urine more acidic. If you can find it, try black currant juice. Stay away from grapefruit juice, however; there's some evidence it might increase your risk of stones. And stop drinking sodas. The phosphoric acid in carbonated drinks can increase your risk of stones.

Eat more fruits and vegetables. They're a great source of a nutrient called phytate, and one major study from Harvard found that the more phytate in women's diets, the fewer kidney stones they developed. However, avoid foods high in oxalates such as spinach and other dark greens, rhubarb, and beets.

Consume more dietary calcium. It sounds counterintuitive, but the more calcium you eat, the less oxalic acid you absorb from food and the less likely you are to develop stones.

Limit salt and sugar, which increase the amount of oxalic acid your body absorbs.

Sip a glass of wine a day. One study found it could cut the risk of stones by 59 percent.

Get 10 to 15 grams of wheat bran (about 1/2 ounce) a day. It decreases the risk of additional stones in people who have already had a calcium oxalate stone.

Lose weight. Being overweight significantly increases your risk of stones.

Supplement with magnesium. Take 300 milligrams a day in one or two doses. If it doesn't make your stool loose, consider increasing the dose to 600 milligrams per day. Magnesium keeps more calcium in your body and less in your urine.

Ask about prescription drugs. Your doctor may prescribe a diuretic such as hydrochlorothiazide, which reduces the rate at which you lose calcium in your urine, or allopurinol, which can decrease uric acid formation.

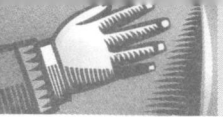

Nausea

The reasons for nausea and vomiting are numerous. They include pregnancy, motion sickness, surgery, chemotherapy, and of course, the stomach "flu."

While there are several prescription drugs for nausea, many have significant side effects and are usually saved for chronic nausea and vomiting, or when you're at risk of dehydration. Even if you're prescribed one of those drugs, some studies find they work better when combined with a complementary therapy like acupuncture.

Do This Now

To quell the queasies, follow these steps.

1. Swallow 500 milligrams dried ginger in capsule form. You can do this four times a day. If you're pregnant, cut the amount in half. If you don't have ginger capsules, chew a piece of ginger candy.

2. Eat a couple of plain, salted crackers or a rice cake (particularly if your stomach is empty).

3. Wear wrist-pressure bands like Sea-Band or ReliefBand, available in drugstores, on each wrist. If you don't have them when you need them, press the thumb of one hand against the inside of the wrist just below the crease of the wrist between the two tendons there and hold firmly for 10 seconds. Release, then repeat on the other side. Continue until the nausea abates.

4. If you're still nauseated, put several drops of peppermint, grapefruit, or spearmint essential oil on a tissue, hold it close to your nose, and breathe in through your nose and out through your mouth until your nausea abates.

Why It Works

Ginger should be one of your first choices if you're pregnant because it is so safe. Numerous clinical studies find it even more effective than Dramamine for motion sickness. It appears to work by blocking receptors in the gut for 5-HT, a form of serotonin, which is responsible for smooth muscle contractions.

The crackers are a tried-and-true remedy for morning sickness. It could be the fact that they're bland, or that salt helps suppress nausea. Plus, they raise your blood sugar slightly, itself a solution.

The wristbands put pressure on the acupuncture point P6. One study of 301 patients found the acupressure band worked as well as prescription medication in relieving nausea after surgery. Even if you're receiving acupuncture for your nausea, you might want to try these bands for relief between visits. The bands are also a better option for pregnant women than acupuncture.

The scent of the essential oils is believed to relieve nausea, and we believe the deep breathing helps too. One study had postsurgical patients sniff peppermint oil, rubbing alcohol, or salt water to treat nausea. All improved, leading researchers to speculate that the act of deep breathing might have been what helped.

❦ Helpful Hint

Motion Sickness Strategies

If you're prone to motion sickness, sit in the front seat of a moving vehicle. If you're on a boat, stand or sit (don't lie down) and focus on the horizon, which allows your eyes to suppress signals from your inner ear that could lead to nausea.

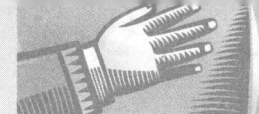

Other Medicines
Herbs and Supplements

Tulsi (*Ocimum sanctum*) is an Ayurvedic herb also known as holy basil. Follow package directions to make a tea and sip several cups a day.

Herbal tea. Mix 1 teaspoon chamomile, 1/2 teaspoon peppermint, 1 teaspoon catnip, 1 teaspoon basil, 2 crushed fennel seeds, and 1/2 teaspoon marjoram. (If you don't have catnip or marjoram, substitute one of the others in the same amount.) Steep in 6 to 8 ounces of boiling water for 10 minutes. Strain and drink three or more cups a day. This mixture contains carminative herbs that aid digestion and antispasmodic herbs that decrease muscle spasms.

Vitamin B_6. The American College of Obstetricians considers this a first-line treatment for pregnancy-related nausea. The vitamin helps break down hormones believed to play a role in morning sickness. Take 25 to 50 milligrams twice a day. For best results, combine with ginger.

Over-the-Counter Drugs

Antihistamines. The most commonly used medication for motion sickness, Dramamine, is actually an antihistamine (hence the reason it makes you so tired). Antihistamines inhibit the actions of histamine and acetylcholine, both of which play a role in nausea. Any antihistamine will do, although most doctors recommend Sudafed for pregnant women because of its safety record. For motion sickness, take it about an hour before you hit the boat, car, or train.

Prescription Drugs

Antiemetics are generally only used to treat severe nausea and vomiting during pregnancy, or to prevent nausea following chemotherapy or anesthesia. There are two main categories:

- **Serotonin antagonists** like Anzemet (dolasetron), Zofran (ondansetron), and Reglan (metoclopramide) block the action of serotonin, a neurotransmitter. They have few side effects, but they are expensive.

- **Dopamine antagonists,** such as Compazine (prochlorperazine) and Phenergan (promethazine), block the action of dopamine, another neurotransmitter. They have a lot of side effects, however.

Other Approaches

Acupuncture. Of all the complementary approaches to postsurgical and chemotherapy-related nausea and vomiting, the evidence is strongest for acupuncture. Studies also find it improves the effectiveness of antiemetic medications. For surgery-related nausea, it's best if the acupuncture occurs in the recovery room. If your hospital has an acupuncture service, you can arrange for this service prior to the surgery. If you're pregnant, stick with acupressure.

Hypnosis. A few small studies found hypnosis effective for "anticipatory" nausea that occurs before a cancer treatment.

Homeopathy. If you think you have food poisoning, try arsenicum. Homeopathy is also a good option for pregnant women. Specific remedies, used alone or in combination, are colchicum (particularly if you're sensitive to odors), ipecac (especially if you're salivating a lot), nux vomica (especially if you have dry heaves or chills), phosphorus (if you're vomiting shortly after eating or drinking), pulsatilla (especially if your nausea comes on later in the day), and sepia (if you're craving tart or spicy foods and your nausea is accompanied by hunger and constipation). Don't eat or drink for at least 15 minutes before and after a dose. For these general remedies, take low-potency supplements: 6X, 12X, or at most 30X.

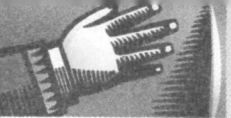

Ulcers

The story of ulcers is a great example of how our understanding of disease continues to evolve. In the early 1980s, when an Australian researcher first proposed that a common bacterium might be an underlying cause of most peptic ulcers (ulcers in the stomach or small intestine), he was nearly laughed out of the medical profession. Today, however, we know that the bacterium *H. pylori* is a primary cause of most peptic ulcers, along with heavy use of nonsteroidal anti-inflammatory drugs (NSAIDs) such as aspirin, naproxen, ibuprofen, and some COX-2 inhibitors.

But these aren't the *only* causes. Even though the medical profession has moved away from the idea of stress as a cause of peptic ulcers, we think the pendulum needs to swing back just a bit. After all, not everyone infected with *H. pylori* or using NSAIDs develops ulcers, and not all people who have peptic ulcers have an *H. pylori* infection or take NSAIDs. In other words, you can't discount stress and lifestyle when it comes to peptic ulcers, which makes them ideal for an integrative treatment approach.

Do This Now

For fast relief, follow these four steps. Read on for longer-term approaches.

1. Eat a few crackers or a few tablespoons of mashed potatoes.

2. Chew two tablets of deglycyrrhizinated licorice (DGL) one-half hour before your next meal (and any meals thereafter until the burning stops). Chew thoroughly and slowly.

TIME TO WORRY

- If you have blood in your stool or a dark, tarry stool.

- If you vomit blood or dark black material that looks like coffee grounds.

- If your abdominal pain is accompanied by weight loss, trouble swallowing, or if you get full very early in a meal. All could be signs of cancer.

- If you have abdominal pain associated with weakness or dizziness, especially when you stand up, or if you've been told you're anemic.

3. Next, drink a cup of slippery elm or marshmallow herbal tea. Continue drinking throughout the day.

4. If you still have the burning feeling, take 2 to 4 teaspoons of a liquid antacid, or an over-the-counter H_2 blocker like Zantac, Pepcid, or Tagamet.

Why It Works

The bland food helps buffer stomach acid, soothing the burning. Stay away from high-fat foods, which can increase the amount of acid your stomach produces.

Licorice has long been used to soothe and speed healing in mucosal tissue like the stomach. Numerous studies in rats show the herb not only helps heal NSAID-induced ulcers, but also protects against their development, most likely because licorice stimulates the lining of the

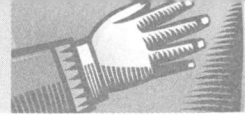

stomach and small intestine to secrete more protective mucus. In fact, a study comparing Tagamet and deglycyrrhizinated licorice in preventing ulcer recurrence found similar results between the two. Additionally, DGL appears to have some antibacterial properties against *H. pylori*. The reason we want you to take the deglycyrrhizinated form is that regular licorice can cause you to retain salt and water and lose potassium.

Slippery elm and marshmallow are demulcents, meaning they soothe and coat the stomach.

Antacids neutralize stomach acid so it doesn't burn. However, antacids won't help heal your ulcer. The H$_2$ blockers, or histamine-2 blockers, work by reducing the amount of acid your stomach produces. Several brands are available, but if you're elderly, avoid Tagamet, which is more likely to cause side effects such as confusion, as well as interfere with how your body metabolizes and eliminates certain drugs.

Other Medicines
Herbs and Supplements

Aloe vera gel. Take 1/4 cup three times a day. Make sure you're taking the gel and not the leaf exudate (sometimes called just "aloe," but check regardless of the name) because the latter is a laxative. The gel-like components in aloe help heal the lining of the stomach or small intestine. Most of the studies on aloe vera gel are in rats, but one early study in humans found it to be an effective treatment for peptic ulcer.

Probiotics. There's some evidence that these friendly bacteria can help your body get rid of *H. pylori* quicker. Plus, we know they help counteract any side effects of antibiotic therapy. We recommend 1 to 2 capsules with each meal and at bedtime for several weeks. Once the ulcer heals, continue taking your usual dose at bedtime for several months. If you might be prone to ulcers

(i.e., you're taking a lot of aspirin or other NSAIDs), continue taking your nighttime dose as long as the risk exists.

Fish oil and black currant or evening primrose oil supplements. Laboratory studies and one clinical trial in humans find that polyunsaturated fatty acids (which these supplements provide) prevent the growth of *H. pylori* and help the body get rid of the bacteria, while other studies find they help the lining of the stomach and small intestine heal from and protect itself against injury. Take 500 milligrams of fish oil twice a day along with 500 milligrams of evening primrose or black currant oil until your ulcer heals, and for one month after.

Turmeric. This herb has long been used to treat peptic ulcers, but there are few clinical

GETTING TESTED

Before your doctor can put together a treatment regimen for your ulcer, he or she needs to confirm that you have an ulcer and if you do, whether *H. pylori* is present. To diagnose the ulcer, the doctor may perform an endoscopy by inserting a flexible viewing tube with a camera on the end into your stomach and small intestine. Or you may undergo a barium contrast X-ray, in which you swallow a dye that shows up on the X-ray film.

During an endoscopy, the doctor may remove a small part of the ulcerous tissue to determine if it's cancerous, and to check for *H. pylori*. The presence of the bacterium may also be revealed through blood, breath, and stool tests. Blood tests detect antibodies to the bacteria. Breath tests, often used to see if a certain treatment worked, involve drinking a solution or swallowing a capsule that contains urea, a chemical made from nitrogen and carbon. The bacteria breaks down the urea, releasing the carbon, which is carried to lungs and exhaled in the breath. Stool tests look for the bacteria in your feces.

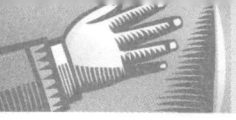

studies on how well it works. One study in 25 people with active ulcers found their ulcers healed in four to eight weeks of treatment with capsules of the dried herb. Take 1 to 2 capsules with meals.

Dragon's blood (*Croton lechleri*). This Amazonian treatment comes from the latex sap of the Amazon rain forest plant *Croton lechleri*. Its Peruvian name, *sangre de grado,* means "blood of the dragon," and is usually what it's called. A 2000 study in rats found it had potent healing effects on ulcers, due primarily to its ability to eradicate *H. pylori*.

Prescription Drugs

Conventional medical treatment for peptic ulcers involving *H. pylori* typically requires several medications. The greatest success comes from the so-called triple therapy: two antibiotics to kill the bacteria and either an acid suppressor, a proton pump inhibitor like Prilosec (these block the production of stomach acid), an H_2 blocker, or a stomach-lining shield, like Tritec (ranitidine bismuth citrate), which is similar to Zantac. Studies find this therapy reduces symptoms, kills the bacteria, and prevents recurrence in more than 90 percent of patients. But it's a pain, requiring that you take as many as 20 pills a day.

Another option is dual therapy, which involves an antibiotic and an acid suppressor. It's not as effective as triple therapy, however. A third option currently under investigation is called quadruple therapy, or bismuth triple therapy. It involves two antibiotics, an acid suppressor, and a stomach-lining or shielding medication. You and your doctor need to discuss the best option for you.

If you don't show any signs of *H. pylori* infection with your ulcer, it will be more difficult to cure. The standard therapy in that case is treatment with a proton pump inhibitor.

Other Approaches

Traditional Chinese Medicine. If you see a TCM practitioner, he or she is most likely to combine these herbal ingredients into one formula: Platycodon (reduces acid secretion), cuttlefish bone extract and/or oyster shell extract (neutralizes acid), *Corydalis rhizome* (relieves pain), and *Bletilla rhizome* (promotes wound healing).

Prevention

Eat less fat, more fiber. Overall, studies find that high-fat diets filled with meat and dairy increase the risk of ulcers. A high-fiber diet, on the other hand, appears to reduce the risk. Because fiber, particularly soluble fiber, slows the emptying of your stomach, it reduces the amount of time the stomach lining remains in contact with stomach acid. Also, soluble fiber (the kind found in oats, dried beans, and many fruits and vegetables) creates a kind of gel-like slurry that protects the lining. Aim to eat small, frequent

✌ What About...

A Bland Diet?

It's a myth. There's no evidence that milk or other "bland" foods heal ulcers. In fact, studies find that people who eat a spicy diet loaded with chile peppers are less likely to develop ulcers, possibly because the chile peppers keep *H. pylori* out of the digestive tract. Chile peppers are also used to treat ulcers in many countries. People who are not used to eating spicy food may, however, find that these foods irritate their stomach—so don't start eating hot peppers at the first sign of an ulcer. You need to develop a tolerance for them. Still, there are dietary changes you should make. In addition to eating less fat and more fiber, avoid alcohol and coffee, which irritate the lining of the stomach.

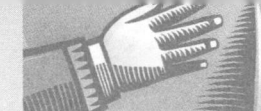

meals, which limits excessive acid production and may help control pain.

Quit smoking. Several population studies find a strong connection between smoking and the development of peptic ulcers. Smoking may also make your ulcer worse. Also, smoking seems to interfere with the action of the H_2 blockers like Zantac, and increase the risk of ulcer recurrence.

Manage your stress. As we noted earlier, the idea that stress and ulcers have nothing to do with each other just doesn't compute. We still believe that stress plays a role, either by promoting unhealthy behaviors (for instance, smoking and drinking alcohol, which irritates the lining of the stomach) or by increasing stress hormones and inflammation, both of which contribute to the development of ulcers. Several studies support our thinking. One Korean study found that the ulcers of people who completed a stress management program healed faster than those who just did muscle relaxation, while a large U.S. study found that people who perceived themselves as stressed were nearly twice as likely to develop ulcers than those who didn't. See Part 2 for suggestions on handling stress.

Take glutathione supplements. Glutathione is a powerful antioxidant found in high concentrations in the stomach. It plays an important role in maintaining the health of the stomach lining. Plus, studies find that when people take their NSAIDs along with glutathione supplements or high doses of vitamin C (which helps your body make glutathione) they are less likely to develop ulcers. Take 500 milligrams three times a day.

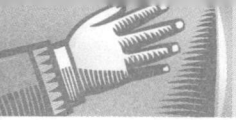

Urinary Tract Infection

UTIs all come down to the same thing: an infection somewhere along the route that carries urine from the bladder out of the body. The infection is most likely bacterial, although fungi, viruses, and parasites can also cause a UTI. These infections are 50 times more common in women than men.

If you're pretty healthy overall, a UTI is just a small bump in the road. But if you have diabetes, spinal cord injuries, urinary tract abnormalities, or you're pregnant, a UTI can be a serious infection, not to be taken lightly. And if you're subject to recurrent UTIs, particularly cystitis, or bladder infection, pay attention to the prevention section in this entry.

Do This Now

To ease the pain of a UTI, take these six steps.

1. Take 100 milligrams of the over-the-counter medication Pyridium (phenazopyridine) four times a day.

2. Drink several large glasses of water.

3. If you have a low fever, take a dose of aspirin or Tylenol (1,000 milligrams) or ibuprofen (400 to 600 milligrams).

4. Go to the bathroom when you need to. If it is too painful to urinate using the toilet, try urinating in a tub of warm water.

5. Add 5 to 10 drops of lavender oil to 1/4 cup castor oil. Massage into your flank (the back of your waist, toward the groin) where you're feeling pain. Cover with a flannel and top with a heating pad.

6. Arrange to give your doctor a sample of urine to test for bacteria so that, if necessary, you can get the right antibiotic.

Why It Works

Pyridium is a kind of aspirin for the urinary tract. It numbs the tissue that lines the urinary tract. Note that it contains a dye that turns your urine bright orange. The dye is a sign that the numbing agent has reached the urinary tract, and you should start feeling better. It is not an antibiotic, however, so it won't address the underlying infection. If the over-the-counter dose helps some, but not enough, call your doctor for a prescription-strength dose. Watch out for the dye: It stains everything it comes in contact with, including clothing and contact lenses.

We want you to drink lots of water because diluting the urine can reduce the burning and pain, while urinating helps flush the germs out of your bladder and urinary tract.

The warm oils will help ease the pain; lavender is a muscle relaxant, while castor oil acts as an anti-inflammatory.

Chances are, you're going to need an antibiotic. If your doctor prescribes one, make sure you finish the full prescription.

Other Medicines
Herbs and Supplements

Goldenrod. This herb helps you urinate, has anti-inflammatory properties, and is safe even in pregnant women. Take one to two capsules two or three times a day.

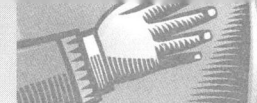

Prescription Drugs

Antibiotics. Expect a one- to three-day course (or 7 to 10 days for recurrent infections or other complications). If you're prone to recurrent UTIs, especially following sexual intercourse, your doctor may prescribe prophylactic (preventive) antibiotics to take after sex.

Herbs and Supplements

Cranberry juice. Studies find that 16 ounces of cranberry juice a day prevents recurrent UTIs. Cranberry juice has potent plant chemicals that prevent bacteria from sticking to urinary tract cells. Drink 16 ounces of juice a day, or buy capsules and take two capsules (500 mg each) 3 to 4 times per day and after sex (this is a minimal dose). Or buy a liquid concentrate, meant to be reconstituted, and take the equivalent of 16 ounces of juice per day.

Bearberry leaf extract. This was traditionally used to prevent UTIs, and it turns out the extract releases an antiseptic substance into the urine. Take 250 to 500 milligrams a day. Don't worry if your urine is discolored while you're taking it.

Lactobacillus capsules. There are excellent clinical trials showing good results using these probiotics to prevent UTIs. They help ensure that the rectum and vagina have enough "good" bacteria to check the growth of "bad" bacteria. Plus, probiotics seem to excrete materials that directly attack "bad" bacteria, as well as stimulate an immune response that helps prevent infection. During an infection, take one to two capsules with meals, then two at bedtime. For prevention, just take two capsules before bed. Various studies also suggest that inserting one or two capsules into the vagina once a week for a year can help prevent recurrent infections just as well as prophylactic antibiotics.

What About...

Vitamin C?

Although it's often recommended, there's no evidence that vitamin C prevents urinary tract infections. Skip it.

Other Approaches

Aromatherapy. Add up to 10 drops of one or more antiseptic essential oils such as lavender, tea tree, juniper, or chamomile to a sitz bath (a shallow bath, usually in a basin) and soak to help prevent recurrent UTIs.

Acupuncture. Women with a history of recurrent UTIs who received acupuncture for six months had half as many episodes of UTIs in the following six months as those who received a fake treatment, and a third as many as those who received no treatment. Certain acupuncture points help tone, or tighten, the kidney and bladder, while increasing urinary flow. This is important because a major cause of UTIs is incomplete emptying of the bladder.

Prevention

Eat foods that promote urination. These include watermelon, parsley, and celery. Avoid caffeine and salty foods, which are dehydrating.

Check your birth control. If you use a diaphragm and are subject to recurrent UTIs, check the fit of the diaphragm and keep it in for as short a time as possible. Or switch to a different form of birth control.

Don't douche. Douching removes beneficial bacteria that keep "bad" bacteria in check.

Urinate after sex. It's a way of washing out the vagina and getting rid of any harmful microbes.

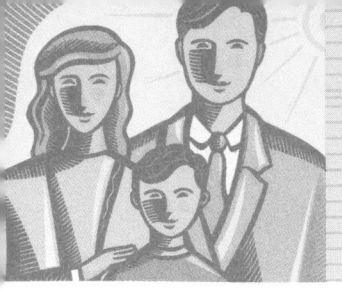

Endometriosis

Endometriosis can devastate a woman's life. This condition, in which the endometrial tissue that normally lines the uterus grows outside the uterine cavity, and sometimes spreads throughout the pelvis, can be tremendously painful and lead to heavy bleeding. There's a bit of overlap between this condition and menstrual cramps (page 151), heavy menstrual bleeding (page 136), and PMS (page 154), so consult those entries as well. It's also common for women with endometriosis to have irritable bowel syndrome (see page 116).

Our remedies focus on pain relief and reducing or stabilizing the production of estrogen, which contributes to the growth of endometrial tissue.

Do This Now

1. Take 220 milligrams Aleve (naproxen) with food. Don't take it on an empty stomach.

2. For cramps and abdominal pain, take 1/2 teaspoon valerian tincture (a liquid) and 1/2 teaspoon cramp bark tincture (both available in natural food stores) every one to two hours.

3. While you're waiting for the herbal tinctures to work, apply heat to your abdomen with a heating pad or a castor oil pack. For the latter, spread castor oil mixed with 10 drops ginger oil over your abdomen, cover with a cotton cloth or towel, then place a heating pad on top.

Why It Works

Aleve is a nonsteroidal anti-inflammatory that reduces the production of prostaglandins, inflammatory chemicals implicated in the development of endometriosis (in fact, studies find higher levels of these chemicals in the abdominal cavity fluid of women with endometriosis than in those without). Prostaglandins also contribute to the production of estrogen, which, in turn, contributes to the production of more prostaglandins in a vicious cycle that increases pain and fosters the growth of more endometrial tissue.

Valerian and cramp bark are smooth muscle relaxants. Smooth muscle is a type of tissue found in the walls of hollow organs such as blood vessels, the gastrointestinal tract, the bladder, and the uterus. So the herbs work quite well when used to relieve abdominal cramps.

Castor oil provides a base for the ginger oil. It also works on its own to relieve the pain by combating inflammation. The warmth of ginger oil not only soothes and relaxes, but ginger also dilates the blood vessels under the skin, helping the oils penetrate more deeply. Moderate dilation of local blood vessels also helps relieve pain by improving circulation, bringing more oxygen and nutrients to the injured cells, and reducing levels of lactic acid and other waste products, which can increase pain.

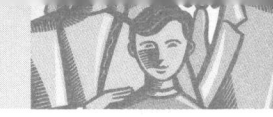

Other Medicines
Herbs and Supplements

Chaste tree berry and other herbs. There is very little research on the use of herbal therapy to treat endometriosis; however, there is a fair amount of research on its use to treat other reproductive conditions, such as painful periods and heavy bleeding. So any of the herbs we recommend for those two conditions, including chaste tree berry, raspberry tea, and shepherd's purse, may help with the symptoms, although they probably won't address the underlying condition.

Other herbs you might discuss with a naturopath or herbalist include yarrow, red root, and calendula, and liver tonic herbs such as dandelion, milk thistle, and artichoke extract to strengthen the liver's ability to metabolize excess estrogen.

Traditional Chinese Medicine (TCM). In the vernacular of TCM, endometriosis is a disease of blood congestion and mass in the lower abdomen. A TCM remedy often prescribed is Neiyi Wan #1, available in this country under the brand names Turtle Shell Tablets and Seven Forests. The formula contains turtle shell herb, vinegar-treated rhubarb, and succinum, a kind of fossil resin.

Prescription Drugs

The goal with conventional medical treatment is to reduce the effect of estrogen on the growth of endometrial tissue. Medications include:

Provera (medroxyprogesterone). This synthetic form of progesterone stops the growth of the uterine lining.

Danocrine (danazol). This drug is a synthetic form of testosterone. It suppresses estrogen production to postmenopausal levels. Like other hormone suppressors, it is only used for a short time. It can also lead to significant side effects, including hair growth, mood changes, voice deepening, and high cholesterol.

Gonadotropin-releasing hormones (GnRH agonists). These drugs, Lupron (leuprolide), Synarel (nafarelin), and Zoladex (goserelin), signal your body to produce less estrogen and progesterone, stemming the growth of endometrial tissue and also effectively putting you into menopause (and potentially causing menopause-related symptoms, such as hot flashes). They can only be taken for a few months, however, because of their menopausal effects, including bone thinning. Once you stop taking them, the endometrial tissue begins to grow again. Ask your doctor about adding progesterone to this treatment; it can help reduce some of the menopausal side effects.

Oral contraceptives. By tricking your body into thinking you're pregnant (at least hormonally), birth control pills stem the growth of endometrial tissue. Ask your doctor about the new, continuous form of birth control pill called Seasonale. It prevents menstruation for three months at a time, eliminating the pain and heavy bleeding many women with endometriosis experience during this phase.

Other drugs. Some doctors are beginning to use other hormonal medications to treat endometriosis, including GnRH antagonists such as Prostap (leuprorelin), and aromatase inhibitors (such as Arimidex [anastrozole] typically used to treat estrogen-receptive breast cancer).

Other Approaches

Omega-3 fatty acids. Increase your consumption of these "good fats," found in fatty fish, flaxseed, and some dark green leafy vegetables. Simultaneously, reduce your intake of omega-6 fatty acids, found in vegetable oils and animal fat. Omega-6 fatty acids contribute to the production of inflammatory prostaglandins, while omega-3 fatty acids have the opposite effect. To get more omega-3s, take 1,300 milligrams of fish or flaxseed oil two or three times a day.

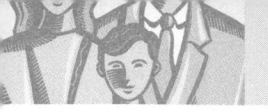

Low-sugar diet. Improving your insulin sensitivity (see Part 2 for a refresher on this important aspect of health) can reduce symptoms of endometriosis, according to one study in 50 women with the disease. So follow a low-glycemic diet, i.e., one high in nonstarchy vegetables, fruit, legumes, nuts, and dairy products.

Low-estrogen diet. That includes animal protein and dairy, which may be high in hormones (unless you buy organic).

Fiber. Fiber reduces the amount of circulating estrogen in your blood by increasing the amount cleared from your body. It also helps the body metabolize existing estrogen into less potent forms. Fiber-rich foods include bran, dry beans, whole grains, most vegetables, fresh fruit with the peel, and berries.

Soy foods. Plantlike estrogens in soy can block the actions of your own estrogen on cells. You'll find soy in many frozen vegetarian burgers. Or buy packaged (not loose) tofu and add to stir-fries or even lasagna. Another option: soy crumbles, found in the frozen food section. They have a meat-like texture and can be added to spaghetti sauce or vegetable stew.

Biofeedback. One very small study in five women found four of the five were better able to manage their pain after training in thermal biofeedback, in which a device on your finger measures your skin temperature. Using guided imagery or other relaxation techniques, you learn to raise the temperature, which can help with pain; eventually you're able to control the temperature without the device.

Surgery. Laparoscopic surgery, in which the surgeon removes excess endometrial tissue via tiny incisions in the abdomen, can provide relief for up to six months. Unfortunately, the tissue, and pain, usually return. In cases of severe pain, the surgeon may sever the nerve transmitting the pain signals.

✂ Helpful Hint

Making Sex More Comfortable

If your endometriosis makes intercourse painful, try getting on top. Women report much less discomfort with this position.

Exercise. Regular exercise improves symptoms of endometriosis, both by helping with pain management and improving insulin sensitivity. It also helps offset the bone loss that can come from GnRH agonists and minimize some side effects of the hormone drug danazol.

Transcutaneous electrical nerve stimulation (TENS). This therapy, which directs electrical current to the painful areas, is often used as part of chronic pain treatment. It has been used with good results in adolescents suffering from endometriosis.

Prevention

Eat plants, not animals. There's some evidence that your diet may affect your risk of endometriosis. One study that compared the diets of 504 women with endometriosis with that of healthy women found that women with endometriosis were much more likely to follow diets low in green vegetables and fruit and high in beef and other red meat, including ham. There's also some evidence that drinking more than 3.5 ounces of alcohol a day might increase the risk.

Watch your waistline. Obese women are more likely to develop endometriosis, possibly because of the additional estrogen production that comes from fat cells.

Be active. There's some evidence that regular exercise, even if you don't start until early adulthood, can help prevent endometriosis.

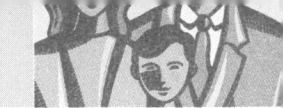

Erectile Dysfunction

To understand what can go wrong in terms of an erection, it helps to understand how an erection works. It starts with either mental or physical stimulation. This, in turn, sends signals to the brain, which tells the nerve endings in the penis to release a chemical called nitric oxide.

Nitric oxide relaxes or dilates blood vessels, enabling them to open up and bring more blood to the penis, swelling the penile tissues and creating an erection. At the same time, the dilated blood vessels entering the penis press up against blood vessels leaving the penis, trapping increased blood and maintaining an erection.

Erectile dysfunction (ED) can have numerous causes, ranging from physical illnesses (including diabetes, vascular disease, high blood pressure, and high cholesterol) to stress to certain medications. That's why it's so important that you get a complete physical examination if you have more than an occasional episode of ED.

Often, however, there's no physical or psychological reason for ED; it just happens.

A word of warning: While pharmacy and health food store shelves fairly burst with products claiming to remedy ED, many products may be contaminated with prescription drugs, which could be harmful. Also, some herbs in these products may be harmful if you have heart disease or high blood pressure. Work closely with your doctor if you want to use natural products, and only use those he or she recommends. Be wary of products sold over the Internet or imported from other countries; many of them are contaminated, expired, or lack the active ingredient advertised.

Do This Now

If your erection isn't related to some underlying medical condition, the following should help.

1. Take a recommended dose of the prescription medication Viagra, Cialis, or Levitra. If you have active angina (chest pain) or get chest pain while taking these medications, don't use them.

2. If you're not taking one of the drugs above, take the recommended dosage on a bottle of Korean red ginseng (*Panax ginseng*) three times a day. Do not take both the prescription medication and the herbal remedy, only one or the other.

3. Throw out your cigarettes.

4. Stay away from alcohol.

Why It Works

Viagra (sildenafil), Levitra (vardenafil), and Cialis (tadalafil) belong to a class of drugs called PDE-5 inhibitors. They prevent the enzyme that normally breaks down nitric oxide from doing its job. The biggest difference among the three is in how long they remain active and how long before intercourse you need to take them. All have similar side effects, including flushing, headache, heartburn, and sinus congestion. Don't take any of these drugs if you're also taking a medication containing nitrates, often prescribed for heart disease.

Several well-designed studies find that Korean red ginseng can improve erectile function, sometimes even more than older pharmaceutical drugs

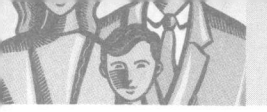
used for ED. Animal studies find the herb increases levels of nitric oxide in the blood, the same mechanism responsible for the benefits of drugs like Viagra. Other possible reasons for the herb's benefits include its ability to reduce fatigue, insomnia, and depression, all of which can affect erections. You can slowly increase the dose of Korean red ginseng, but only with your doctor's knowledge, because this herb can raise blood pressure in people with poorly controlled hypertension. It can also result in jitteriness, shakiness, and insomnia if you take it with other stimulants like coffee or amphetamines.

Despite the movie images of men smoking a cigarette after sex, smoking reduces blood flow to the penis and causes long-term damage to blood vessels. And alcohol, which is a central nervous system depressant, can make it difficult to have and maintain an erection, even if you think it gets you in the mood.

Other Medicines
Herbs and Supplements

Ginkgo. Although the studies on this herb are mixed, it seems to benefit many men, particularly those whose ED is related to the use of antidepressants. One well-designed clinical trial on 24 participants (men and women) with sexual impairment attributed to antidepressants found "spectacular individual responses" in both groups, even though there were no statistically significant differences between the men taking the supplement and a placebo group. Another study of 63 men and 33 women with antidepressant-related sexual dysfunction, which didn't compare the herb to a placebo, found ginkgo improved erections in 76 percent of the men.

L-arginine. This amino acid is a precursor to nitric oxide, so you can understand why it might work for ED. Studies suggest that high doses may particularly benefit men who have low

amounts of nitric oxide. One small study found that 40 percent of men taking 2.8 grams a day for two weeks had more erections than those taking placebos, while another found statistically significant benefits in men taking 5 grams a day for six weeks for ED related to diabetes or clogged arteries. One caution: It may lower blood pressure.

Try 2 grams a day for two weeks to see if your erections improve. You may gradually increase the dose up to 5 grams, taken in a divided dose two or three times a day. Simultaneously get more food sources of L-arginine, including legumes, whole grains, and nuts.

Pycnogenol. This antioxidant stimulates the production of nitric oxide. One study found that adding it to L-arginine worked better than the L-arginine alone, with 1.7 grams a day of L-arginine plus 80 milligrams of pycnogenol improving erectile function in nearly all of the 40 men involved.

Prescription Drugs

Testosterone. Occasionally, erectile dysfunction is related to low levels of testosterone. In those instances, testosterone patches or injections usually help.

Other Approaches

Acupuncture. Several studies suggest that acupuncture may be a good treatment for ED. One study of 22 men with ED unrelated to any

❦ Helpful Hint

Taking Viagra? Eat Salad

Skip the high-fat hamburger and fries before taking Viagra or Levitra. Consuming a heavy meal may slow the drug's effect, meaning it takes longer to have an erection.

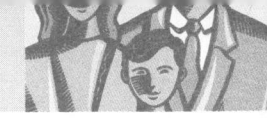

physical problem found that nearly 70 percent of those receiving real acupuncture improved, compared to just 9 percent of men who received a fake treatment.

Vacuum constriction device. If you don't want to take medication or you've had prostate surgery and can't get an erection even with medication, try a vacuum constriction device. You slip a relatively large plastic tube with a band around the bottom over the penis, pushing it firmly over the skin at the base, then use an attached pump to create a vacuum. The suction draws blood into the penis, resulting in an erection. You then slip the band around the bottom of the tube down around the base of the penis, trapping the blood and maintaining the erection.

Surgery. Performed rarely and only in the most extreme cases of ED, surgical procedures involve placing an implant into the penis to restore erection.

Kegel exercises. You don't usually see these pelvic floor exercises recommended for men, but since the pelvic floor muscles are active during normal erection, it makes sense to consider that weak muscles could interfere with erection. One study of 55 men with ED had half the men do Kegels and biofeedback. They also received recommendations on ways they could better manage stress. The other half only received recommendations about stress management. After three months, the control group also received the treatment. Overall, 40 percent of the men had normal erections, while 35 percent had improved erections, leading the researchers to conclude that pelvic floor muscle exercises and biofeedback were effective treatments.

To do Kegels, squeeze your pelvic floor muscles as if you were trying to stop the flow of urine or keep from passing gas. Count to 10 as you hold the contraction. Relax, then repeat 10 times. Perform 10 sets a day.

Prevention

Lifestyle changes are essential. Specifically:

Lose weight. ED is much more common in obese men.

Manage chronic health conditions. ED can be a sign that your diabetes, high cholesterol, vascular disease, or high blood pressure is poorly controlled. All affect the health of your blood vessels, which is critical to having and maintaining an erection.

Get a handle on stress. See Part 2 for specific recommendations on stress management.

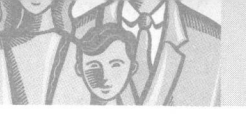

Heavy Menstrual Bleeding

Heavy bleeding during your period (known as menorrhagia) can be a condition in and of itself, or a symptom of another condition, such as uterine fibroids, perimenopause, cancer, or endometriosis. It may also signify a blood-clotting disorder. Your doctor should conduct a thorough physical examination before treating you, possibly including a biopsy of the uterine lining, to rule out other medical problems.

If nothing else is wrong, heavy bleeding is likely caused by an imbalance between estrogen, which thickens the lining of the uterus, and progesterone, which firms up the lining and prepares it for a clean separation from the wall of the uterus during menstruation. In most cases, estrogen levels are too high and progesterone levels are too low, usually because you're not ovulating. This thickens the endometrial lining. When the lining does slough off, it tends to separate irregularly or incompletely. The result is heavy and/or irregular periods.

If you have too much progesterone (as can happen if you're taking a progesterone-only birth control pill), then you may have regular periods and be ovulating, but menstrual flow will be very heavy, or you may bleed unexpectedly.

We've aimed our remedies at normalizing hormone levels while helping you maintain iron levels so you don't develop anemia due to excessive blood loss.

Do This Now

For fast, short-term relief during your period, follow these steps.

1. Put an ice pack on your abdomen over a thin cloth. Leave it there for 10 minutes at a time.

2. Take 20 drops shepherd's purse tincture two or three times a day while you're bleeding.

3. Take 400 to 600 milligrams ibuprofen every four hours.

Why It Works

Although you may have heavy cramps with your heavy bleeding, don't put heat on your abdomen, because it dilates blood vessels, which may increase bleeding. Ice can help ease the pain and may slightly reduce bleeding.

Shepherd's purse is a traditional remedy for heavy menstrual bleeding. It was used during World War I to stem bleeding from injuries. Although it hasn't been studied for use with heavy periods, it contains several flavonoids, which one small study suggests may help reduce menstrual bleeding. Try it for two cycles; if it works, begin taking it on a daily basis two weeks before your period and continue until you stop bleeding.

NSAIDs such as ibuprofen interfere with the production of prostaglandins, hormone-like chemicals involved with blood clotting. Levels are often high in women with heavy bleeding.

Other Medicines
Herbs and Supplements

Chaste tree berry. You'll see this herb recommended quite often for menstrual problems, including PMS. It's thought to work by reducing the release of the follicle-stimulating hormone (FSH) and increasing the release of luteinizing hormone (LH), which then reduces the amount of estrogen and increases levels of progesterone.

Good brands are Agnucaston and Cyclodynon. (See Resources, page 365, for buying information.) Follow the dosage instructions on the label. Take chaste tree berry for at least three months; it may take six or more cycles for you to feel its full effects. This herb is especially appropriate if you're not ovulating (you'll know by the pattern of your period—your cycle is usually longer than 28 days and irregular).

Vitamin C. Vitamin C is a powerful flavonoid that can strengthen blood vessels. In one small study, heavy menstrual bleeding in 14 of 18 women (88 percent) treated with 200 milligrams vitamin C and 200 milligrams of other flavonoids three times a day improved.

Vitamin E. Vitamin E seems to decrease the growth of new blood vessels in the uterine lining, thus helping to reduce bleeding. Most studies on the benefits of vitamin E for heavy bleeding were in women taking progesterone or those with heavy bleeding related to the Norplant birth control implant or an IUD, but we think it's worth trying even if you don't fall into either category. Start with 200 milligrams a day of vitamin E with mixed tocopherols for at least three months, or until bleeding slows, to see if it helps.

Iron. Ironically, low iron levels can *increase* menstrual bleeding. Make sure you're getting 18 milligrams of iron with your multivitamin. Also have your hemoglobin levels checked to make sure you're not anemic. Check with your doctor before taking iron supplements.

Prescription Drugs

Birth control pills. For women with no sign of endometrial cancer or other health problems, doctors often prescribe estrogen/progesterone birth control pills to normalize hormone levels and minimize bleeding. If you already have normal estrogen levels, you may need a progesterone-only birth control pill.

Copper IUD. A copper IUD that releases small amounts of progesterone may be a good option not only for birth control and to reduce bleeding, but also to increase iron levels.

Other Approaches

Surgery. If your bleeding doesn't respond to conservative measures, your doctor may recommend surgery. Options include:

- **Dilatation and curettage (D and C).** In this procedure, the doctor scrapes away the lining of the uterus. It grows back, but this should provide some relief temporarily.

- **Endometrial ablation.** The lining of the uterus is permanently destroyed with heat, freezing, microwaves, or radio waves.

- **Hysterectomy.** This should be a last-ditch option. If it's the first thing your doctor recommends, get a second opinion.

Exercise. When you're bleeding heavily, take it easy. Exercise can stimulate the flow. Otherwise, exercise regularly to maintain your weight. Heavy bleeding is more common in overweight women.

Prevention

Watch your diet. Eat plenty of dark, leafy greens and other good food sources of vitamin K, which aids in blood clotting. Other foods that may help with blood clotting include green drinks, such as those made with wheatgrass, chlorophyll, and seaweed. There's also some evidence these foods may reduce estrogen levels. Limit meat and dairy products unless they come from animals that have not been given hormones.

Avoid estrogenic herbs. Some herbs, such as ginseng, flax, and licorice, may act like estrogen.

Watch out for aspirin. Aspirin makes blood platelets less sticky, leading to increased bleeding.

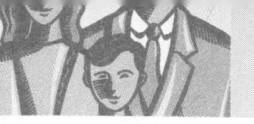

Herpes, Genital

Herpes, whether genital or oral (see Cold Sores, page 170), is a chronic, lifelong viral infection that can flare up at any time, often when you're stressed or your immune system is weak.

You usually get a warning of an outbreak—tingling, discomfort, itching or aching in the groin, in the same place as the initial outbreak. This is when we want you to begin using the remedies described here. Don't wait until the blisters erupt; by then, it's probably too late to reduce the severity or duration of the outbreak.

Although you can use antiviral drugs to prevent outbreaks, we don't recommend them for prevention unless you have six or more outbreaks a year, because they can lead to viral resistance. Instead, try the integrative therapies discussed here first, most of which have some pretty good evidence behind them.

Finally, keep in mind that even if you aren't having any acute symptoms, you may still be "shedding" the virus, meaning you're infectious and could pass it on to others. Your sexual partners need to know you're infected, and if you're male, you should always use a condom. You should, of course, avoid sex when you have an outbreak.

Do This Now

To reduce the duration and severity of an outbreak, initial or recurrent, follow this advice at the first tingling.

1. If this is your first outbreak, see a doctor immediately for an antiviral prescription.

2. Apply an ice pack to the affected area. Keep the ice on for at least 15 minutes, three or four times a day.

3. After each ice application, thickly apply lemon balm ointment (70:1 concentration) to the area. Lemon balm is sold in health food stores and online under the brand name Cold Sore Relief (but don't worry, it works on genital "cold sores" too).

4. Take 1 gram lysine along with 1,000 milligrams vitamin C that also contains 1,000 milligrams flavonoids. Take up to five times a day until the recurrence ends.

Why It Works

The first outbreak of herpes is usually the worst, and the one for which we definitely recommend an antiviral medication (described below) as soon as possible. The earlier you start it, the more likely it is that you can reduce the length and severity of the outbreak.

Meanwhile, you want to deal with the pain and discomfort. The ice numbs the pain, and it may also decrease the amount of virus created, reducing the severity and duration of the attack. Lemon balm is our favorite remedy for a herpes outbreak. Test tube studies suggest that the herb (*Melissa officinalis*) prevents the virus from attaching to cells, thus blocking its ability to replicate. One well-designed study of 116 people with oral or genital herpes found those treated with the balm recovered much quicker than those receiving a placebo. Plus, there's some evidence that using lemon balm during the initial outbreak (the very first time you realize you have herpes) may reduce the risk of recurrence.

The vitamin C with flavonoids enhances your immune system. One study treated 20 episodes of a herpes outbreak with 600 milligrams flavonoids

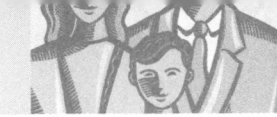

Lemon Balm Alternatives

If you don't have any lemon balm, try these alternatives:

• **Tea tree oil gel 6%.** Spread the gel over the affected area as soon as you feel the first tingling. Laboratory studies find tea tree oil slows viral activity, specifically against herpes viruses. One tiny study found it might lead to a quicker healing time—not as quick as with lemon balm, but still better than nothing. Use five times a day.

• **Black tea bag.** Moisten the tea bag and apply to the affected area. We only have anecdotal reports about this remedy, but it seems to help with pain and reduce the duration of an outbreak. Its benefits may be related to the effects of antioxidant compounds called catechins.

• **Vitamin E.** Puncture a vitamin E capsule and squeeze the liquid onto the sore. If started at the first tingling, it may help reduce healing time. It will definitely help soothe the pain, although we're not quite sure why.

---

and 600 milligrams vitamin C three times a day, 20 outbreaks with 1,000 milligrams of each vitamin five times a day, and 10 with a placebo. The vitamin regimen worked best, reducing the number of blisters and preventing their bursting, particularly when used during the pre-outbreak, "tingling" phase.

Lysine is an amino acid that works as an antiviral by blocking the activity of another amino acid, arginine. Arginine-rich proteins provide "food" for the virus, enabling it to replicate. So cutting off this fuel source reduces the amount of virus in your system. One study of 53 people with oral and genital herpes found those who received lysine supplements and cut out arginine-rich foods (nuts, chocolate, and gelatin) had an average of 3.1 outbreaks over six months, compared to an average of 4.2 in the control group. Only take the supplemental lysine until the outbreak fades (unless you have frequent outbreaks, in which case, see the advice under "Prevention"). Then, to prevent another outbreak, increase the amount of lysine-rich foods (cheese, eggs, chicken, milk, lima beans, fish, potatoes, brewer's yeast, and soy) and decrease the amount of arginine-rich foods (nuts, chocolate, raisins, and gelatin) in your diet.

Other Medicines
Herbs and Supplements

Niu Huang Shang Qing Wan. This Chinese herbal patent medicine is used to treat open sores and ulcers. From a Chinese medicine standpoint, its primary actions are to "clear heat," "disperse fire," and reduce inflammation, which makes sense when you consider the burning pain of a herpes outbreak. You can get it through a Traditional Chinese Medicine practitioner. It is recommended for viral conditions, including herpes.

Aloe vera cream or extract 0.05% strength. Apply to the affected area three times a day for five days during outbreaks. Studies find it reduces healing time.

Esberitox. This German herbal remedy (see Resources, page 365, for buying information) contains two types of echinacea as well as white cedar and wild indigo extracts. Numerous studies have found that it increases immune response. One study specific to herpes found that taking it at the beginning of an outbreak not only reduced the length of the outbreak but also prevented another outbreak in 80 percent of the patients for the four months they were followed. Take three pills three times a day at the beginning of the outbreak, then take three pills once a day for four months. You can also apply the liquid form to the affected area several times a day.

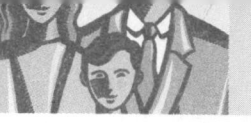

Zinc. Take 25 milligrams along with 250 milligrams vitamin C twice a day. One study found the combination either completely suppressed an outbreak (when taken at the first sign) or healed the outbreak in 24 hours. At the same time, you can apply a topical zinc sulfate cream (or zinc oxide, which is much more widely available) several times a day to the affected area. Another study found this not only helped heal herpes blisters, but also reduced the rate of recurrence.

Prescription Drugs

Doctors prescribe antivirals such as Zovirax (acyclovir), Famvir (famciclovir), and Valtrex (valacyclovir) to treat initial and recurrent outbreaks. These drugs prevent the virus from replicating, but they're most effective if you start taking them within 48 hours of an infection. If you're prone to outbreaks, use with caution; the more you use them, the more likely the virus will become resistant to them.

Prevention

Avoid triggers. Two primary ones are a weak immune system and stress. Review Part 2 for our advice on handling stress and maintaining a strong immune system. Also avoid any trauma to the skin in the genital area—too-hot baths and rough intercourse, for instance.

Follow a high-lysine/low-arginine diet as described under "Why It Works."

Eat seaweed. Laboratory studies find that seaweed has antiviral properties. Consider adding seaweed salads, sushi rolls, or green drinks containing seaweed extracts to your diet.

Take a daily aspirin. One small study found participants who took an aspirin at the first sign of an outbreak, then continued taking it for several months, had far fewer outbreaks than a control group that didn't take aspirin. Take 83 milligrams a day, the amount found in a baby aspirin.

Think zinc. Take 25 milligrams by mouth every day. Zinc enhances immunity, helping prevent recurrences.

Supplement with selenium. Take 200 micrograms a day to help maintain a healthy immune system. One study in women with genital herpes found higher levels of the virus in women with low blood levels of selenium.

Rely on lysine. Take 1 gram a day to prevent recurrences, but don't take if you have high cholesterol, because long-term use of lysine can increase levels of "bad" LDL cholesterol.

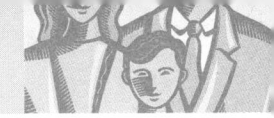

Infertility, Female

Although it's not life-threatening or even physically harmful, infertility can be devastating for a woman, particularly if she's spent most of her life trying *not* to get pregnant. And with more women putting off childbearing until their late thirties or forties, the incidence of infertility is growing.

Luckily, numerous medical treatments have been developed in the past 20 years to help women have a baby, from in vitro fertilization (IVF) to sperm injection. Integrative medicine can also play an important role. Studies find that incorporating natural approaches such as acupuncture and mind-body therapies can significantly increase the success of these medical treatments, leading many infertility clinics to add them to their menu of options.

Don't pursue any alternative therapies on your own, however, without your doctor's knowledge. The hormonal system is very sensitive; the therapy you're following on your own may render the medical treatment you're undergoing ineffective, and vice versa. This truly needs to be an integrative approach.

Also, anything that affects your period can affect your fertility. So see Endometriosis (page 130) and Uterine Fibroids (page 160) if these conditions apply to you.

Do This Now

Although most infertility treatments require considerable medical expertise or time, there are a few things you can try on your own before turning to the experts.

1. Stop drinking alcohol.

2. Stop eating fish.

3. Take your basal body temperature for several cycles to see when you're ovulating, and make sure you have intercourse during ovulation. To chart your cycle: Each morning before getting out of bed or eating or drinking, place a basal body temperature thermometer under your tongue. Record the temperature on a grid, with temperature on the vertical axis and date on the horizontal axis. When your temperature rises, you're ovulating. You should have intercourse at least every other day during your fertile period.

4. Stop using vaginal lubricants.

5. Stop taking all nonsteroidal anti-inflammatory (NSAID) medications (with your doctor's permission).

6. Start taking a daily multivitamin.

Why It Works

Numerous animal and human studies find that mild to moderate alcohol use can disrupt normal menstrual cycles and affect hormonal levels, possibly affecting fertility. Plus, if you do conceive, it may be several weeks before you know for sure that you're pregnant. Alcohol is toxic to the baby. Best to stop altogether in the trying stage.

Although we still want you to get your omega-3 fatty acids from fish oil supplements (which are purified), several studies suggest that eating fish from the Great Lakes and other local waters exposes women to certain toxins, like mercury, that can affect fertility.

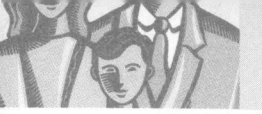

Tracking your basal body temperature is key. Obviously, the best way to get pregnant is to have intercourse when you're ovulating.

We want you to stop using vaginal lubricants because some brands can interfere with sperm motility, and to stop using NSAIDs because some evidence suggests they may interfere with the ability of a fertilized egg to implant in the uterine lining.

As for the multivitamin, a large Hungarian study in which more than 4,000 women were instructed to take a multivitamin while trying to become pregnant found that those who took the vitamins had more regular menstrual cycles and were more likely to conceive than those who didn't. On average, women who took the vitamins got pregnant 5 percent faster than those who didn't. Plus, if you do get pregnant, you'll be getting the supplemental folate you need to help prevent neural tube birth defects in the baby.

Other Medicines
Herbs and Supplements

Chaste tree berry (*Vitex agnus-castus*). This herb normalizes the menstrual cycle and hormone levels, which may help restore fertility. Good brands are Agnucaston and Cyclodynon. (See Resources, page 365, for buying information.) Take for three full cycles if your cycles are irregular. Don't take if you're also taking the prescription fertility drug Clomid (clomiphene).

N-acetyl-cysteine (NAC). This nutritional supplement is a precursor to glutathione, the most powerful antioxidant in the body. We recommend it as an adjunct to conventional treatment for polycystic ovary syndrome (PCOS), a common cause of infertility. Studies find it softens cervical mucus, making it easier for the sperm to get to the egg, and improves insulin sensitivity, which helps you get pregnant. One study of 150 infertile women with PCOS found those receiving the drug clomiphene plus NAC were more likely to ovulate and to get pregnant than women receiving only the drug. Take 1,200 milligrams daily in two divided doses.

L-arginine. This is another good nutritional supplement to use in conjunction with conventional medical treatment. An Italian study found that women taking the supplement had more eggs collected and more embryos transferred back into their uterus while undergoing ovarian stimulation than those taking a placebo, with three pregnancies in the L-arginine group compared to none in the placebo group.

Prescription Drugs

Several prescription drugs are available to help with various causes of infertility.

Clomid (clomiphene). This drug stimulates ovulation. It, along with the progesterone derivative medroxyprogesterone, is typically the first drug used for infertility, particularly if you haven't ovulated in several months.

Parlodel (bromocriptine). This drug prevents production of prolactin, high levels of which can prevent ovulation.

Follicle-stimulating hormone (FSH) drugs. These are injectable hormones that help the egg follicles in the ovaries mature and produce an

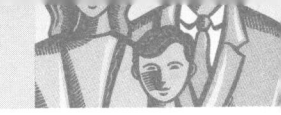

egg. They include Gonal-F, Follistim, Bravelle, and Repronex (Pergonal).

Human chorionic gonadotropin (HCG). This injectable hormone triggers ovulation after egg follicles mature.

GnRH agonists (Lupron). This drug blocks production of estrogen, reducing the amount of endometrial tissue. It's often used if endometriosis is an underlying cause of infertility.

Progesterone. This hormone helps the endometrium develop properly to support an embryo, particularly if you're undergoing IVF.

Corticosteroids. These treat immune disorders that result in sperm-destroying antibodies.

Metformin. This drug increases insulin sensitivity in women with PCOS.

Other Approaches

Mind-body therapies. There is very good evidence that stress significantly interferes with fertility. Several studies find that high stress levels prior to IVF can result in a lower pregnancy rate, and that stress-reduction techniques (many of which are described in Part 2) can improve pregnancy rates.

Surgery. Several reproductive surgeries can help with infertility, including laparoscopic surgery to unblock the fallopian tubes, and other procedures to remove endometrial tissue that may be interfering with conception.

Assisted reproduction techniques. Artificial insemination and IVF are the most common procedures used in infertile women. If you aren't ovulating, you can consider donor eggs. If carrying the baby is the problem, a surrogate mother is an option.

Acupuncture. A growing body of evidence points to the benefits of acupuncture as an adjunct therapy to conventional treatment for infertility, and some practitioners are beginning to specialize in acupuncture for this condition. One study

found that women with PCOS who underwent electrical acupuncture ovulated more frequently—by a factor of four—than women who didn't. Another compared pregnancy rates in women undergoing IVF. Those who received acupuncture had a pregnancy rate of 42.5 percent, compared to 26.3 percent in the control group.

Researchers speculate that acupuncture's ability to trigger the release of stress-reducing endorphins plays a role. These hormones appear to affect the secretion of certain reproduction-related hormones, such as GnRH, affecting the menstrual cycle and ovulation. Make sure you see a qualified practitioner and don't be surprised if he or she wants to work with your partner too.

Homeopathy. One study had 67 women with fertility disorders take a homeopathic preparation called Phyto Hypophyson L, which contains chaste tree berry, or a placebo, three times a day over three menstrual cycles. The women taking the remedy were more likely to menstruate without drugs, to ovulate, and to get pregnant.

Prevention

Protecting your fertility is a lifelong endeavor. These lifestyle approaches will help:

Maintain a normal body weight. Obesity and being underweight are both strongly associated with infertility, and many women who struggle to get pregnant while they are overweight or underweight find they have no problem once they reach a normal weight.

Practice safe sex. A major cause of infertility is pelvic inflammatory disease (PID), an infection resulting from sexually transmitted diseases that can scar the fallopian tubes or other reproductive organs.

Don't overexercise. Very strenuous exercise, such as running marathons, may affect your menstrual cycle, making pregnancy difficult.

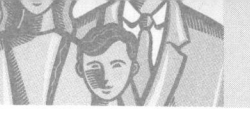
Infertility, Male

Although women seem to get most of the attention when it comes to infertility, about one in five men have fertility problems. The most common causes are low sperm count, high numbers of abnormal sperm, or problems with sperm motility (the little guys just can't get to the egg fast enough). Other, less common, causes include infections, disease, or even certain drugs. Lifestyle also plays a role, as you'll see below. Something as simple as wearing boxers instead of briefs really *can* affect fertility.

One major cause of sperm-related problems is oxidation, which damages the membrane of the sperm cell. So several of our remedies are designed to increase antioxidant levels.

Do This Now

To boost your fertility:

1. Start taking 2 to 3 grams of Panax ginseng root or 100 milligrams of a Panax ginseng extract.

2. Ask your doctor for a B_{12} shot.

3. Ditch your briefs for boxers.

4. Steer clear of all hot tubs, hot baths, and steam rooms.

Why It Works

We don't know for sure that it will help you get a woman pregnant, but one study evaluating Panax ginseng in 30 men with an unknown cause of low sperm count, and 16 men with low sperm count related to abnormal dilation of the veins surrounding the testicles, found taking the herb for three months increased the quantity of sperm and

improved sperm motility. It also increased testosterone levels, as well as levels of other reproductive hormones, leading researchers to speculate that the main chemicals in ginseng may affect a crucial hormonal pathway critical to men's fertility.

Note that quality control has been a problem with this herb in the past, so choose a high-quality brand. One of the best-researched brands (although not for this particular indication) is Ginsana, standardized to contain 4 percent ginsenosides.

On the vitamin front, anecdotal evidence finds that once-a-month B_{12} shots can increase sperm counts in infertile men.

As for the underwear, high temperatures in the testicular region suppress sperm production. So keep it cool for a while by wearing boxers.

Other Medicines
Herbs and Supplements

Antioxidants. The evidence is very strong for the benefits of antioxidant supplementation on sperm quality and quantity. The most important antioxidants are described below. Try to find a high-potency multivitamin that contains these amounts of vitamins E and C, selenium, and zinc. The fish oil and the L-carnitine you'll have to get in separate supplements.

TIME TO WORRY

If you're having trouble with fertility and you find a swelling in your testicle, whether painful or not and no matter how fast it's growing, see your doctor immediately. It could be a sign of testicular cancer.

- **Vitamin E.** Several studies find this antioxidant can improve sperm motility as well as increase the number of live and normal sperm. Take 600 to 800 IU of mixed tocopherols in the short term (i.e., four to six months). For long-term use, take no more than 400 IU a day.

- **Selenium.** Studies in rats find a dietary deficiency of selenium leads to deformed sperm with motility problems and infertility in rats. Take 100 to 200 micrograms daily.

- **Vitamin C.** Take 500 milligrams of vitamin C twice a day, gradually increasing up to 2,500 milligrams total daily. If you develop diarrhea, cut back.

- **Zinc.** Zinc seems to improve the number and motility of sperm and may also increase testosterone levels (critical to making sperm). Take 25 to 30 milligrams of zinc per day.

- **Fish oil supplements.** So far studies have only been conducted on animals (actually, fowl), but they clearly show that supplementing with essential fatty acids like those contained in fish oil supplements can help both the health of the sperm and its fertilizing ability. Take 2 to 3 grams a day.

- **L-carnitine.** Sperm contains more of this amino acid than any other cells, leading researchers to suspect it plays a role in sperm motility. One study on 30 men with poor sperm motility found that supplementing with 2 grams of L-carnitine a day for three months improved sperm motility compared to placebo. Other studies show it may also improve sperm count. Take 3 to 4 grams a day for three to six months.

Other Approaches

Surgery. One of the most common causes of infertility in men is varicocele, in which the veins wrapped around the testicles are overly dilated, increasing the temperature in the scrotum and reducing fertility. Minor surgery can loosen the vessels, although the success of this treatment is mixed, with pregnancy rates after surgery between 30 and 50 percent.

Stress reduction. In a kind of chicken-and-egg conundrum, one study found that the stress from infertility can negatively affect sperm quality. So review Part 2 for our stress reduction techniques.

Assisted reproductive techniques. Several techniques, including artificial insemination and intracytoplasmic sperm injection (ICSI), in which a sperm is directly injected into the egg, can be pursued if an integrative approach doesn't work.

Prevention

Limit alcohol. Alcohol is a sperm suppressor.
Don't smoke. Nicotine reduces antioxidants in semen.
Avoid pesticides, herbicides, and radiation.

✌ What About...

Less Frequent Sex?

The idea that you can "store up" your sperm until the timing is right doesn't pan out in studies. While it's obviously important that you have intercourse while your partner is ovulating, there's no evidence that less frequent intercourse at other times results in higher levels of sperm or better-quality sperm. In fact, studies find that having sex at least every other day supplies more viable sperm that remain active in the woman's reproductive tract for two to three days. However, having sex several times a day isn't going to improve your chances either; it does take a while to make a fresh batch of sperm.

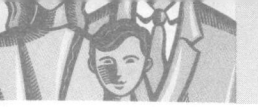

Jock Itch

You can probably tell by the name that this condition, known medically as tinea cruris, is common in men. But that doesn't mean it doesn't also affect women. Jock itch is a fungal infection more common in warm weather. It's also more common in people with diabetes or those with compromised immune systems. Pay attention to the prevention section; if you get one tinea infection, you're more likely to get another.

Do This Now

1. Apply over-the-counter Lotrimin Ultra cream to the affected area and about an inch around it, following the package directions.

2. Soak in a sitz bath infused with 10 drops of tea tree oil.

3. To control itching, use Benadryl cream or an over-the-counter hydrocortisone cream (only use for one week before seeing a doctor).

4. After cleaning and drying the area thoroughly, sprinkle with a medicated powder or cornstarch.

Why It Works

Lotrimin is an antifungal cream. Mild cases should clear up within about a week, while a more difficult or chronic infection might take up to two weeks to resolve. Continue using for a week after the infection clears to prevent a recurrence.

The sitz bath helps soothe the itching, while the tea tree oil fights fungus. The powder or cornstarch helps absorb moisture, a fungal infection's best friend.

Other Medicines
Herbs and Supplements

Antifungal tea. Put 1 to 2 tablespoons of thyme, eucalyptus, or lavender in a cup, cover with 8 ounces of boiling water, and steep for 10 to 15 minutes. Strain and cool. Wash the affected area with tea tree soap (available in health food stores), then soak a cotton ball in the tea and apply twice daily, after showering and before bed.

Prescription Drugs

If an over-the-counter cream doesn't do the trick, you may need something stronger. Prescription drugs include Nizoral (ketoconazole) and drugs that combine antifungals with steroids, such as Lotrisone (clotrimazole/betamethasone).

Other Approaches

Bitter orange oil. Mix five drops of bitter orange oil with 25 drops of a carrier oil like castor oil and test on a small area of skin. Apply three times a day for four weeks or until the infection clears. If you see no response in a week, increase the strength to 5 drops per 20 drops of carrier oil.

Tea tree lotion, soap, and diluted oil. Use regularly to cure mild to moderate infections.

Prevention

Follow good hygiene. Wear loose-fitting cotton clothing, and change out of wet clothes as soon as possible. Wash all sports clothes, including your jockstrap, in hot water.

Maintain a healthy weight. Skin folds are ideal areas for breeding fungus.

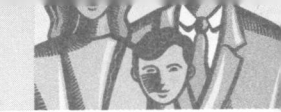

Menopause

Few conditions lend themselves quite so well to an integrative approach as the menopausal transition. Although hormone therapy can help with many of the symptoms, recent studies have raised concerns about its safety, sending millions of women searching for other options.

Let's be clear about what we mean when we talk about menopause. Menopause itself is just one day in a woman's life—the day on which she has gone 12 months without menstruating. The bulk of so-called menopausal symptoms, such as hot flashes, headaches, vaginal changes, urinary problems, mood swings, fatigue, etc., occur during perimenopause, which can last for years before true menopause arrives.

Although menopausal women need to be concerned with bone strength and heart health, we deal with those chronic conditions elsewhere in the book. Here we've focused on the menopausal symptoms—primarily hot flashes and vaginal changes—that aren't addressed anywhere else.

Do This Now

For fast, non-drug relief of hot flashes, do the following. Longer-term approaches to menopause symptoms are discussed later in this entry.

1. Wear all-natural materials that breathe, and dress in layers.

2. Several times a day, use your breath to release tension in your body by taking a deep breath in and, with the exhalation, releasing tension from the part of your body that is holding it in (often the back of your neck and shoulders).

3. Take a yoga class.

4. Make an aromatherapy spritz bottle. Mix 1 ounce water and 1/4 ounce alcohol (vodka or other odorless alcohol is best; isopropyl or rubbing alcohol will smell of the alcohol, but you can use it in a pinch). Add 10 to 15 drops of one or more of the following essential oils: chamomile, clary sage, geranium, peppermint, or lavender. Shake the bottle and spray over your body whenever you feel a flash coming on. You can also pat it on your face, chest, arms and neck.

5. Mix 1 cup pomegranate juice with 1 teaspoon sugar and 1/2 teaspoon lime juice. Refrigerate and drink every time you feel a hot flash coming on.

6. Sleep with a fan blowing on you.

Why It Works

It's important that you dress in layers, i.e., a camisole, then a T-shirt, then a jacket or sweater, so you can take off and put on clothing as necessary. Natural fibers breathe more than synthetics.

The deep-breathing technique helps you maintain your cool when you get upset or anxious. Anxiety can precipitate or aggravate hot flashes. One study found that women with moderate anxiety experienced three times the hot flashes of women with normal anxiety scores; those with high anxiety had five times the number of hot flashes. That's why yoga is a good idea. Several studies find yoga helps reduce anxiety and depression, as well as reduce levels of stress-related hormones.

The spritz won't stop a hot flash, but it can cool you down fast thanks to the evaporation of

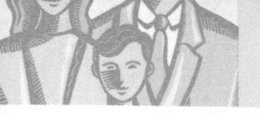

the water and alcohol (recall that rubbing alcohol is often used to bring down a fever). The aromatherapy oils all have calming effects. A warning: The oils can stain cotton.

The pomegranate juice mixture is a centuries-old Ayurvedic remedy for hot flashes. There aren't any published studies on it, but pomegranates contain large amounts of phytoestrogens, which could help moderate some menopausal symptoms. Also important, the powerful antioxidants in pomegranate juice can provide cardiovascular protection—something every menopausal woman should be concerned with.

Finally, keeping your bedroom as cool as possible at night will help you sleep. A fan not only cools you down but dries you off after sweaty flashes. This is also a good time to invest in some high-quality, 100 percent cotton sheets. You'll find them much cooler to sleep on than synthetic fabrics. Ditto for your nightgown or pj's.

Other Medicines
Herbs and Supplements

There are numerous herbs and supplements touted for menopausal symptoms. The following have good clinical evidence behind them and/or have had good results with patients.

Black cohosh for hot flashes. This is probably the most studied and most recommended herb for menopausal symptoms. Almost all clinical studies on this herb use a standardized extract, either Remifemin or Klimadynon. Three out of four well-designed clinical trials found these remedies effective for treating hot flashes. They may even be appropriate for women who have had estrogen-sensitive breast cancer who can't take hormone therapy. (See Resources, page 365, for buying information.) Be patient; it may take six to eight weeks before you see full results.

Chaste tree berry extract for irregular periods. This herb helps regulate menstruation.

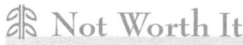

Not Worth It

Dong Quai

This Chinese herb is often touted as the ideal supplement to prevent hot flashes. However, clinical evidence shows otherwise; when given as a single herb, it has no benefit. Skip it.

Some patients say it also has a positive effect on their libido, and some studies suggest it may help relieve breast pain. Chaste tree berry is thought to work by increasing progesterone levels, which helps prevent the heavy menstrual cycles so common during this time. There really are no good clinical studies on its use, but integrative practitioners have had years of positive results using it. This herb is also helpful if you develop PMS as part of your perimenopause. Preparations vary considerably, so follow the instructions on the package.

St John's wort for mood swings and mild depression. Europeans consider St. John's wort to be a treatment for menopause as well as depression, and you often find it combined with black cohosh in herbal supplements. Studies find its benefits are comparable to those of Prozac and older antidepressants for mild to moderate depression. Take 300 milligrams of a preparation standardized to 0.3% hypericin and 2% to 5% hyperforin (or hyperforin only) three times a day. If you take a product standardized to hyperforin only, take 10 to 15 milligrams three times daily. *Caution:* There are several herb/medicine interactions with St. John's wort. Check with your doctor first if you're taking other drugs.

Wild yam cream for dry vaginal tissue. Despite the hype, this cream does not contain progesterone and is not a replacement for progesterone. However, it is often used in herbal medicine to heal wounds, and can help with the irritation and pain that often results from vaginal dryness, protecting the vagina from tears.

Ginkgo for forgetfulness. Ginkgo appears to help mental functioning by improving blood flow and protecting blood vessels. Take 60 milligrams of standardized ginkgo extract once or twice a day.

Prescription Drugs

Hormone replacement therapy. HRT, either with estrogen alone or estrogen plus progesterone (for women who still have their uterus) is the only drug approved for the treatment of hot flashes and vaginal and urinary changes related to menopause. Although HRT has become extremely controversial in recent years, it remains a good option for some women with severe hot flashes. If you decide to take it, take the estradiol form of estrogen for the shortest time possible at the lowest effective dose.

Also consider non-oral forms of estradiol, such as EstroGel (rubbed on your arm), Estrace (a vaginal cream best used for vaginal and/or urinary tract symptoms), Estring (inserted into the vagina), and estrogen patches. Because they aren't broken down by the liver, researchers suspect they may be safer than oral estrogens.

While there is a lot of interest in "natural" plant-based hormones dispensed by compounding pharmacies (pharmacies that mix up preparations not available in other pharmacies), there is no scientific evidence that they are any safer or more effective than pharmacologic hormones.

Testosterone. Although it's not approved for this purpose, many doctors today prescribe small doses of testosterone to help women boost a sagging libido. Ongoing studies find it can be beneficial, but watch out for side effects like acne and excess hair growth.

Progesterone cream. One study found a significant improvement in hot flashes in women using the cream versus a placebo. You'll need to go to a compounding pharmacy to get it.

Paxil (paroxetine). Low doses of this antidepressant can help with hot flashes, with few side effects. The dose commonly prescribed is 10 to 20 milligrams once daily.

Other Approaches

Sage tea. This is a traditional remedy that many women find helpful. Pour 8 ounces of boiling water over 2 to 3 teaspoons of the fresh herb and steep for 10 minutes. Strain and, if necessary, add a small amount of honey to taste. Sip one cup several times during the day, especially in the evenings, to help with nighttime flashes and sweats.

Acupuncture. One study of 45 women comparing acupuncture to oral estrogen therapy or a fake acupuncture treatment found that while the oral estrogen had the greatest effect, the women receiving acupuncture still had significantly fewer hot flashes. The fake acupuncture treatment worked too (there's often a large placebo effect with hot flash remedies).

Prevention

Obviously, there is no way to prevent menopause! So we've focused on ways to prevent hot flashes. Also see Incontinence, Urinary (page 110), Headache (page 228), Urinary Tract Infection (page 128), Insomnia (page 235), and Depression (page 272) for tips on managing and preventing other common menopausal symptoms. Other entries to review are High Cholesterol (page 284) and Coronary Artery Disease (page 268). More women die of heart disease than any other illness, and their risk increases sharply at menopause.

Stay away from spicy foods and alcohol. Both of these can trigger a hot flash.

Add soy foods to your diet. While the evidence on soy as a prevention or treatment for hot flashes is mixed, soy does seem to help some women. And it definitely benefits your heart and bones. Ideally get some of your soy fermented, as

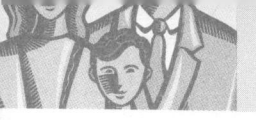

in miso, tempeh, soy sauce, and fermented tofu. The fermented type is easier for your body to absorb. Aim for one serving (about 2.8 ounces) of low-fat soy foods a day.

Avoid hot baths or showers, which increase your core body temperature. Instead, opt for tepid or cooler baths and showers.

Lose weight. A study that followed women over 10 years as they moved through the menopausal transition found that overweight women were much more likely to experience hot flashes. Researchers aren't sure why, particularly since fat cells secrete estrogen, which should,

theoretically, offset any increased body temperature from the weight, but the evidence was clear.

Quit smoking. The same study noted above also found that women who smoked had nearly twice as many hot flashes as nonsmokers.

Get 30 minutes a day of moderate exercise. Several studies find regular exercise can reduce the frequency and severity of hot flashes. Make sure some of your physical activity includes weight-bearing exercise, like weightlifting, to help preserve bone and increase muscle mass so your body burns more calories.

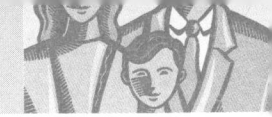

Menstrual Cramps

Menstrual cramps affect about half of all women every month, and some women have cramps so severe they can't work, exercise, or keep up with other routine activities. Most often cramps occur without any other obvious condition, but sometimes they are the result of premenstrual syndrome (PMS), endometriosis, fibroids, or heavy bleeding. See those entries as well. If you have one of them, your doctor should treat that underlying condition as well as addressing the cramps.

Do This Now

When you're in the midst of the cramps and need relief fast, try these steps. For longer-term approaches, keep reading.

1. Take 220 milligrams of naproxen (Aleve) or 400 to 600 milligrams of ibuprofen. For severe pain and to improve the cramp-relief benefit of these drugs, add 500 to 1,000 milligrams of acetaminophen (Tylenol).

2. Take 1/2 teaspoon valerian tincture (a liquid) and 1/2 teaspoon cramp bark tincture (both available in natural food stores) every one to two hours until the cramps abate.

3. While you're waiting for the tinctures to work, apply heat to your abdomen with a heating pad or a castor oil pack. For the latter, spread castor oil mixed with 10 drops ginger oil over your abdomen, cover with cotton or wool flannel, then apply a heating pad. If your lower back also hurts, apply the castor oil spread there.

4. Now draw yourself a warm bath and soak until the water cools.

5. Afterward, lie on your side with your legs drawn up into your abdomen or with a pillow under your legs to elevate them, especially if you have back pain along with your cramps.

Why It Works

Nonsteroidal anti-inflammatory drugs (NSAIDs) remain the first-line treatment for menstrual cramps and are effective in up to 70 percent of women. These drugs, including ibuprofen, naproxen, aspirin, COX-2 inhibitors, and others, reduce production of pro-inflammatory prostaglandins (hormone-like chemicals). Studies find taking acetaminophen with NSAIDs is better at relieving severe pain than taking either alone.

The valerian and cramp bark are thought to relieve cramps by relaxing the smooth muscle around the uterus. The castor oil counters inflammation and also helps the ginger oil penetrate the skin. Ginger's warmth soothes and relaxes (as does the warm bath), and ginger also dilates the blood vessels under the skin, helping the castor oil penetrate more deeply.

Getting into the fetal position shifts the position of the uterus so it doesn't press on the bundle of nerves at the front of the pelvis known as the sacral plexus.

Other Medicines
Herbs and Supplements

Chaste tree berry extract (*Vitex agnuscastus*). Because cramps are more common in women who have heavy bleeding and a long menstrual cycle, they are likely related to an imbalance of estrogen and progesterone. This herb helps

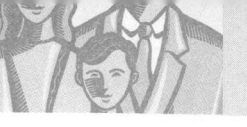

normalize estrogen levels. Good brands are Agnu-caston and Cyclodynon. (See Resources, page 365, for buying information.) Although it will start to work sooner, it can take up to three months to see the full effect of this herb.

Fennel. This herb is an antispasmodic, meaning it relieves muscle spasms. Although you can buy fennel tea in health food stores, we recommend you try the more potent essential oil preparation. Buy a fennel oil of sufficient purity to be taken internally (it should say on the label that it can be taken internally) and add 1 drop of the oil to 20 drops olive oil, or put 1 drop on a charcoal tablet (available in drugstores) and swallow. Take up to three times a day while you have cramps, but stay out of the sun because it may increase sun sensitivity.

Anti-cramp tea. Pour 8 ounces of boiling water over 1/4 teaspoon each of raspberry leaves, chamomile, crushed fennel seeds, and spearmint, steep for 10 minutes, strain, then drink when the cramps hit (you can drink it warm or refrigerate it and drink it cool). Ginger or chai teas can also help.

Vitamin/mineral regimen. Several studies, along with clinical experience, suggest the following vitamin/mineral supplements can reduce menstrual cramps.

- **Vitamin E.** Although best known as an antioxidant, vitamin E also acts as an anti-inflammatory. Take 400 IU per day beginning two days before your period and continue for the first three days of bleeding. At this dose, vitamin E shouldn't thin the blood enough to cause any additional bleeding.

- **Magnesium pidolate.** Take 300 to 500 milligrams of this or another magnesium salt, daily beginning the day before your period is due. Cut back the dose if you find you have loose stools. This form of magnesium appears to reduce inflammatory prostaglandins.

- **Calcium.** Take 1,000 or more milligrams per day, in two divided doses (500 or 600 milligrams each) throughout the month. Calcium helps ease muscle spasms. Some supplements contain both calcium and magnesium; we suggest you look for one.

Omega-3 fatty acids. As you've heard before, these are excellent anti-inflammatories. Small studies find that women with low daily intake of these "good fats" are more likely to experience cramps. Take 1 to 3 grams a day of fish oil, flaxseed oil, or evening primrose supplements throughout the month for the first three months—six months if your symptoms are severe. Then decrease as you are able. You may find you can get relief simply by taking it for 10 days before your period. However, we recommend this supplement for numerous other conditions, especially heart disease, so it's fine to take every day.

Prescription Drugs

Oral contraceptives. Birth control pills can reduce the severity of menstrual cramps by suppressing ovulation. Without ovulation, there's less progesterone, which can contribute to cramps.

Nitroglycerine patch. Although it's not approved for this use, a large clinical trial found that applying a patch that releases nitric oxide (a form of nitroglycerine) to the lower abdomen just before menstruation begins can relieve cramping. The study involved 88 women from six countries who wore the patch for two menstrual cycles. Before wearing the patch, most women said their pain was bad enough to require painkillers. After using the patch, the majority of women reported using less medication. Nitric oxide halts the uterine contractions that cause cramps. The main side effect is headache.

Other Approaches

Biofeedback. Several studies find that thermal or EMG biofeedback can help. With thermal biofeedback, a device on your finger measures your skin temperature. Using guided imagery or other relaxation techniques, you learn to raise the temperature, which can help with pain; eventually you're able to control the temperature without the device. EMG biofeedback uses electrodes that measure muscle tension or brain-wave function. Using guided imagery or other relaxation techniques, you learn to reduce muscle tension or alter your brain waves to reduce the pain.

Acupuncture. In the 1990s a National Institutes of Health panel on acupuncture found it might be beneficial for menstrual cramps. Since then, several small studies have backed up the idea.

Transcutaneous electrical stimulation (TENS). Several good studies find that TENS, in which mild electrical current is delivered to the painful area, can relieve menstrual pain better than a placebo. It's thought to work by altering the body's ability to receive or perceive pain signals. Make sure you receive high-intensity TENS; studies find few benefits with the low-intensity form.

Prevention

Follow an anti-inflammation diet. This type of diet is one that's low in meat, animal fat, and fried foods, and higher in fish, fruits, soy, vegetables, and legumes. One study found a lower risk of painful periods in adolescents who ate more fruit, eggs (look for eggs high in omega-3 fatty acids for additional benefits), and fish. Other studies find that a low-fat, vegetarian diet is associated with a lower incidence of cramps and less severe cramps, possibly because it increases the amount of sex hormone binding globulin—a fancy way of saying there's less estrogen floating around, so the uterine lining doesn't grow as thick.

Try yoga. Several studies find moderate physical exercise throughout the month can prevent menstrual cramps. We recommend yoga because of physical conditioning and stress-reduction benefits.

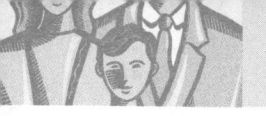
Premenstrual Syndrome (PMS)

Most women who experience PMS get it every month. So while our "Do This Now" advice is meant to offer quick relief from some symptoms (cramping, bloating, nausea, and mood swings), most of the remedies we recommend are long-term treatments designed to eventually prevent many of the symptoms, or at least make them less severe. They need time to work; don't expect your moodiness or breast pain to disappear overnight.

As for the herbal therapies and supplements, we suggest taking them every day for at least three full cycles. If your symptoms are under control by then, you can try to gradually cut back to taking them daily during the two weeks before your period is due. But taking these remedies every day will not hurt you, and many (like calcium) have other important functions, like protecting bones.

PMS overlaps with several other menstrual-related entries, such as Menstrual Cramps (page 151), as well as with Depression (page 272) and Anxiety (page 216). Also, the first sign of menopause for some women is changes in the menstrual cycle length or interval accompanied by PMS symptoms, even if you've never had them before. So also see the Menopause entry on page 147.

Do This Now

For fast relief of cramps, nausea, and bloating, follow these steps.

1. Take 220 milligrams naproxen (Aleve) or 400 to 600 milligrams ibuprofen (Motrin). For more relief, you can add 500 to 1,000 milligrams acetaminophen (Tylenol).

2. Apply heat to your abdomen with a heating pad or a castor oil pack. For the latter, spread castor oil mixed with 10 drops ginger oil over your abdomen, cover with cotton or wool flannel, then apply a heating pad. If your lower back also hurts, also apply the castor oil spread there.

3. If you're feeling nauseated or bloated, make a castor oil spread with 10 drops grapefruit oil instead of ginger oil and massage over your abdomen as described above.

4. For bloating and water retention, take 1 capsule nettle and/or dandelion leaf and root three to four times a day.

5. Run a hot bath and add 10 to 15 drops of lavender, geranium, or clary sage essential oil (or all three) and soak until the water cools. If you're retaining fluid, add juniper oil to the bath as well.

6. For nausea, suck on ginger candy or sip a cup of ginger tea.

Why It Works

Nonsteroidal anti-inflammatory drugs (NSAIDs) remain the first-line treatment for painful menstrual cramps, and are effective in up to 70 percent of women. These drugs reduce production of the prostaglandins that contribute to inflammation and cramps. Studies find that combining an NSAID with acetaminophen provides better pain relief. Don't combine them on a regular basis, however—just for occasional severe pain.

Castor oil combats inflammation (which contributes to cramps) and is an excellent carrier oil

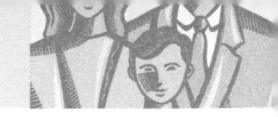

for essential oils. For cramps, we recommended ginger oil mixed into the castor oil because ginger's warmth soothes and relaxes. Ginger also dilates the blood vessels under the skin, helping the castor oil penetrate more deeply. Grapefruit oil is often used for nausea.

Nettle and dandelion both act as diuretics.

The hot bath has several benefits. The heat along with the essential oils soothes cramps and backache. And just spending some time alone, in a quiet place, focusing on *you* for a change, can also improve your mood.

Ginger is a traditional—and effective—remedy for nausea and the bloating that comes from gas.

Other Medicines
Herbs and Supplements

Chaste tree berry. This is our most highly recommended PMS remedy, along with calcium and magnesium (described below). It's thought to work by reducing the release of follicle-stimulating hormone (FSH) and increasing the release of luteinizing hormone (LH). Together, they reduce estrogen levels and increase progesterone levels, helping balance hormones and mood. Several studies support our faith in chaste tree berry for PMS. Good brands are Agnucaston and Cyclodynon. (See Resources, page 365, for buying information.) Take for at least three months; it may take six or more cycles for you to feel its full effects. Don't take with oral contraceptives; it may make them less effective.

Calcium and magnesium. Studies find that reproductive hormones affect your body's ability to absorb and use calcium and magnesium. That could be why several large studies found that supplementing with these two minerals improved PMS symptoms. Calcium reduces the irritability of smooth muscles during PMS, which helps decrease cramping, while magnesium enhances

muscle relaxation and reduces levels of pro-inflammatory prostaglandins.

The studies for calcium are so strong that a 1999 review on calcium as a PMS treatment determined that doctors should recommend it for women with PMS.

We recommend 1,000 to 1,200 milligrams calcium citrate (it's the form that's absorbed best) along with 200 to 400 milligrams magnesium divided in two doses daily. If you have trouble taking large calcium pills, look for liquid calcium or calcium-fortified foods for part of your daily dose (orange juice or chews). These may not have enough magnesium, but you can add that separately.

Evening primrose oil. Although the scientific literature isn't as strong for this herbal remedy as it is for chaste tree berry, we (and many patients) think it's helpful. Take 3,000 milligrams a day. You can also substitute the same amount of fish oil.

Ginkgo. Although ginkgo is primarily used as a memory aid, there's good evidence of its benefits for PMS. One study of 165 women found those who took an extract of ginkgo called EGb761 for two months showed significant improvement in all PMS symptoms, especially breast tenderness and fluid retention, compared to women who took a placebo. The extract is sold as Ginkgo Gold by Nature's Way and is available in most drugstores. Take 120 to 180 milligrams a day.

St. John's wort. It's well known that low levels of serotonin, a mood-regulating neurotransmitter, play a role in PMS symptoms. St. John's wort, a well-studied remedy for mild depression, also seems to benefit mood in women with PMS, at least according to one preliminary trial. Take 300 milligrams of a product standardized to 0.3% hypericin or 2% to 5% hyperforin three times a day.

A word of warning here: St. John's wort can interact with certain drugs, including cyclosporine and protease inhibitors, so check with your doctor before taking it. Also, don't take it if

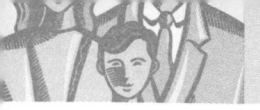
you're immunocompromised in any way or use blood thinners. If you're taking birth control pills, you may have some spotting with St. John's wort, and it may make you more sensitive to the sun, particularly if you're fair-skinned.

Vitamin B$_6$. This vitamin is involved in numerous chemical reactions that produce mood-related neurotransmitters such as dopamine and serotonin. Several studies find that doses of 50 to 100 milligrams a day can help relieve breast pain and depression related to PMS. Don't exceed 100 milligrams a day, however; higher doses may cause nerve damage.

Optivite. This vitamin formulation contains high levels of vitamin B$_6$ and magnesium, both of which have been shown to reduce PMS symptoms. This is an easy way to get both supplements in one pill. Several studies conducted on Optivite showed it significantly improved PMS symptoms. Take 2 tablets a day during the first half of your cycle, then 4 a day during the second half. If that doesn't result in any improvement in one or two cycles, double the dosage to 4 and 8 tablets.

Prescription Drugs

Progesterone. Given alone or with estrogen via oral contraceptives, progesterone prevents the release of an egg from the ovaries, stemming the hormonal cascade that results in PMS. You can also take a natural progesterone vaginal or rectal suppository, 200 to 400 milligrams twice a day beginning 14 days before the first day of your period. Progesterone creams and suppositories are available through compounding pharmacies, special pharmacies that make these medications from scratch.

Sarafem (fluoxetine). You know it as Prozac, but this selective serotonin reuptake inhibitor (SSRI) has also been approved to treat the severe form of PMS, premenstrual dysphoric disorder (PMDD). You take it only during certain parts of the month rather than every day.

Other Approaches

Stick to a low-dairy, low-sugar, low-salt diet. Studies find that women who suffer from PMS are more likely to have diets high in dairy, sugar, and salt. If you're willing, you might want to consider a vegetarian diet. One study found a low-fat, vegetarian diet not only improved physical PMS symptoms like water retention but also mood.

Increase dietary manganese, calcium, and vitamin D. Studies find diets low in these nutrients increase PMS symptoms. Good sources of manganese include pineapple, nuts, oatmeal, brown rice, tea, spinach, and legumes. Good calcium sources include any form of dairy, calcium-fortified juices and soy products, and deep leafy green vegetables like spinach. Good sources of vitamin D include skim milk, as well as about 15 minutes of sunshine a day.

Decrease caffeine. Not only do several small studies suggest that cutting down on caffeine can help with PMS symptoms, it's often recommended for women with fibrocystic breast disease, which can be a cause of premenstrual breast pain.

Eat less red meat and more fiber. This will help reduce the levels of circulating estrogen in your body. One study in particular showed that adding 10 to 20 grams of wheat bran a day decreased circulating estrogen in premenopausal women. Also lose weight if you need to, since fat cells produce estrogen.

Progressive muscle relaxation therapy. We describe this technique in Part 1 (page 25), and a couple of small trials found that women who practiced it found more relief from the physical symptoms of PMS than women who didn't.

Cognitive-behavioral therapy (CBT). CBT is essentially talk therapy that helps you reframe difficult situations so you can better cope with them. One study found that women who received 12 weekly sessions of CBT for PMS symptoms had an almost complete remission of their physical and psychological symptoms compared to women in the control group who merely documented their symptoms. Most therapists are trained to provide this type of therapy. You can find a practitioner certified by the National Association of Cognitive-Behavioral Therapists by logging on to www.nacbt.org/searchfortherapists.asp.

Aerobic exercise. Studies find that doing any kind of aerobic exercise, such as walking or biking, for an hour three times a week helps with PMS symptoms.

Acupuncture. There's good evidence that acupuncture can be beneficial for PMS, especially for pain associated with menstruation. Plus, it doesn't take that long to work—two or three treatments may show results. One study comparing acupuncture to a placebo treatment found a nearly 80 percent success rate in treating PMS symptoms with up to four acupuncture sessions, compared to 6 percent in the placebo group. Researchers suspect acupuncture affects levels of serotonin and opioids in the brain, chemicals that affect mood.

Massage therapy. Massage, particularly reflexology (massaging certain points on the feet, hands, or ears thought to correspond with other parts of the body) has been found to be particularly helpful in relieving symptoms of depression, anxiety, and pain in women with PMS compared to control groups. Try to get a regular massage twice a week for one menstrual cycle, or a reflexology treatment once a week for two cycles, and see if things improve.

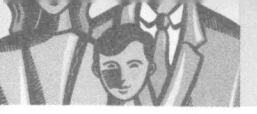

Prostate Enlargement

Prostate enlargement, or benign prostatic hypertrophy (BPH), will affect nearly every man over 50 at some point in his life. Because an enlarged prostate puts pressure on the urethra, the tube that travels from the kidney to the penis, the primary symptoms have to do with urination—being unable to urinate, urinating too much, retaining urine. The condition often co-exists with erectile dysfunction (see page 133).

It's important to see your doctor if you're having any urinary problems. While BPH is an annoying condition, it's not life threatening; but prostate cancer, which may have similar symptoms, is.

Do This Now

The following steps will help with some of the urinary problems you're probably experiencing.

1. Start taking 160 milligrams of a standardized extract of saw palmetto twice a day, or 320 milligrams once a day.

2. Practice deep breathing (breathe in deeply through your nose until your stomach expands, then breathe out through your mouth) when you're trying to urinate.

3. If this doesn't get the urine flow started, put your hand under warm running water.

4. If you're still having trouble urinating, ask your doctor for a prescription for Flomax (tamsulosin).

5. If you're urinating frequently at night, don't drink anything for at least four hours before you go to bed.

Why It Works

With more clinical trials and more use in clinical practice than any other natural remedy for prostate enlargement, saw palmetto is usually the first non-drug choice. This herb is thought to work by reducing levels of an enzyme required to convert testosterone to its more potent form, dihydrotestosterone, or DHT. This hormone stimulates prostate cell growth and is linked to both BPH and prostate cancer.

Studies find saw palmetto is just as effective as Proscar (finasteride), the most commonly prescribed drug for BPH. Unlike Proscar, it doesn't suppress levels of PSA (a blood chemical used as a marker for prostate cancer), so men can still get accurate prostate cancer screenings. Note that the benefits can take several months to fully kick in.

The deep breathing helps you relax, allowing the pelvic floor muscles to drop, which may help start the flow of urine. If not, the running water may do the trick.

Flomax and other alpha blockers cause blood vessels to relax and expand, enabling blood to pass through more easily. This, in turn, relaxes prostate and bladder neck muscles, making it easier to urinate. These drugs work faster than saw palmetto or Proscar. However, they may affect libido and your ability to have an erection.

❦ Helpful Hint

Lay Off the Cold Medicine

Certain medications, particularly decongestants and some antihistamines, may prevent the muscles in the prostate and bladder neck from relaxing enough to allow the free flow of urine.

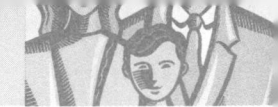

Other Medicines
Herbs and Supplements

You can take saw palmetto alone, but you may also see it combined with any of the following herbs in formulas designed for BPH.

African plum (*Pygeum africanum*). More than a dozen trials have been conducted on extracts from the bark of this tree. A review study found that men using the supplement were more than twice as likely to say their symptoms improved than those taking a placebo. Overall, African plum improved symptoms of frequent nighttime urination by 20 percent, and increased urinary flow by 23 percent. Supply may become a problem, however, since the bark is being overharvested. Take 75 to 200 milligrams a day. If you're taking a combination supplement, follow the label instructions.

Beta-sitosterol. This plant chemical mimics the structure of cholesterol. It and other plant sterols are often used to reduce the amount of cholesterol your body absorbs. There's some evidence that lowering cholesterol may reduce the activity of DHT and enzymes that stimulate the growth of prostate cells. One study of 75 men with BPH found that urinary symptoms significantly improved in those taking the supplement for nine weeks. Another study found it worked slightly better than Flomax. This is a particularly good supplement to take if you also have high cholesterol. Take 60 to 130 milligrams divided into two or three daily doses.

Nettle root. This herb has been used since ancient times to treat prostate conditions. It's thought to work by interfering with the activities of several hormones and reducing inflammation. One German study found those who took the herb had twice the improvement in symptoms after three months as those who took a placebo. Take 300 milligrams two or three times per day. Take the last dose with dinner, so you won't have to get up at night (nettle root is a diuretic).

Flower pollen. Several clinical trials have found the flower pollen product Cernitin has a benefit in treating BPH. It probably works by reducing the inflammation that leads to swelling in the prostate. Take two 63-milligram tablets three times a day. Give it at least 12 weeks to work.

Prescription Drugs

In addition to alpha blockers like Flomax, the other primary class of drugs prescribed for BPH are 5-alpha reductase inhibitors such as Proscar and Avodart (dutasteride). Like saw palmetto, they work by inhibiting the 5-alpha reductase enzyme. Unlike saw palmetto, however, there's some evidence they can reduce the size of the prostate gland. As noted earlier, they also reduce PSA levels, making it more difficult to screen for prostate cancer. They can also take several months to reach their full benefit. Sometimes doctors prescribe these drugs along with alpha blockers.

Other Approaches

Surgery. Transurethral resection of the prostate, or TURP, is the most common surgery for BPH. The surgeon cuts away excess parts of the prostate, reducing pressure on the urethra. The main risk is retrograde ejaculation, in which the ejaculate flows up the urethra instead of out.

Prevention

Eat less saturated fat and more antioxidants and fiber. There's good evidence that such a diet can reduce the risk of BPH and other prostate diseases, including cancer. In fact, diet is thought to be the primary reason for rates of prostate cancer in American men, which are up to 10 times those in Japanese men.

Exercise regularly. This significantly reduces the risk of BPH.

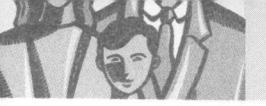

Uterine Fibroids

The good news about these noncancerous uterine tumors is that they usually go away after menopause (unless you take hormone replacement therapy). The bad news is that until then, the pain and heavy bleeding they cause can make your life miserable. Here we mainly discuss an integrative approach to removing or shrinking fibroids. See also Heavy Menstrual Bleeding (page 136) and Menstrual Cramps (page 151).

One study showed how powerful an integrative treatment approach can be. The study, conducted at the University of Pittsburgh, involved 74 women with fibroids. Twenty-seven received weekly Traditional Chinese Medicine (TCM), including herbal therapy, acupuncture, Chinese massage, and guided imagery for up to six months. The control group received conventional treatment, including hormones to stop excessive bleeding and nonsteroidal anti-inflammatories for pain.

The fibroids of 29 women in the TCM group either shrank, stopped growing, or grew more slowly, compared to those of 12 women in the conventional group. Three women in the TCM group reported a complete cure, compared to none in the control group. An added bonus: Women receiving TCM were more satisfied with their treatment.

Do This Now

For immediate pain relief, follow this sequence of actions. To treat the fibroid itself, talk with your doctor about which combination of treatment approaches, discussed later, is right for you.

1. Take 400 to 600 milligrams of ibuprofen every four hours. If you still have severe pain after two doses, add one or two 500-milligram doses of acetaminophen (Tylenol).

2. Put an ice pack on your abdomen.

3. Take 20 drops of shepherd's purse tincture two or three times a day during your period.

4. To relieve cramps and abdominal pain, take 1/2 teaspoon valerian tincture (a liquid) and 1/2 teaspoon cramp bark tincture every one to two hours.

5. Lie on your side with your legs drawn up into your abdomen or with a pillow under your legs to elevate them, especially if you have back pain along with your cramps.

Why It Works

Ibuprofen relieves pain and also reduces production of prostaglandins, hormone-like chemicals that contribute to inflammation and cramps. It also interferes with the production of progesterone, which contributes to heavy bleeding. The acetaminophen bumps up the pain relief, while the ice numbs the area and may slightly reduce bleeding.

Shepherd's purse is a traditional remedy used to slow menstrual bleeding. Although there aren't any studies on its use in fibroids, it does contain several flavonoids, plant chemicals that one small study suggests may help reduce heavy menstrual bleeding. Try it for two cycles; if it works, begin taking it on a daily basis two weeks before your period is due and continue until you stop bleeding. Use with caution if you have a history of kidney stones or vulvodynia (pain around the opening of the vagina) because this herb contains oxalates, salts that form kidney stones and con-

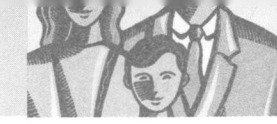

TALK TO YOUR DOCTOR

Three things to ask:

- Am I anemic? Heavy menstrual bleeding can lead to iron deficiency.
- Do I have a thyroid problem? Heavy bleeding may be related to hypothyroidism.
- Should I continue on hormone therapy? The additional hormones feed the fibroids so they keep growing.

tribute to vulvodynia. Also don't use if you are, or think you might become, pregnant.

Valerian and cramp bark are two herbs traditionally used to relieve abdominal cramps, whether menstrual or gastrointestinal.

Getting into the fetal position moves the position of the uterus so it doesn't press on the bundle of nerves at the front of the pelvis known as the sacral plexus.

Other Medicines
Herbs and Supplements

We don't have any studies to report on the following three herbs, but this regimen seems to work with patients who have fibroids.

Chaste tree berry. If your menstrual cycle is irregular, take chaste tree berry extract to help normalize estrogen levels and restore a regular cycle. Good brands are Agnucaston and Cyclodynon. (See Resources, page 365, for buying instructions.) Follow the dosage instructions on the label and take for at least three months.

Milk thistle. Also take a standardized extract of milk thistle, 175 milligrams two or three times a day. Milk thistle strengthens the liver, which breaks down estrogen for removal.

Yarrow. Put 1 tablespoon yarrow in a nonreactive pot and cover with 8 ounces boiling water. Simmer for 10 minutes, then remove from heat and steep for 15 minutes. Strain, allow to cool, then drink up to 3 cups per day. Don't make more than two days' worth at a time and rewarm before drinking.

Traditional Chinese Medicine. Several herbal formulas show good success in treating fibroids, either with or without conventional treatment. In one study, researchers treated 30 women with fibroids with the remedies Keishi-bukuryo-gan (KBG) and Shakuyaku-kanzo-to. More than 60 percent of the women who had fist-size fibroids found their heavy bleeding and painful periods improved, although women with larger fibroids experienced no benefit.

Another study, this one using Kuei-chih-fu-ling-wan in 110 women with fibroids, found heavy bleeding and painful periods improved in more than 90 percent of the women taking the herb, and fibroids shrank in about 60 percent.

Toki-shakuyaku is useful for women with mild anemia related to heavy menstrual bleeding from a fibroid because it improves iron levels without the side effects commonly seen with iron pills (nausea, constipation, dark tarry stools).

Flaxseed. Take 1 tablespoon a day of ground flaxseeds (mix them into a glass of water and drink, sprinkle them over cereal or yogurt, or add to muffin mix) or 1,000 milligrams flaxseed oil. This plant contains estrogen-like compounds that may block or modify the action of your own estrogen.

Fish oil supplements. Take 2,000 milligrams per day to reduce the inflammation that is often the cause of menstrual pain.

Prescription Drugs

Gonadotropin-releasing hormones (GnRH agonists). These drugs, Lupron (leuprolide), Synarel (nafarelin), and Zoladex (goserelin), signal your body to produce less estrogen and progesterone, effectively putting you into

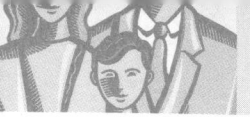

menopause. They shrink fibroids and reduce bleeding, and are often used before fibroid surgery. They're only prescribed for a few months, however, because of their menopausal side effects, including bone thinning. Once you stop taking them, the fibroids return. Studies find that adding progesterone while taking a GnRH agonist can minimize hot flashes.

Low-dose estrogen oral contraceptives. These don't seem to increase the size of fibroids and can be quite helpful in reducing bleeding.

Mifepristone. Although not approved for treating fibroids, this drug, also known as RU-486, or the "abortion pill," is showing promise as a treatment. One potential negative: There's some evidence it might cause an overgrowth of the endometrial lining.

Other Approaches

Surgical procedures. In addition to hysterectomy, surgical options include:

- **Myomectomy.** In this procedure, the fibroids are removed, leaving the uterus. Downside: The fibroids may return.

- **Endometrial ablation.** This minimally invasive procedure uses electrical energy, heat, or cold to destroy the lining of the uterus and may minimize or stop heavy bleeding associated with fibroids.

- **Uterine artery embolization.** One of the newest, nonsurgical methods of treating fibroids, this still-investigational procedure uses heat to destroy the blood supply to the arteries feeding the fibroids. The procedure is risky, however, with infection or massive bleeding possibly resulting.

- **Myolysis or cryomyolysis.** Also investigational, myolysis uses lasers, electric current, or, in the case of cryomyolysis, freezing to destroy fibroids during minimally invasive surgery.

Prevention

Although there is no known way to prevent fibroids, some studies suggest they may be related to certain lifestyles. We recommend that you:

Think Mediterranean. One study found that women with fibroids were more likely to eat diets high in red meat and ham, and lower in fruit, fish, and leafy green vegetables.

Decrease dietary estrogen. That includes animal protein and dairy, which may be high in hormones.

Bump up your fiber intake. Fiber increases the amount of estrogen cleared from your body. It also helps your body metabolize existing estrogen into less potent forms.

Start eating soy. Plantlike estrogens in soy can block the actions of your own estrogen on cells.

Keep off extra weight. Every 20 pounds of excess weight increases your risk of fibroids 20 percent, possibly because fat cells not only store hormones but also manufacture estrogen.

Use oral contraceptives for birth control. The longer you've used them, the lower your risk of fibroids. You might also want to skip an IUD: One study found women who had infections related to IUD use were more likely to have a fibroid.

Practice safe sex. One study found a significantly increased risk of fibroids in women who had pelvic inflammatory disease (an infection resulting from sexually transmitted diseases) or chlamydia.

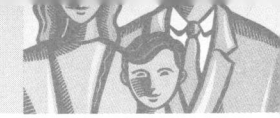

Vaginal Pain

There are several types of vaginal pain. There's pain due to atrophic vaginitis—thinning of the vaginal lining—which is typically related to low levels of estrogen and most common during menopause. There's also pain due to vaginal scarring after trauma or childbirth, which is fairly rare.

Then there's the most common cause of vaginal pain, vulvodynia, or vulvar vestibulitis syndrome (VVS), a type of vulvodynia. These conditions involve pain at the opening of the vagina and in the vulva, the various tissue and organs outside the vagina. We don't know what causes vulvodynia, although we know it is often associated with vaginismus, in which the muscles at the opening of the vagina go into spasm, usually during intercourse.

There is little available in terms of conventional medicine to treat these conditions (except topical or vaginal estrogen for atrophic vaginitis due to menopause), but they do respond quite well to nonmedical approaches such as biofeedback. Having said that, you should still undergo a comprehensive medical examination. Many other conditions, including endometriosis, sexually transmitted diseases, skin problems, and infections can cause similar pain, and some medications can contribute to vaginal dryness, resulting in painful intercourse.

Do This Now

Try these self-care measures for fast relief. For longer-term treatments, see our suggestions in the rest of this entry.

1. Light an aromatherapy candle or essential oil burner to fill the room with a relaxing scent like lavender, clary sage, or geranium. Then take a deep breath and practice several minutes of deep breathing or progressive muscle relaxation (see pages 60-61 for instructions).

2. If you have atrophic vaginitis, rub a water-based herbal cream containing wild yam, chamomile, or calendula on the affected area. The creams are available in health food stores or online.

3. Apply a cold compress or ice to the vulva for 10 minutes at a time. Wrap the ice in a thin towel to avoid freezing the skin.

4. Fill a peri bottle (a 6- to 8- ounce plastic bottle with a spray spout on the top) with tap water and several drops each of lavender, rosemary, and tea tree oils. Shake, then squirt on the painful vaginal area in between ice treatments, and especially after urinating or intercourse.

5. Use a water-based vaginal lubricant, such as K-Y jelly, Vagisil Intimate Moisturizer, or Replens Vaginal Moisturizer, during sex.

Why It Works

Remember the mind-body connection? Deep breathing and other relaxation techniques not only take your focus off the discomfort, but also help relax clenched muscles that may be contributing to the pain. Inhaling a soothing aromatherapy scent like lavender, shown to exert a relaxing effect, can enhance the results.

During menopause, vaginal tissue becomes thin and easily irritated. These creams are soothing and help heal and prevent tears or irritation.

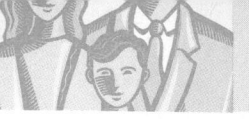

The cold compresses or ice cool the burning many women say they feel with vulvar pain. The spray is soothing thanks to the lavender, and also has anti-inflammatory properties and antibacterial properties to help fight off infection.

If vaginal dryness contributes to pain during intercourse, a lubricant will help.

Other Medicines
Over-the-Counter Drugs

Yeast infection treatment (like Monistat). Infections can cause irritation of the vulva. Use a cream or suppository if you suspect a yeast infection might be behind your pain or itching.

Cortisone cream (1/2 percent). Use this for vaginal itching without discharge.

Prescription Drugs

Lidocaine ointment. Try this painkilling cream at night. You may feel some burning initially, but that fades quickly as the cream numbs the vulva. While the cream doesn't address any underlying cause of vulvar pain, in one small study in which 61 women used the cream nightly for seven weeks, 76 percent said they could have intercourse after treatment, compared with 36 percent before the treatment.

Tricyclic antidepressants. Low doses of these drugs, particularly Elavil (amitriptyline) and Norpramin (desipramine), are often used to treat nerve-related pain and are a first-line medical treatment for vulvodynia. Ask your doctor if you can start on Norpramin first; it has fewer side effects than Elavil.

Antiseizure medication. Although it's not approved expressly for this purpose, the antiseizure medication Neurontin (gabapentin) is sometimes used for women who don't respond to antidepressants. But it can be very sedating, so use it with caution.

Interferon alfa. This anti-inflammatory immune system substance is injected into the vulvar vestibule, the folds around the vagina, three times a week for four weeks. Studies find some benefits in some women. This is not an easy treatment, however; it's painful, produces flulike side effects, and may take up to a year before you see significant improvement.

Other Approaches

Diet. Cut out seeds, nuts, leafy plants like spinach and other dark greens, chocolate, and tea. These foods contain high amounts of oxalic acid, which tends to bond with minerals in the body, forming oxylate salts. While researchers don't think oxalates cause vulvar pain syndrome, they suspect the salts may irritate the vulva and vagina when levels are high in urine.

Calcium. Take two tablets of calcium citrate (such as Citracal) three times a day to neutralize oxalates in the urine, and drink lots of water. If you're still feeling pain, try adding Ox-Absorb, a nutritional supplement available in drugstores and online, which absorbs oxalates in the digestive tract. Only take it with your doctor's supervision, however, as it may cause some nutritional deficiencies. Take as directed.

Sitz bath with Aveeno oatmeal. If you have bothersome itching along with pain, mix 1/2 cup of the oatmeal into a small amount of warm water and soak.

Kegels. A couple of small studies find that strengthening the pelvic floor muscles can help alleviate vaginal pain. See our description of Kegels in Incontinence, Urinary (page 110). Perform 10 repetitions at least twice a day.

Surgery. In severe cases, doctors may remove the vulvar vestibule in women with VVS, even areas that aren't painful. However, the pain can return in some women, few surgeons are experi-

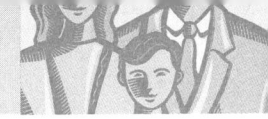

Exercising Without Pain

Severe vulvar pain may make exercise difficult. If that happens, try riding a recumbent bicycle (on which you lean back as you pedal, taking pressure off the genital area), or swimming. You don't want to give up all physical activity, because regular exercise contributes to a healthy sense of appreciation for your body and improves mood and relaxation, all of which can help when you're coping with chronic pain.

enced in this procedure, and the procedure itself is quite painful.

Biofeedback. Biofeedback may help with involuntary muscle contraction and improve the effectiveness of Kegel exercises. One study in women with vulvar vestibulitis who also suffered from painful intercourse found that 12 weeks of biofeedback worked just as well as 12 weeks of cognitive-behavioral therapy or surgery to improve the condition. Another study found that after 16 weeks of biofeedback, 83 percent of the 33 women in the study had less pain and were able to resume intercourse, with the benefits lasting at least six months.

Cognitive-behavioral therapy. As noted above, cognitive-behavioral therapy—a type of psychotherapy that helps you change detrimental thinking patterns and learn how to better handle situations that trigger negative reactions and contribute to the physical problem—can be as effective as surgery. Sometimes, sexual counseling for both partners might be required.

Prevention

Because we don't know what causes vulvodynia, we really don't know how to prevent it. The following are approaches that have helped individual patients or have been reported helpful in the medical literature.

Check your environment for irritants. If your symptoms are intermittent, think about what you're exposing that area to. Are you using a lubricant during intercourse? Have you switched laundry soap? Are symptoms worse when you wear a certain kind of underwear, or use a certain brand of sanitary pad? Try changing one thing at a time and see if it helps. If you do use lubricants to help with intercourse, stick to high-quality, water-soluble brands like Aqua-Lube, Astroglide, or K-Y jelly.

Consider probiotic supplements. If you're prone to recurrent yeast or nonspecific vaginal infections, try probiotics. Start with 2 capsules with each meal. At night, mix the powder in two capsules with a small amount of plain yogurt and use a medicine syringe to insert into the vagina.

Try cutting out gluten. There is one case report of vulvodynia associated with celiac disease, an allergy to gluten, a protein found in wheat products. If you suspect this might be your problem, try eliminating all gluten products (*Warning:* This is much easier said than done) and see if your pain improves.

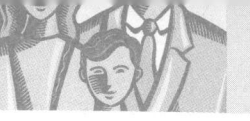

Yeast Infection

With over-the-counter remedies readily available, yeast infections (caused by an overgrowth of fungi) have gotten more convenient to deal with. Just make sure that a yeast infection is really your problem before treating it. A visit to your doctor is in order if this is your first occurrence. Aside from yeast infection, your symptoms could result from a different type of infection, such as bacterial vaginosis (BV) or the sexually transmitted disease trichomoniasis.

In most instances, the symptoms and treatment of yeast infection and BV are the same (you will definitely need prescription medication for trichomoniasis).

One way to preventing recurrent yeast infections is to strengthen your immune system, so revisit Part 2 for tips on how to do it.

Do This Now

To soothe the discomfort of a yeast infection or bacterial vaginosis, follow these steps.

1. If you have a yeast infection, begin using an over-the-counter antifungal treatment like Gyne-Lotrimin (clotrimazole), Monistat (miconazole), or Terazol (terconazole). If you have BV, skip this step; instead, get a prescription for antibiotics from your doctor.

2. Sit in a warm sitz bath (a basin of warm water or shallow bath) to which you've added 15 drops of one or more of these oils: chamomile, lavender, tea tree, and thyme essential oils. Other options to add to the sitz bath instead of the oils are 1/2 cup oatmeal or Domeboro, an over-the-counter soothing powder. Dissolve one packet in 16 ounces of water.

TIME TO WORRY

- If you have more than three to five yeast infections a year, you may have diabetes.
- If you have fever, a foul-smelling discharge, or severe pain associated with vaginitis, this could signify a serious infection that may lead to pelvic inflammatory disease (PID).
- If you have discharge and a fine red rash, especially if you are having your period, this could signify toxic shock syndrome.

3. If you don't like sitz baths, make a compress. Soak a soft cloth in a bowl of cool water with 10 drops of any of the essential oils named above or the Domeboro solution and press against the vaginal area.

4. Insert 2 capsules of lactobacillus (probiotics) into the vagina with each meal and two at bedtime (you can find gelatin capsules or uncoated tablets that dissolve in vaginal fluids). Another option is to mix the powder in 2 capsules with a small amount of plain yogurt and use an applicator or medicine syringe to insert in the vagina.

5. Keep a peri bottle, a 6- to 8-ounce plastic bottle with a spray spout on the top, filled with tap water and 10 drops of lavender essential oil. Shake, then squirt on your vaginal area after using the bathroom or having intercourse.

Why It Works

All over-the-counter yeast infection preparations work about equally well. Studies find that they cure about 80 percent of infections.

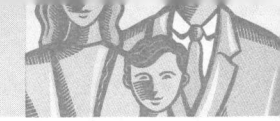

The sitz baths and compresses help relieve the itching.

The probiotics and yogurt contain live bacteria, which help relieve infections by restoring normal bacterial levels in the vagina.

We want you to use the peri bottle to keep the vaginal area clean, which helps clear the infection quicker.

Other Medicines
Over-the-Counter Drugs

Boric acid gelatin capsules. Available in drugstores, these capsules are inserted into the vagina. Several large studies find they're very effective at clearing up yeast infections, even in women who already tried antifungal medications.

Prescription Drugs

Oral medications. If your infection doesn't clear up with over-the-counter treatments, your doctor may prescribe stronger drugs, such as Diflucan (fluconazole) or Nizoral (ketoconazole).

Other Approaches

Tea tree oil. Put 1 drop tea tree oil in 19 drops of a carrier oil like almond oil. Test on a small patch of skin to make sure you're not allergic or sensitive. If there's no reaction in several hours, apply to the external vaginal area several times a day. Stop if any irritation develops. In health food stores you may also be able to find tea tree capsules you can insert into the vagina. Studies find tea tree oil is an excellent antibacterial and antifungal therapy.

Prevention

Continue your probiotics at night. After your yeast infection clears, continue with the nighttime dose of lactobacillus for weeks or even months to prevent a recurrence. Begin taking probiotics during the day again if your risk of an infection increases (e.g., you're using antibiotics).

Try AciGel. This prescription medication is inserted into the vagina daily at bedtime for several weeks after a vaginal infection clears to prevent a relapse. Also use at least a week before those times during which you're prone to infection (if you get them during your period, for instance). A form of vinegar, AciGel makes the vagina more acidic, preventing overgrowth of yeast.

Eat more fiber and fewer simple carbs. One study found that women with recurrent yeast infections have subtle abnormalities in their ability to use insulin, the hormone that enables your cells to turn glucose into energy. So avoid simple carbohydrates like crackers, cookies, and chips, and stick with high-fiber foods like vegetables, legumes, and whole grains.

Eat yogurt with active cultures every day. They contain beneficial bacteria that help prevent yeast infections.

Wear cotton underwear and loose clothing. They help keep the vaginal area dry and cool.

Cut out or decrease oral sex. It may make you more likely to have recurrent yeast infections. Also have your partner checked for any transmissible infections if you're not using condoms.

Ask your doctor for an oral antifungal drug when you need to take antibiotics.

✌ What About...

Douching?

We don't recommend it. Douching strips out everything in the vagina—the good bacteria as well as the bad, and increases the risk of complications from vaginal infections, including pelvic inflammatory disease (PID), endometriosis, and tubal pregnancy.

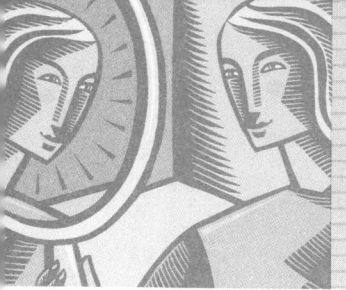

Bad Breath

Your teeth and gums provide wonderful hiding places for bacteria, where they multiply, creating sulfur compounds and nitrogen gases that, well, stink. Add postnasal drip from a cold or allergies, which deposits more bacteria on the back of the tongue, and you can understand why breath is sometimes less than sweet.

A dry mouth can also lead to odor, since saliva is your body's natural mouthwash. So also see the Dry Mouth entry on page 174.

Do This Now

To quickly get rid of bad breath, try any one of these steps.

1. If you have access to a toothbrush, brush your teeth and floss.

2. Dip your toothbrush in mouthwash and stroke your tongue from the back to the front.

3. Chew on parsley or a few fennel seeds.

4. Chew a piece of sugarless gum with xylitol.

Why It Works

Brushing your teeth and tongue dislodges the bacteria that create bad breath and temporarily adds the fresh scent of toothpaste and mouthwash.

Parsley is high in chlorophyll, a natural breath freshener, so start chewing those sprigs on your plate. Fennel seeds, often provided at Indian restaurants, are also natural breath fresheners. In addition to improving digestion, they keep bad breath in check until you can brush.

Xylitol, a food additive, kills bacteria that can lead to bad breath. Plus, as you chew, you create saliva, which also helps freshen breath.

Other Medicines
Herbs and Supplements

Chlorophyll tablets. The substance that lends plants their green color is a natural deodorizer and breath freshener. You can find chlorophyll tablets at pharmacies and health food stores.

Ginger tea or peppermint tea. Both lend a fresh scent to your mouth and can help soothe breath-souring indigestion. Sip a cup after eating, and keep a pitcher of iced tea in the fridge.

Digestive enzymes like Beano and others help break up gas-forming foods, reducing breath-souring indigestion.

Prevention

Brush your teeth twice a day with toothpaste that contains tea tree oil, mint, or baking soda.

Floss every day.

Skip odor-producing foods such as garlic, onions, broccoli, canned tuna, and strong spices.

After meals, gargle with a glassful of water with 1 to 3 drops tea tree oil (a natural antibacterial) to remove food and other debris from your mouth as well as kill bacteria.

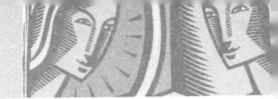

Canker Sores

These small mouth sores can surface anywhere in your mouth, like painful minefields. Hormone fluctuations, trauma (such as biting your tongue or cheek), nutritional deficiencies, stress, as well some inflammatory diseases may trigger flare-ups, although we don't know what causes them. They may even be triggered by viruses.

You can take a minimalist approach—do nothing and the sores will disappear on their own within 10 to 14 days. Or you can take a more active approach with these remedies.

Do This Now

To ease pain and speed healing, take these steps.

1. Mix 1 teaspoon Benadryl liquid (found in the children's section of the drugstore) with 1 teaspoon milk of magnesia, swish it in your mouth for one minute, then spit out. Repeat four to six times a day.

2. Mix a painkilling gel (such as Anbesol) with deglycyrrhizinated licorice powder, available in natural food stores. Apply to the sore hourly while you're awake.

3. If that doesn't help, also take 400 to 600 milligrams ibuprofen.

Why It Works

The anti-inflammatory benefits of Benadryl help speed healing, while the milk of magnesia coats the sore and neutralizes acid in the mouth, helping reduce pain. Don't eat or drink anything for a half-hour after this treatment.

We recommend licorice powder for its wound-healing properties. One Indian study found it healed canker sores within three days. The powder doesn't numb the pain, however, which is why we suggest mixing it with Anbesol. The gel also helps the powder stick to the sore.

Although it won't make the sore go away any faster, the ibuprofen does help with pain.

Other Medicines
Herbs and Supplements

Zinc lozenges. Sucking on a zinc lozenge four to six times a day may help tame any virus associated with the sore and minimize pain.

Prescription Drugs

Kenalog (triamcinolone 0.1%). Applying this anti-inflammatory cream two to four times a day coats the canker sore, speeding healing.

Prevention

Take a daily multivitamin. Low levels of certain nutrients may trigger outbreaks.

Take 25 to 50 milligrams of zinc daily. Studies suggest zinc may help prevent canker sores. Take in addition to the multivitamin.

Eliminate gluten and dairy. A wheat or dairy allergy may contribute to outbreaks. Try cutting out gluten (a component of wheat). If that doesn't work, add it back and try eliminating dairy.

Learn to relax. One study found a hypnosis-like relaxation program decreased the frequency of canker sore outbreaks. For more on relaxation techniques, see Part 2.

Change your toothpaste. Avoid brands that contain sodium laurel sulfate.

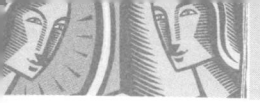
Cold Sores

There's nothing worse than a painful cold sore, which always seems to appear just when you least want one. Cold sores are caused by a herpes simplex virus similar to the virus that causes genital herpes. It hides out in the nerves and becomes active as a result of stress, overexposure to sunlight, or hormonal changes, or when your immune system is weak.

You usually get a warning of a cold sore—tingling, discomfort, itching, or aching. This is when we want you to begin using the remedies described here. Don't wait until a blister erupts; by then, it's often too late.

Do This Now

To reduce the duration and severity of an outbreak, follow this advice at the first tingling.

1. Apply a damp black tea bag to the area where the outbreak typically occurs. Keep it on for 10 minutes. Repeat three or four times a day.

2. Next, apply an ice pack to the same area. Keep the ice on for 15 minutes, and repeat three or four times a day.

3. After each ice application, thickly apply lemon balm ointment (70:1 concentration) to the area. Lemon balm is sold in health food stores and online under the brand name Cold Sore Relief.

4. Now take 1 gram lysine along with 1,000 milligrams vitamin C that also contains 1,000 milligrams of flavonoids. Take up to five times a day until the recurrence ends.

5. Also take a baby aspirin (83 milligrams) once a day with food.

❦ Helpful Hint

Stop the Spread

Wash your hands after applying anything to your cold sore so you don't spread the virus to your nose or eyes or to other people.

Why It Works

Tea bags contain tannic acid, an astringent that has antiviral properties (which is why tannic acid is often an ingredient in over-the-counter cold sore remedies). Ice numbs the pain, and there's some evidence it may also reduce the amount of virus created.

Test tube studies suggest that lemon balm (*Melissa officinalis*) prevents the virus from attaching to cells, thus blocking its ability to replicate. One well-designed study of 116 people with oral or genital herpes found those treated with the balm recovered much quicker than those receiving a placebo. Plus, there's some evidence that using lemon balm during the initial outbreak (the very first time you realize you have a cold sore) may reduce the risk of recurrence.

Lysine is an amino acid that works as an antiviral by blocking the activity of another amino acid, arginine. Arginine provides "food" for the virus, enabling it to replicate. Cutting off this fuel source reduces the amount of virus in your system. One study of 53 people with oral and genital herpes found those who received lysine supplements and cut out arginine-rich foods had an average of 3.1 outbreaks over six months, compared to an average of 4.2 in the control group.

Take lysine only until the outbreak fades (unless you have frequent outbreaks, in which

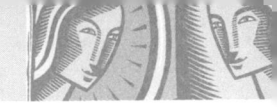

case, see the advice under "Prevention"). Then, to prevent another outbreak, increase the amount of lysine-rich foods (cheese, eggs, chicken, milk, lima beans, fish, potatoes, brewer's yeast, and soy) and decrease the amount of arginine-rich foods (nuts, chocolate, raisins, and gelatin) in your diet.

The aspirin helps relieves the pain of a cold sore and may also reduce healing time. One small study found participants who took an aspirin at the first sign of an outbreak, then continued taking it for several months, had far fewer outbreaks than a control group that didn't take aspirin.

Other Medicines
Herbs and Supplements

Quercetin. Take 500 milligrams twice a day of this flavonoid, which laboratory studies find blocks cold sore viruses from replicating.

Over-the-Counter Drugs

Aloe vera cream or extract 0.05% strength. Apply three times a day for five days during outbreaks. Studies find it reduces healing time.

Zinc. Apply a topical zinc sulfate cream (0.01% to 0.025%) several times a day. This helps heal the sore and reduces the risk of a recurrence.

Abreva (docosanol). This is the only over-the-counter, FDA-approved treatment for cold sores, with studies finding it can clear an infection quicker than using nothing. It works by changing the membrane of skin cells, blocking access by the virus.

Prescription Drugs

Denavir (penciclovir). This is the only prescription-strength topical treatment found to be effective, with studies showing it helps cold sores heal about a day faster than placebo.

Oral antivirals. As with genital herpes, you can take an oral antiviral such as Zovirax (acyclovir), Famvir (famciclovir), or Valtrex (valacyclovir) at the first sign of an outbreak to prevent the virus from replicating.

Other Approaches

Aromatherapy. Dilute 1 drop lavender, lemon balm, chamomile, bergamot, or rose oil in 10 drops jojoba oil (which serves as a carrier oil) and smooth over the affected area several times a day.

Prevention

Avoid triggers. Two primary ones are a weak immune system and stress. Review Part 2 for our advice on handling stress and maintaining a strong immune system. Also avoid overexposure to sunlight and any trauma to the skin around the mouth, such as rough kissing.

Follow a high-lysine/low-arginine diet. (See details above.) Also add seaweed salads, sushi, or green drinks containing seaweed extracts (available in health food stores). Laboratory studies find that seaweed has antiviral properties.

Zinc. Take 25 milligrams of zinc by mouth every day. Zinc enhances immunity, helping to prevent cold sore recurrences.

Selenium. Take 200 micrograms a day to help maintain a healthy immune system.

Lysine. If you have frequent recurrences of cold sores, take 1 gram a day to prevent outbreaks, but don't take if you have high cholesterol, because long-term use can increase levels of "bad" LDL cholesterol.

Sunblock. Wear a high-SPF sunblock on your face, and apply zinc oxide to areas prone to cold sores.

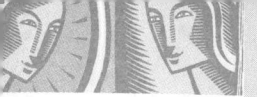

Conjunctivitis

More commonly known as pinkeye, this red, itchy, crusty eye condition stems from inflammation of the conjunctiva, the membrane that covers the white part of the eye and lines the inner eyelids. It can be caused by viruses or, less commonly, bacteria, or by seasonal allergies. If you have the infectious type, don't relax just because it's only in one eye; it will likely spread to the other eye. If allergies are to blame, you probably have it in both eyes simultaneously. (An oral antihistamine and/or antihistamine eye drops are your best bets in this case.)

Do This Now

Viral pinkeye will go away on its own, but to relieve the discomfort and crustiness, follow these steps.

1. Take out your contact lenses, if you wear them, and clean them thoroughly.

2. Buy a commercial eyewash and add 1/4 teaspoon raw honey. If you don't have eyewash, put 3 tablespoons honey in 2 cups boiling water, stir to dissolve, and let it cool. Dip a makeup remover pad into the mixture and use it to wash the crust and pus from your eyes, using a different pad for each eye. Repeat several times a day.

3. Place a warm, wet black or chamomile tea bag over your infected eye for five minutes, followed by a cool, wet tea bag for two minutes. Repeat several times a day with a fresh tea bag.

4. Throw away any eye makeup you've been using and don't wear eye makeup again until the pinkeye disappears.

Why It Works

Removing your contacts allows your eye to heal faster and prevents reinfection (as does throwing away your eye makeup).

Studies show that applying raw honey to the eyes reduces the swelling, pus, and redness. Make sure you use raw honey; pasteurization destroys honey's antibiotic properties. (Even though the honey hasn't been sterilized, its very high sugar content prevents bacteria from surviving in it.)

The tannins in the tea bags help reduce swelling. Alternating hot and cold allows the area to be pumped out to help remove toxins and cellular debris without too much swelling.

Other Medicines

Pink Eye Relief. These homeopathic drops contain eyebright (traditionally believed to combat pinkeye) and belladonna, an anti-inflammatory. Apply 2 to 3 drops in each eye as needed.

Antibiotic ointment or drops. If symptoms drag on for 6 to 10 days, these may be advisable.

Prevention

Wash your hands several times a day.

Thoroughly clean your contact lenses before wearing to prevent spread of the infection to the other eye. Better yet, switch to glasses.

Don't share towels, eye drops, tissues, eye makeup, washcloths, or pillowcases with family members who have pinkeye.

Launder sheets, pillowcases, and towels of infected family members in hot water separately from those of the rest of the family.

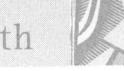

Dry Eyes

Tears aren't just for crying. They also remove dirt, microbes, and other debris from the surface of your eyes, as well as lubricate your eyes. As you age, however, your tears evaporate more easily, and you produce fewer of them.

Dry eyes can also be caused by drugs like blood pressure medications, antidepressants, heart medications, antihistamines, decongestants, muscle relaxants, and sleeping pills, as well as conditions like allergies, diabetes, and Parkinson's disease.

Do This Now

To relieve dryness and irritation, do the following.

1. Remove your contact lenses if you wear them.

2. Rinse your eyes with water.

3. Place a few drops of artificial tears in each eye.

4. Before you go to bed, use an eye ointment with paraffin such as Lacri-Lube.

Why It Works

Contact lenses are drying, so removing them helps. Rinsing your eyes removes any dirt or other irritants. Artificial tears are just what their name implies. At first, use the drops every half-hour until you feel better; then just once or twice a day as needed. Look for preservative-free brands, which are less irritating.

You may not realize that you don't make tears while you're sleeping (the gunk you rub from your eyes in the morning is a clue). The eye ointment, which is thicker than artificial tears, protects your eyes while you sleep. Because it blurs your vision, it's not suitable for daytime use.

Other Medicines

Fish and flaxseed oil. One reason for dry eyes is inflammation on the surface of the eye that may decrease tear production. Fish and flaxseed oil contain anti-inflammatory omega-3 fatty acids. They may also boost the oil content of your tears, allowing them to more effectively coat your eyes. Take 2 to 3 grams fish oil and 1 tablespoon flaxseed oil daily.

Restasis (cyclosporine ophthalmic emulsion 0.05%). These drops suppress inflammation on the eye's surface, increasing tear production. Place one drop in each eye every morning and night.

Other Approaches

Punctal plugs. These tiny plugs are placed in the opening through which tears drain, preventing tears from escaping. Ask your ophthalmologist about starting with dissolvable, temporary collagen plugs; some people don't like the plugs because their eyes become *too* moist. Once you have the permanent plugs, they can't be removed.

Acupuncture. Although we don't know why it works, numerous studies find acupuncture can increase eye moisture.

Prevention

Blink frequently, especially when watching television or working at the computer.

Drink 8 to 10 glasses of water a day.

Run a humidifier in your house, particularly in the winter.

Wear glasses, not contacts. If you must wear contacts, remove them daily.

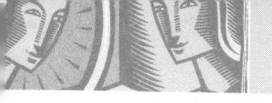

Dry Mouth

Dry mouth can be caused by something as simple as mouth breathing or medications—or as serious as diabetes, Sjögren's syndrome, or cancer. It's often a side effect of cancer treatment, particularly radiation to the head and neck.

Not only is dry mouth uncomfortable, it can cause dental problems, including cavities and mouth sores. It can also interfere with your ability to absorb nutrients from food.

Do This Now

When your mouth feels like the Sahara, follow these four steps.

1. Take small sips of a low-sugar drink (water is ideal). Avoid very hot or very cold beverages.

2. Chew sugarless gum or suck on a piece of sugar-free candy.

3. If your mouth is still dry, suck on a lemon slice.

4. If you still can't work up a good mouthful of saliva, use an over-the-counter saliva substitute like the gel Biotene Oral Balance, Oasis (discs that slowly dissolve in your mouth), or MEDOral Dry Mouth Treatment (a spray).

Why It Works

Drinking is the first step. Stay away from extreme temperatures because they can irritate mouth tissue that's sensitive because of the dryness.

Chewing gum, sucking on a piece of hard candy, or sucking on something sour triggers the salivary glands to release more saliva. Stick to sugarless because sugared gum or candy can increase your already increased risk of cavities.

Over-the-counter saliva substitutes work in various ways. Some release chemicals that lubricate the mouth, some rewet the mouth, while others contain enzymes that maintain moisture. If the first one you try doesn't work, try another.

Other Medicines
Herbs and Supplements

Slippery elm lozenges or tea. Slippery elm soothes and coats the mouth. Some brands of lozenges also contain apple pectin, which also helps coat the mouth. To make the tea, pour 6 to 8 ounces of boiling water over 1 tablespoon of the herb and steep until cool. Strain, and sip.

Prescription Drugs

Salagen (pilocarpine hydrochloride). This drug is the primary treatment for people with severe dry mouth. It works on the parasympathetic nervous system, which controls involuntary movements like breathing, heartbeat, and saliva release. It may take weeks to begin working, so be patient. Major side effect: sweating.

Prevention

Avoid salty or spicy foods. Both of them soak up saliva.

Cut down on caffeine and alcohol, which are drying. Also avoid mouthwashes that contain alcohol or peroxide.

Run a humidifier near your bed at night.

Stop your snoring. If you're a mouth breather at night (and you'll know if your partner says you snore), check out the Snoring entry on page 90.

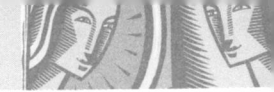

Ear Infection

This probably won't soothe your frayed nerves after you've been up all night with a screaming child, but we'll tell you anyway: Ear infections are extremely common, striking three out of four children at least once before age three. They develop when the same viruses or bacteria that triggered your child's runny nose migrate up the tube that connects the nose to the ear (most infections are actually caused by viruses). When the tube (or the adenoids at its base) swells, it traps fluid in the inner ear, causing pressure and pain and enabling an infection to fester.

Here's the good news: Most children outgrow ear infections by age three, when the eustachian tubes become large enough and the adenoids small enough to keep infections in check.

How can you tell whether your child has an ear infection? Look for tugging at the ears, a piercing cry (especially when lying down, which intensifies the pain), and balance and hearing difficulty.

Now for the not-so-good news: Older children and adults can still get ear infections, although they're far less common. They can be very painful and are more likely to require antibiotic treatment. If you have an ear infection, you may also have a sinus infection (see page 88) or a cold (see page 82).

Do This Now

Most ear infections resolve on their own without antibiotics. Meanwhile, to reduce the pain, whether it's you or your child with the ear infection, take these steps.

1. Take 500 to 1,000 milligrams (follow the package directions based on your child's age) of acetaminophen (Tylenol).

2. Following the package directions, take the recommended dose of homeopathic earache tablets by Boiron, Hyland, or Source Natural every 15 minutes for the first hour and then less frequently during the first 24 hours until the pain resolves. If there is no response within 24 hours or the pain worsens, see your doctor.

3. Apply a warm compress (a washcloth dipped in hot water and then wrung out, or a hot water bottle wrapped in a thin towel) to the ear.

4. Blow up a balloon (don't have a child do this unless he's more than six).

Why It Works

The Tylenol and the warm compress ease the pain immediately, while the homeopathic ear preparations relieve pain and speed healing through a combination of ingredients.

Blowing up a balloon opens the eustachian tubes, allowing fluid to drain from the ears, speeding healing, restoring hearing, and reducing discomfort. If you're having your child do this, however, make sure you watch carefully; children have been known to suck balloons into their windpipes.

Other Medicines
Herbs and Supplements

Otikon Otic Solution. These drops contain several antibiotic and antiviral herbs, including garlic, mullein, calendula, and St. John's wort, in an olive oil base. Studies show this combination of herbs can work just as effectively as anesthetic ear drops to relieve pain. Before using it, however,

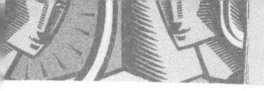

consult your pediatrician to make sure your child's eardrum is intact. If it's broken, anything you put in the outer ear can go directly into the middle ear, possibly damaging the small bones that vibrate as part of the hearing process, affecting hearing.

Prescription Drugs

Antibiotics. Doctors used to prescribe antibiotics routinely to treat ear infections. Because many ear infections clear up on their own and because some are caused by viruses that don't respond to antibiotics, however, the American Academy of Pediatrics and the American Academy of Family Physicians now recommend watchful waiting—not offering antibiotics for 2 to 3 days to see if the infection clears up on its own. If your doctor feels antibiotics are needed, he or she will probably prescribe high doses of amoxicillin, taken twice a day for 5 to 10 days. Make sure you complete the entire course, even if you start to feel better. Otherwise the germs may strike again.

Other Approaches

Allergy testing. Numerous studies have linked food allergies with an increased incidence of ear infections. In one study of 25 children with chronic ear infections, the infections improved for all but three children when their parents eliminated eggs and milk, common food allergens, from their children's diets. When parents reintroduced these foods, the infections returned. Other common trigger foods include beans, citrus, and tomatoes. See an allergist, who can use a skin prick test or blood test to help determine whether your child has food allergies. (Skin tests for food allergies tend to work better in children than in adults.)

☙ Helpful Hint

Probiotics

Use these tablets, sold at most health food stores, in conjunction with antibiotics. Antibiotics reduce amounts of all bacteria in the body—friendly or otherwise—allowing unfriendly organisms such as yeast to get a foothold, causing diarrhea and other side effects. Probiotic preparations contain healthful bacteria, alleviating these side effects. Follow package instructions for your child's age. For adults, take 1 or 2 tablets with each meal and at bedtime while you're taking an antibiotic.

Ear tube surgery. If your child suffers chronic ear infections that don't respond to antibiotics, this procedure (called myringotomy) might help. A surgeon places a small tube through an opening in your child's eardrum, relieving pressure, restoring hearing, and allowing fluid to drain more easily. After a few months, the tubes fall out. Because the operation requires anesthesia, only consider ear tubes if fluid has remained in your child's ears for several months, triggering recurrent ear infections and hearing difficulty.

Adenoidectomy. Surgical removal of the adenoids at the base of the eustachian tubes may help children between ages four and eight who suffer recurrent ear infections. It's not worth considering this surgery for children younger than four, however, many of whom outgrow the infections when their adenoids shrink.

Osteopathic manipulation. An osteopathic physician can gently massage your child's face and head, opening up ear passages and allowing fluid to drain more easily. In a study of 57 children with recurrent ear infections, osteopathic treatment significantly reduced the need for antibiotics and surgical procedures compared to children who received routine pediatric care. It also improved the health of the inner ear. Look for an osteopath who is trained in and uses the Galbreath technique, the manipulation used for ear problems.

Prevention

Breast-feed your baby. Breast milk contains protective compounds that keep bacteria in check. The sucking action also keeps your baby's eustachian tubes open.

Vaccinate your children against the flu. In one study, the flu vaccine reduced the incidence of ear infections in children by 30 percent during flu season.

Add plums, strawberries, and raspberries to your, and your child's, diet. These fruits contain xylitol, a natural sweetener used in many chewing gums, which, studies find, stems recurrent ear infections by preventing viruses and bacteria from migrating up the nose.

Don't smoke around your children. Studies show that children who live in houses with smokers are more likely to have ear infections than children who live in smoke-free homes.

Try a daily teaspoon of fish oil. In a small study of eight children who suffered chronic ear infections, 1 daily teaspoon of fish oil cut the need for antibiotics by 12 percent. You can use fish oil supplements as directed for your child's age.

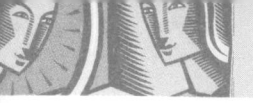

Glaucoma

Glaucoma is one of the leading causes of blindness. Most frightening about the condition is that you rarely have any symptoms until the disease is already fairly advanced. Although there are several forms of glaucoma, the most common is open-angle, in which the eye's drainage canals become clogged and fluid builds up within the eye, creating pressure and eventually damaging the optic nerve.

This pressure is called intraocular pressure (IOP), and most treatments focus on lowering it. Other treatments aim to strengthen the eye's collagen, a protein that contributes to the strength of those all-important drainage canals. Since uncontrolled allergies can increase IOP, also see Allergies (page 72). If you have the form of glaucoma called normal tension glaucoma, in which IOP remains normal, you may also be prone to migraines (see page 245).

Our Best Advice

There's no cure for glaucoma, only treatments to try to arrest its progress, primarily by lowering the IOP (for open-angle glaucoma). Our best recommendations in that area are to:

1. Begin taking prescription medications as directed by your physician.

2. Stop taking any over-the-counter antihistamines, decongestants, motion sickness medication, or sleeping aids.

3. Make sure you're getting at least 30 minutes of daily exercise.

Why It Works

There are dozens of medications available to lower IOP. They work by either reducing the amount of fluid produced in the eye or increasing drainage of fluid. Xalatan (latanoprost), a drug that increases drainage of fluid, is likely to be the first prescribed because it's the most effective at lowering pressure, according to several large clinical trials. The second most commonly prescribed drugs are beta-blockers, such as Betoptic (betaxolol) or Betagan (levobunolol), which reduce fluid production and increase drainage.

At the same time you're taking your eye medication, stop taking the drugs listed in item 2 above, because they can worsen existing glaucoma. So can antidepressants, corticosteroids, cholesterol-lowering drugs, asthma medication, and medication for vertigo, so if you're on one of these medications, talk to your doctor about whether or not something else can be substituted.

As for the exercise, there's good evidence that IOP drops after exercise, reaching its lowest level 60 minutes afterward. One study conducted in people with normal eyes who exercised for three months found a consistent drop in IOP.

TIME TO WORRY

- If you have severe pain in one eye, especially if you have any loss of vision in that eye.
- If you have redness in one eye, especially if accompanied by nausea and vomiting.
- If you have changes in your vision, such as new blind spots in your side vision or rings around light sources.
- If your pupil enlarges and doesn't shrink when you shine a light on it.

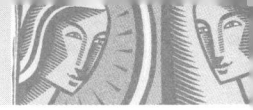

Other Medicines
Herbs and Supplements

Ginkgo. Several clinical trials on the use of this herb in glaucoma patients showed some benefits, primarily improving vision. Laboratory studies find ginkgo significantly increases blood flow to the ophthalmic artery, which feeds the optic nerve, helping it remain healthy. Take 120 milligrams of a standardized ginkgo extract (such as Ginkgold or Ginkai) twice a day. Don't take it if you're also taking prescription anticoagulants or antiplatelet drugs or are about to undergo surgery.

Vitamin C. The concentration of vitamin C in the fluid of your eye is 25 times higher than in your blood—signifying the importance of this antioxidant vitamin in maintaining eye health. Part of its role is to help build collagen. During one trial in which participants received high doses of vitamin C for two weeks, the IOP dropped in all but one. Start with 1,000 milligrams a day taken in two to three doses. If there is no change in your IOP after one month, gradually increase the amount up to 3,000 grams. Increase it slowly; otherwise, you may have diarrhea and other stomach upset. If you don't have any improvement after this dose, don't increase without first talking to your health-care provider.

Magnesium. This mineral may help if you have a mild form of the type of glaucoma in which your IOP is normal. This form is primarily treated with calcium channel blockers, and magnesium is a natural calcium channel blocker, so if you want to avoid medications as long as possible, you could start here. If you're already taking a calcium channel blocker, it's safe to add to the regimen with your doctor's okay—it might enable you to reduce the amount of calcium channel blocker you're taking. Take 200 to 300 milligrams a day.

Glutathione boosters. Glutathione is the most powerful antioxidant in the body. Some evidence suggests that low levels may contribute to changes in the eye that lead to glaucoma. In one Russian trial of 45 glaucoma patients, supplementing with alpha-lipoic acid (a precursor to glutathione) for two months improved peripheral and central vision in 45 percent of the participants. To increase your body's ability to manufacture glutathione, take one of the following: 600 milligrams N-acetyl-cysteine (NAC) twice a day, 1,000 milligrams methyl sulfonyl methane (MSM) once a day, 200 milligrams S-adenosyl-L-methionine (SAMe) twice a day, or 250 milligrams alpha-lipoic acid twice a day.

Other Approaches

Stress reduction. There's some evidence that high levels of stress can affect IOP in acute closed-angle glaucoma, and some suspicion it may also affect open-angle glaucoma. Review our recommendations for reducing stress in Part 2.

Acupuncture. One small study of 8 glaucoma patients found one session of acupuncture reduced IOP up to 24 hours after the treatment.

Cholesterol control. Studies in rats have revealed that high cholesterol levels can increase IOP. See High Cholesterol (page 284) for our advice on lowering cholesterol.

Prevention

Bump up your intake of omega-3 fatty acids. Eskimos who follow their native diet, which is very high in omega-3 fatty acids, have very low rates of glaucoma. It's no wonder: Laboratory studies find that fish oil can reduce IOP. Take 2 to 3 grams of fish oil a day, and eat more fatty fish and ground flaxseed. Also reduce the amount of omega-6 fatty acids in your diet (primarily found in vegetable oils). This helps lower inflammation in the eye, making it easier for fluid to flow out.

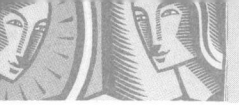

Gum Disease

The bacteria, mucus, and food debris that make up dental plaque do more than eat away at your teeth. Over time, plaque hardens into a substance called tartar at the base of the tooth, irritating and inflaming the gums. The gums may swell, bleed easily, and appear reddish-purple. They can also hurt, and may become infected. Left untreated, your teeth could fall out.

Suddenly flossing doesn't seem so bad, does it?

Do This Now

Although gum disease takes a long time to develop and an even longer time to reverse, these remedies will help when your gums are swollen and sore.

1. Brush your teeth thoroughly.

2. Pour 8 ounces boiling water over two bags of green tea and steep 10 minutes. Add 5 drops tea tree oil. Dip a string of dental floss in the mixture and floss, slowly and gently moving the floss between the teeth and into the gum.

3. Gargle 2 to 5 minutes with the leftover green tea mixture.

Why It Works

Brushing and flossing help loosen and remove any plaque irritating your gums. Green tea contains catechins, plant chemicals that can reduce gum-irritating bacteria and shrink swollen gums. One study found that gargling with green tea for 2 to 5 minutes significantly increased the amount of catechins in the saliva and reduced levels of gum-irritating bacteria for an hour afterward.

We suggest adding the tea tree oil because it's a natural anti-inflammatory and antibiotic. When 49 people with severe gingivitis smeared a tea tree oil gel on their gums twice a day for two weeks, the gel significantly reduced gum bleeding and plaque much better than a placebo gel. A similar study found that using tea tree oil as a mouthwash provided the same benefits.

Other Medicines
Herbs and Supplements

Liquid probiotic supplements such as acidophilus. Studies show the beneficial bacteria in these supplements, sold in health food stores, help crowd out harmful bacteria in your mouth, improving gum disease. Rinse your mouth with water, then swish the liquid supplement around your mouth for one minute before swallowing. Wait 15 to 30 minutes after brushing your teeth before using this remedy because most toothpastes contain ingredients that suppress bacteria in the mouth, rendering probiotics worthless if taken just after brushing. Note that liquid probiotics must be refrigerated or they lose potency. Don't buy them if the expiration date is near. You can also buy a probiotic powder and dissolve in a small amount of water.

Coenzyme Q_{10}. This supplement may boost immunity, helping your body fight off gingivitis. In a small study of eight patients with gum disease, CoQ_{10} significantly reduced plaque and improved gum health within seven days. For mild to moderate cases of gingivitis, take 60 milligrams once or twice a day. For severe gingivitis, take 100 milligrams three times a day.

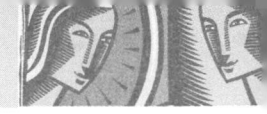

Other Approaches

Propolis powder. Bees use this sticky plant resin to line the insides of their hives because its natural antiseptic properties create a germ-free environment in which their eggs can hatch. This "bee glue" can also kill the bacteria that lead to gingivitis, according to various studies. Mix a pea-size amount into your toothpaste for twice-daily brushing.

Hydrogen peroxide and salt water. Gargling and swishing with a solution composed of equal parts of these liquids halts bacteria growth and reduces swelling.

Xylitol gum. This sugar substitute reduces *Streptococcus mutans*, the main bacterium responsible for gum disease. Switch from sugary gum to those sweetened with xylitol.

Tea tree oil toothpastes and gel. Twice-daily brushing with a gel that contained tea tree oil reduced gum swelling and bleeding in 49 people with severe gingivitis compared to a placebo.

Sugar-free 100 percent cranberry juice. Cranberry, a natural antiseptic, prevents a thick, bacteria-laden film—called biofilm—from sticking to your teeth and eventually turning into plaque and then tartar. In one unpublished study conducted at the University of Rochester, researchers submerged artificial teeth twice a day in cranberry juice. The juice prevented most of the bacteria from binding to the teeth.

Relaxation therapies. Stress elevates levels of cytokines, proteins that trigger inflammation throughout the body, including the gums. A study of 140 routine dental care patients found that stress and depression could increase gum bleeding and plaque formation, making gum disease worse. Check in Part 2 for relaxation therapies to integrate into your daily life.

Massage. Improve blood flow to your gums (and speed healing) by gently massaging them in a circular motion with your finger after brushing or even while sitting in front of the TV for 5 or more minutes a day.

Prevention

Brush your teeth at least twice a day, preferably with an electric toothbrush, which helps prevent the overbrushing that can irritate gums.

Floss at least once a day.

Get a professional dental cleaning every six months. If the cleaning makes your gums swell temporarily, swish salt water, or the green tea and tea tree oil mixture mentioned above, around your mouth.

Visit a dentist to repair misaligned teeth or update ill-fitting dental or orthodontic devices that can irritate your gums.

Take a daily multivitamin that contains 100 percent of the Daily Value for vitamins C and D, folic acid, riboflavin, zinc, and magnesium. Follow with a separate calcium supplement of 600 milligrams taken twice a day. Deficiencies in these vitamins and minerals have been linked to gum disease. In particular, your body needs vitamin C to heal wounds and bind teeth to bone.

Switch from coffee to green or black tea. Tea contains catechins that reduce plaque buildup.

Avoid sugary drinks.

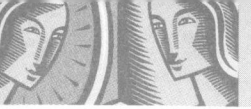
Macular Degeneration

Eye doctors call macular degeneration an "epidemic" for good reason: It's a progressive eye disease that occurs with age, and we're all living longer.

The condition primarily affects the macula, the part of the retina responsible for sharp central vision. The macula is a small cluster of light-sensing pigment cells. Even a little damage can lead to serious vision loss. We don't really know what causes macular degeneration, but researchers suspect some kind of immune response to inflammation. It's the leading cause of blindness in older Americans.

There are two forms of age-related macular degeneration (AMD). Dry macular degeneration, affecting about 90 percent of people with AMD, occurs slowly, over years, as fatty deposits collect under the macula cells. Your first symptom is blurred vision. As fewer cells in the macula function, you see details less clearly, although the blurriness may disappear in bright light. As you lose more light-sensing cells, a blind spot in the middle of your field of vision will develop, growing larger and larger. Our advice focuses on slowing down vision loss. There is no treatment for the dry form of AMD.

The other form of AMD, wet macular degeneration, begins as the dry form but can progress very rapidly to the wet form, considered advanced AMD. In this form, new blood vessels grow into the macula, breaking and bleeding and causing very fast, severe vision loss. The classic early symptom is that straight lines appear crooked; this happens because fluid from the leaking blood vessels gathers and lifts the macula, distorting your vision. A small blind spot may also appear in wet AMD, resulting in the loss of your central vision.

Our Best Advice

Since there are no acute symptoms related to macular degeneration, our best advice relates to slowing the progression of the disease.

1. Begin taking 500 milligrams vitamin C, 400 IU vitamin E, 15 milligrams beta-carotene, and 80 milligrams zinc with 2 milligrams copper, 6 milligrams zeaxanthin and lutein combined, and 80 milligrams of a standardized extract of bilberry (standardized to 25 percent anthocyanidins). You may be able to find this combination in a single supplement marketed for eye health.

2. Begin taking 120 milligrams of a ginkgo biloba standardized extract twice a day.

3. Wear polarized sunglasses whenever you are outside or in very bright light, even if you are inside.

Why It Works

A study called the Age-Related Eye Disease Study, which followed 3,600 people with AMD, found that this combination of vitamins and minerals cut the risk that the disease would progress to the advanced stage by about 25 percent. Additionally, in people with intermediate AMD or advanced AMD in one eye but not the other, the nutrients reduced the risk of vision loss 19 percent. We're not sure if these supplements could also slow the progression of early to intermediate AMD, but they certainly won't hurt.

Lutein and zeaxanthin are powerful plant-based antioxidants that are major components of the macula, helping protect underlying cells from

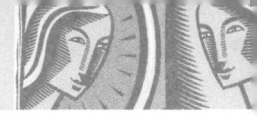

damage. Their presence is the reason the macula looks yellowish (stare into someone's eye and you'll see what we mean). One study found that people with low levels of these nutrients, also called carotenoids, had a much greater risk of developing AMD. There's also some evidence that getting more of these antioxidants, through diet or supplements, can make the macula slightly thicker, protecting the underlying cells and, theoretically at least, slowing progression of the disease. Good food sources include leafy green vegetables such as spinach, collard greens, and kale.

We recommend bilberry extract because it has a high concentration of anthocyanidins, powerful antioxidants that can improve the delivery of oxygen and blood to the eye and scavenge free radicals that contribute to macular degeneration. These antioxidants have a special attraction for pigment cells in the back of the retina. Good food sources of anthocyanidins are cherries, cranberries, and pomegranates.

Although the evidence is still preliminary, one small well-designed study in 10 patients with macular degeneration found that those who took ginkgo had statistically significant improvements in their vision compared to those who took a placebo. Researchers suspect ginkgo's ability to improve blood flow, and its strong antioxidant properties, are responsible for its benefits. Don't take ginkgo if you're also taking any antiplatelet drugs, aspirin, or anticoagulants, and stop taking it two weeks before any surgery.

We recommend sunglasses because there's clear evidence that ultraviolet light contributes to the free-radical damage that leads to AMD.

Other Medicines
Herbs and Supplements

Folate and pyridoxine. Studies find low levels of these B vitamins in people with AMD. Take a vitamin B50 complex (a supplement that provides significant levels of all the important B vitamins) daily.

Fish oil supplements. The anti-inflammatory effects of fish oil may help reduce the inflammation believed to be behind AMD. Take 2 to 3 grams per day for the dry form, half that amount if you have the wet form, because fish oil can thin the blood, which could increase the possibility of inner-eye bleeding.

Glutathione. Glutathione is the most powerful antioxidant in the body, and studies find it can protect against damage to the cells that make up the macula, possibly preventing AMD or slowing its progression. To increase your body's ability to manufacture glutathione, take 600 milligrams NAC (N-acetyl-cysteine) twice a day, 1,000 milligrams MSM (methyl sulfonyl methane) once a day, 200 milligrams of SAMe (S-adenosyl-L-methionine) twice a day, or 250 milligrams alpha-lipoic acid twice a day.

Prescription Drugs

All prescription drugs are for the wet form of AMD only.

Macugen (pegaptanib sodium injection). This is the first drug approved to treat the wet form of AMD. It works by preventing the action of growth factors that enable blood vessels to form and grow. It's administered every six weeks by injection into the eye.

Thalidomide. Infamous as the drug responsible for the birth defects of thousands of infants in the 1960s, thalidomide has been reborn as a cancer treatment. Although it's not approved for treating macular degeneration, some doctors use it for the wet form because it can stop the formation of new blood vessels. However, it can have serious side effects that lead some patients to stop using it.

Estrogen therapy. Although AMD is not reason enough to take estrogen therapy, one study

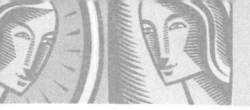

did find that women with the eye disease who had taken supplemental estrogen after menopause were less likely to have their disease progress to the advanced stage. Only take it, however, if you also need it for hot flashes and other menopausal symptoms, because it increases your risk of other serious health conditions like breast cancer.

Other Approaches

Laser therapy. In this treatment, a high-energy beam of light is aimed at the abnormal blood vessels, destroying them. However, it may also affect your remaining vision, depending on where the leaky blood vessels are. This procedure is only appropriate for a small percentage of people with the wet form of AMD, and repeat treatments are often required.

Photodynamic therapy. In this treatment, a special dye is administered intravenously. The dye "sticks" to the abnormal blood vessels. Then a light is shined onto the eye, activating the dye and destroying the blood vessels. This treatment may need to be repeated every three months.

Radiation therapy. This treatment destroys the abnormal blood vessels while sparing normal blood vessels in the retina, which are relatively resistant to radiation. It doesn't cure the disease, only slows its progression.

Acupuncture. There is some evidence that acupuncture affects the macula, although no studies have been published on its use in treating AMD.

Prevention

Take the same mix of nutrients mentioned under "Our Best Advice".

Stop smoking. The longer and more you smoke, the greater your risk of macular degeneration will be.

Wear sunglasses. There's some evidence that exposure to ultraviolet light may increase the risk of AMD, possibly because the light contributes to the formation of free radicals, which can damage delicate cells in the eye.

Get more omega-3 fatty acids. One study found people with diets high in anti-inflammatory omega-3 fatty acids (found in fatty fish) and low in omega-6 fatty acids (primarily found in vegetable oils and processed foods) were significantly less likely to develop AMD than those whose ratios of the fatty acids were reversed. In the study, if a person's diet was high in omega-6 at all—even if he still ate plenty of fish—the protective effects of the omega-3 fatty acids disappeared. You can also supplement with 2 to 3 grams of fish oil a day.

Eat more leafy green vegetables. Studies find people with diets high in these foods have a lower risk of developing AMD, possibly because the vegetables contain lutein and zeaxanthin.

Drink a glass of wine several days a week. There's some evidence that moderate consumption of wine can reduce the risk of AMD. Beer, on the other hand, may increase your risk.

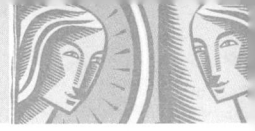

Temporomandibular Joint Disorder (TMJ)

The temporomandibular joint is one of the most complex joints in your body. Because it connects the lower jaw to the skull, it has to move in all directions—up and down, forward and back, and side to side—so you can chew, talk, and make facial expressions.

Over time, these movements can make the jaw joint and surrounding muscles and tissues swell, especially if your mouth and jaw aren't properly aligned. This swelling puts pressure on nearby nerves, causing facial, ear, and head pain. Symptoms of the disorder, which is referred to as TMJ or TMD, may also include clicking and popping noises, and lockjaw, when the joint gets stuck in one position, often forcing your mouth partially open.

Stress is often a major factor in TMJ, causing you to clench or grind your teeth, irritating the jaw joint. So if we haven't convinced you yet to manage your stress through relaxation techniques (see pages 59-61), maybe your jaw pain will.

Other factors that contribute to TMJ include jaw injuries, problems with your bite, arthritis (see page 333), hormonal changes, and infections. Even poor posture, such as holding the head forward of the neck like a turtle, can irritate jaw muscles.

Do This Now

When TMJ pain strikes, eat only soft foods, don't chew gum, and follow these steps.

1. Apply an ice pack to your jaw joint (just in front of the ear) for 10 to 15 minutes.

2. Follow with a warm, moist washcloth to the same area, also for 10 to 15 minutes.

3. Use your fingers to gently massage your face, shoulders, and neck muscles with hard, slow, short strokes for several minutes.

4. Place your thumb on the outside of your cheek on the side that hurts, with the fingers of the same hand inside the cheek. Squeeze your cheek between your fingers and move it in a circular, massaging motion for several minutes.

5. If you still have pain, take 240 milligrams Aleve (naproxen) twice a day or 400 to 600 milligrams ibuprofen three times a day with food.

6. Repeat steps 1 through 3 throughout the day as needed,

Why It Works

The ice numbs the pain and reduces swelling, while the heat increases blood circulation to the area, bringing healing oxygen and nutrients and relaxing tight face and jaw muscles. Alternate between the two—ice and then heat—for best results.

Massage further reduces muscle tension and pain, while the pain relievers reduce swelling and the soft food diet gives your jaw the rest it needs to recover.

Other Medicines
Herbs and Supplements

Nervine tea. Nervine herbs, such as chamomile and valerian, relax the nervous system, soothing stress and muscle tension that trigger TMJ pain. Mix 1/2 teaspoon chamomile, 1/4 teaspoon valerian root, 1/2 teaspoon oat straw, 1/4 teaspoon passionflower, and 1/4 teaspoon skullcap into 6 to

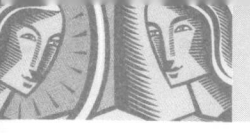

8 ounces of boiling water. Steep for 10 minutes, strain, and drink several times a day.

Calcium and magnesium. These minerals reduce muscle spasms, which may contribute to TMJ pain. Take 500 milligrams of calcium and 250 milligrams of magnesium twice a day.

Other Approaches

Injections. A dentist or ear, nose, and throat doctor can inject steroids or numbing medication into the jaw joint, decreasing pain and inflammation. You'll need local anesthesia for the procedure, but you'll experience near immediate pain relief.

Relaxation techniques. Often, once you reduce stress and muscle tension, TMJ pain disappears quickly. One study found that six months of relaxation training significantly reduced tooth grinding and TMJ discomfort in 33 children. Any relaxation technique—including biofeedback, visualization, progressive muscle relaxation, and hypnosis—will work.

Jaw exercises. In a small study of 20 patients with TMJ, a combination of jaw exercises, relaxation therapy, and improved posture reduced TMJ pain within six months. First apply a warm compress for 15 minutes to loosen and relax your jaw muscles. Then open and close your jaw and move it from side to side repeatedly for 5 minutes, increasing your range of motion with each movement. Repeat three to five times a day for two to four weeks.

Bite block. Also called a splint, this plastic guard fits over your teeth, preventing grinding or clenching. Bite blocks may also correct bite abnormalities that lead to jaw pain. In a study of 122 teenagers with TMJ, 60 percent experienced significantly less pain within six months after wearing a dental device.

Although bite blocks work well for most people, they can magnify pain for others. If your dentist suggests you wear a bite block but it doesn't work, make another appointment. There are many different types (some fit over the top of the teeth and others over the bottom), and one may work better than another.

Posture improvement. Repeatedly jutting your head forward of your shoulders can stress muscles in and around the jaw. So organize your workstation to enable good posture, with your head directly over your shoulders. Also sleep on a contoured pillow designed to keep your head and neck relaxed during sleep.

Chiropractic. In a small study of nine patients, a chiropractic technique that used a small device called an activator to make a controlled, light, and fast thrust to the jaw joint in addition to standard chiropractic care improved jaw alignment and relieved jaw pain within two weeks. Several case studies support these results.

Acupuncture. In a study of 89 patients with TMJ, acupuncture and a bite block relieved TMJ symptoms in 85 percent of patients within six visits. Another study found acupuncture as effective as splints at relieving TMJ pain. For best results, see an acupuncturist weekly for six weeks. Because acupuncture soothes pain but does not treat the underlying cause of TMJ, it's best combined with other treatments, such as a bite block.

Prevention

Avoid problem foods. That includes chewy foods like taffy and steak. Don't chew gum, or crunch ice or hard candy.

Keep your chin out of your hand. Repeatedly resting your chin in your hand can push your jaw out of alignment, triggering TMJ pain.

Use a headset when you talk on the phone to reduce strain on your neck and jaw muscles.

Relax your face. Every hour, stop what you're doing and consciously relax your facial muscles.

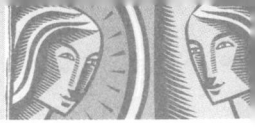

Tinnitus

Although experts don't know what causes tinnitus, the leading suspect is loud noise, such as a gunshot blast, that damages the auditory nerve in the inner ear, leading to the ringing that is the hallmark of the condition. Normal aging and even some drugs may also fray the endings of this nerve.

Other theories include poor blood flow to the ear, caused by narrowed blood vessels (which is why managing high cholesterol and heart disease is so important), wax buildup, jaw misalignment (see Temporomandibular Joint Disorder on page 185), and swelling from allergies and infections. Benign tumors that grow on the auditory nerve may also cause tinnitus, which is why it's a good idea to get a doctor involved if you have symptoms.

Do This Now

Unfortunately, there's no cure for tinnitus (it sometimes goes away on its own). But the following steps can help you cope when the ringing is driving you nuts.

1. Listen to your favorite music, or a recording of nature sounds or white noise, through headphones. Turn up the volume until it's slightly louder than the noise you hear inside your head. Alternatively, turn on a white-noise machine or even a loud fan.

2. Close your eyes and breathe deeply and slowly, bringing the air deep into your abdomen and releasing through your mouth.

3. With your eyes still closed, imagine a bright light enveloping, filling, and warming your whole body.

Why It Works

The music, sounds, or white noise help mask the sounds inside your head.

We suggest the deep breathing and visualization to help distract you from the annoying sounds, as well as to help you to relax. There is evidence that distracting yourself makes the ringing more bearable. Plus, studies find stress triggers tinnitus, while relaxation eases it. In one German study, 40 tinnitus patients reported they felt significantly less annoyed and disabled by their condition when they distracted themselves by listening to white noise or imagining a bright light.

Other Medicines
Herbs and Supplements

Vinpocetine. Although there are no clinical studies on its benefits, some tinnitus sufferers report that this supplement, isolated from a Madagascar periwinkle, reduces the ringing, possibly by dilating blood vessels and improving blood flow. Take 5 to 10 milligrams three times a day.

Ginkgo. Because it dilates blood vessels, ginkgo may improve symptoms. Take 120 milligrams of a standardized ginkgo extract (such as Ginkgold and Ginkai) twice a day. Don't take if you're also taking prescription anticoagulants or are about to undergo surgery.

TIME TO WORRY

If you suddenly experience ringing sounds along with hearing loss, slurred speech, vision changes, or numbness, seek medical attention immediately. You may be having a stroke.

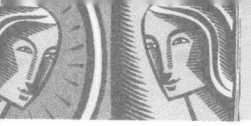

Melatonin. A 30-day study of 30 people with tinnitus found that supplementing with this hormone daily helped improve sleep and reduce symptoms. Because the effective dose, 3 grams, is extremely high, we recommend you take this amount for just one month, then taper down until you find the minimum amount required to suppress symptoms.

Prescription Drugs

Antidepressants and antianxiety medications. Drugs like Xanax and nortriptyline can help you relax, lift your mood, and aid sleep. They may also ease symptoms.

Other Approaches

Tinnitus retraining therapy (TRT). This therapy trains your brain to tune out the tinnitus, so you're no longer aware of the sounds unless you focus on them. It involves wearing an ear device that emits low-level, constant noise (this noise does not drown out the tinnitus noise). A counselor also works with you to teach you skills to help you ignore the ringing. Physicians at Emory University in Atlanta report this therapy resulted in an 80 percent improvement in symptoms in their patients.

Tinnitus maskers. Your doctor can fit you with a hearing aid-like device that constantly emits a white-noise sound, drowning out the ringing. In one study of 30 tinnitus patients, such a device significantly reduced participants' distress. If you have hearing loss, you can also be fitted with a combination hearing aid/masker.

Biofeedback. By teaching you to relax, biofeedback can help decrease the stress associated with tinnitus. In one small study, slightly more than half the participants experienced less tinnitus discomfort and psychological distress after learning biofeedback.

Cognitive-behavioral therapy. Cognitive-behavioral therapy involves changing the way you react to events. When 77 people with tinnitus learned this technique through an Internet-based program, their symptoms decreased.

Acupuncture. In Traditional Chinese Medicine, the ear and kidneys are connected by meridians (energy pathways), so for tinnitus, an acupuncturist focuses on meridians that cleanse the kidneys. Although research has yielded mixed results on acupuncture for tinnitus, studies find it does help alleviate the stress associated with the condition.

Diet. Cut back on alcohol, caffeine, and nicotine, all of which can make tinnitus worse.

Prevention

Eat less fat, cholesterol, and salt to maximize blood flow to the ears.

Wear earplugs or protective earmuffs when exposed to sounds above 85 decibels (such as a lawn mower or rock concert).

Avoid aspirin and ibuprofen, which studies find can both trigger and worsen tinnitus.

Take 25 milligrams of zinc daily. Studies find a deficiency in this mineral may trigger tinnitus.

GETTING TESTED

If you have tinnitus, don't pass it off as just a nuisance. It could be a sign of a serious health condition. Ask your health-care provider to check your:

- Ears for wax buildup or possible infection.
- Levels of thyroid hormone, cholesterol, and blood sugar. Low thyroid hormone levels, high cholesterol levels, and diabetes are all linked to tinnitus.
- Blood pressure. Hypertension may trigger tinnitus.

If all tests are negative, ask your doctor whether a CT scan is warranted to rule out benign tumors on the auditory nerves. If you have any jaw pain, see your dentist to rule out TMJ as a cause.

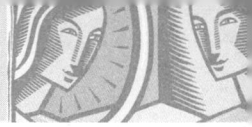

Toothache

Most toothaches stem from cavities, abscesses (an infection around the tooth or gum), or gum disease (an inflammation of the gum around a tooth), so you'll need to consult your dentist to treat the underlying problem. (And check out the entry on gum disease on page 180). Temporomandibular joint disorder (page 185) and sinusitis (page 88) can also cause toothache.

Do This Now

These remedies can help ease the pain while you're waiting for your appointment with the dentist.

1. Place a couple of drops of clove oil on a cotton ball. Place the cotton ball over your sore tooth and bite down gently for several minutes, then discard.

2. Mix 1/4 teaspoon salt and several drops clove oil into 6 ounces water. Swish around your mouth and spit.

3. Take 500 to 1,000 milligrams Tylenol along with 400 milligrams ibuprofen.

Why It Works

Dentists have long used clove oil to soothe dental pain. In addition to numbing the ache, this pleasant-tasting antiseptic also kills bacteria and other germs, preventing an abscess from getting worse. You don't want to swallow the oil, however, which is why we suggest you rinse your mouth with salt water and clove oil after biting on the cotton ball. The salt in the mouthwash decreases swelling and relieves pain, while the clove oil bathes your mouth with a small amount of the nat-

ural antiseptic. Don't use clove oil on children younger than two, because they might swallow it.

Both the Tylenol and ibuprofen further relieve the pain. Take them together; one study found taking both provided more pain relief than taking either separately.

Other Medicines
Herbs and Supplements

Vanilla extract. It's a good alternative if you don't have clove oil.

Other Approaches

Ice. Place an ice pack on your cheek, outside the sore area, to numb the nerves that transmit pain from the tooth.

Toothpaste. Rub a small amount of toothpaste designed for sensitive teeth (such as Sensodyne) on the sore tooth to calm the nerves triggering the pain.

Dental wax. You'll find it in emergency dental kits sold in drugstores. Pack it around your tooth to temporarily seal off a cavity while you wait for a dental appointment. Beeswax also works.

Prevention

Preventing toothache means maintaining a healthy mouth. Specifically:

Brush and floss your teeth at least twice daily. Do it religiously!

See a dentist at least twice a year for professional cleanings.

Get fitted for a bite block to wear at night if you grind your teeth during your sleep.

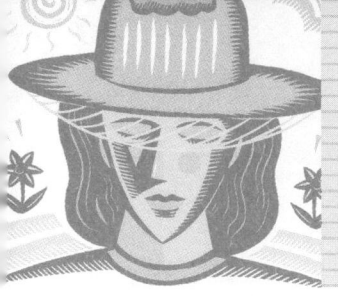

Your Skin

Acne

What do teenagers and perimenopausal women have in common? Wild hormone levels—and, not coincidentally, acne. Hormonal imbalances contribute to the overproduction of sebum, the oily stuff that blocks pores and creates a breeding ground for bacteria. This bacteria, along with inflammation, causes acne. (Contrary to popular belief, chocolate's not the culprit.)

Acne can be a side effect of hormonal treatment for conditions like endometriosis, and a sign of polycystic ovary syndrome (PCOS), which involves elevated levels of androgens, "male" hormones that contribute to acne. More recently, we're beginning to see evidence that acne can also be related to insulin resistance (common in women with PCOS). What's the connection? Abdominal fat—one sign of insulin resistance—produces inflammatory compounds. It also churns out androgens. Everything you can do to control inflammation (see page 38 in Part 2) and insulin resistance (see page 48 in Part 2) should help rein in the pimples.

Do This Now

Acne won't disappear overnight. But the following steps will get you started on the road to recovery, with more treatment options described below.

1. Clean your face thoroughly using a tea tree oil cleanser, either pads or soap, available in health food stores. Don't use a washcloth.

2. Apply an over-the-counter product that contains benzoyl peroxide.

3. If you have severe acne (i.e., large cysts and red, painful areas), add 2 to 3 drops lavender and eucalyptus or tea tree essential oils to 4 ounces very warm water. Soak a cotton ball in this mixture and apply to serious problem areas. Then reheat the water and repeat several times a day. If a larger area is involved, soak a washcloth in the water and gently apply—don't scrub.

4. Apply any topical medication your doctor has prescribed, such as an antibiotic or retinoid.

5. Apply sunscreen if you're going outside after using these prescription medications.

Why It Works

Tea tree oil is a perfect acne-fighter because it combats both bacteria and inflammation, which contribute to the redness and swelling of pimples. In Australia it's used to treat and prevent everything from fungal infections to drug-resistant staph infections. In studies, it seems to work almost as well as benzoyl peroxide lotion in reducing pimples (although it takes longer to work), and it causes less skin irritation. It's particularly beneficial for large areas of acne, like the back or chest, which are hard to treat with topical benzoyl peroxide. We don't want you to use a

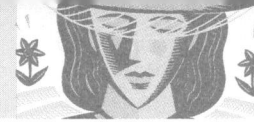

washcloth to apply it, because scrubbing can further irritate the skin, making your acne worse. For more serious infections, directly applying a tea tree or lavender solution can soothe the skin, decrease inflammation, and reduce bacteria on the skin.

Benzoyl peroxide (available in over-the-counter and prescription strengths) is an antibacterial that improves acne in as little as five days. It fights bacteria differently than tea tree oil, so don't be afraid to use both.

Antibiotic creams such as erythromycin or tetracycline are usually the first prescription treatment recommended (often used in conjunction with benzoyl peroxide). They are sometimes prescribed along with retinoid creams such as Retin-A or Retinol. Retinoid creams contain a synthetic form of vitamin A that unclogs pores by regulating the growth of skin cells. If you're using a retinoid cream, skip the tea tree oil, since the combination might be too irritating. And stay out of the sun, because these creams make your skin more sensitive to sunlight.

Other Medicines
Herbs and Supplements

Brewer's yeast. There's some evidence that this medicinal yeast supplement can help boost insulin sensitivity, probably because it is high in the mineral chromium. Although there's only one published study on its use for acne, that study of 139 patients found significant improvements in nearly 75 percent of those who took the supplement, compared to just 22 percent of those who took a placebo. Take 2 grams a day, but don't take it if you're susceptible to migraines or you're taking a monoamine oxidase (MAO) inhibitor.

Guggulipid. This supplement, from the resin of a myrrh tree, is more often used to lower cholesterol, but it works for acne and inflammation too. In fact, in one study of 20 patients with acne,

🌿 Helpful Hint

Reduce Drug Side Effects With Supplements

If you're taking oral retinoids for acne, add 100 milligrams a day of L-carnitine for every 2.2 pounds you weigh (that's 7 grams for a 160-pound person) to reduce the muscle pain that is a side effect of the drug. Take in two or three divided doses. If you're taking oral antibiotics, take 1 to 2 capsules of probiotics a day with meals to maintain a healthy balance of bacteria in your stomach and intestines. If you're taking oral contraceptives for acne or birth control, also take 400 to 800 micrograms folic acid. The pill causes you to lose folic acid.

it worked as well as the oral antibiotic tetracycline when taken for three months. Take 500 milligrams (standardized to 25% guggulsterones) three times a day.

Prescription Drugs

If topical treatments aren't enough to get rid of your acne, your doctor might prescribe oral drugs. Prescription drugs for acne are often prescribed in combination. Options include:

Oral antibiotics. If your skin doesn't improve with topical treatments, your doctor may prescribe oral antibiotics, such as tetracycline or erythromycin. Antibiotics are often prescribed together with topical retinoids.

Oral retinoids. If you have severe acne, your doctor may prescribe oral retinoids, but they have significant side effects, including muscle pain, depression, and birth defects (if used during pregnancy).

Azelex (azelaic acid). This topical cream is made of a naturally occurring acid found in rye and wheat. It may lighten dark skin, however, and isn't as effective as topical antibiotics or retinoids.

Oral contraceptives. If you need a form of birth control and you have acne, consider using Ortho Tri-Cyclen, Ortho-Cyclen, or Desogen brands, all of which have been shown to improve acne.

Other Approaches

Relaxation techniques. It's not coincidental that your face breaks out when you're under stress. One of the few studies to examine this correlation found that university students' acne got worse during exams. Whether this is due to the actual stressful event itself, or to the fact that during stress you're less likely to get enough sleep, eat right, and exercise, isn't known. But several relaxation techniques, including biofeedback and mental imagery, have been shown to improve acne.

Aromatherapy. After cleaning your face, give yourself a steam treatment by adding 10 drops tea tree and lavender oil to a pot of hot (not boiling) water. Lean over the pot and cover your head with a towel to keep the steam in. Stay until the water cools, then rinse your face with cool water.

Prevention

Follow a diet higher in protein and lower in simple carbohydrates and fat. Avoid sugary foods and foods made with white flour. This type of diet improves insulin sensitivity, and some studies find it can reduce acne.

Consume foods rich in vitamin A. These include sweet potatoes, carrots, spinach, and other greens.

Load up on omega-3 fatty acids. These fatty acids reduce inflammation and therefore may help with acne. Get them in fatty fish and ground flaxseed (try sprinkling it over yogurt or salads) or take 1 tablespoon flaxseed oil a day.

Change your sheets and pillowcase every few days, and wash them in hot water with a non-irritating soap. You can add lavender or tea tree oil (5 drops in the rinse water) to kill more bacteria.

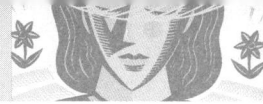

Athlete's Foot

Despite the name, you don't have to work out to have athlete's foot, just as you don't have to be a man to have jock itch. The two are the same—fungal infections that are more common in warm weather and in men.

Do This Now

1. Soak your foot in a pan or basin of water with 20 drops tea tree oil.

2. After cleaning and drying the area thoroughly, sprinkle with either a medicated powder or cornstarch, then sprinkle your socks and shoes with the powder too.

3. Apply Lotrimin Ultra cream to the affected area and about an inch around it.

4. Apply Benadryl cream or hydrocortisone cream (only for up to a week before seeing a doctor).

Why It Works

The footbath with tea tree oil, which fights fungus, helps soothe the itching. The powder or cornstarch helps absorb moisture, a fungal infection's best friend.

Lotrimin (sold over the counter) is an antifungal cream that usually clears up mild cases within a week or so; a more difficult or chronic infection might take up to two weeks to improve. Continue using the cream for a week after the infection clears to prevent a recurrence.

The Benadryl or hydrocortisone cream won't kill the fungus, but it will give you relief from the annoying itching.

Other Medicines
Herbs and Supplements

Antifungal tea. Put 1 to 2 tablespoons of thyme, eucalyptus, or lavender in a cup, cover with 8 ounces boiling water, and steep. Strain and cool. Wash the foot with tea tree soap, then soak a cotton cloth in the tea and apply twice daily.

Antibacterial salve. Add 10 drops lavender oil, 10 drops tea tree oil and a bit of aloe vera gel to an ounce of calendula salve and rub in. These oils have antifungal and antibacterial properties, and are very helpful if your feet are cracked.

Over-the-Counter Drugs

Burow's solution. If you have a blistering rash on your foot, soak your feet in this solution (sold under several brand names, including Domeboro) twice a day before applying antifungal creams.

Prescription Drugs

Nizoral (ketoconazole). This antifungal is also effective against some bacterial infections.

Lotrisone (clotrimazole/betamethasone). This combination drug and others like it combine an antifungal with a steroid.

Oral antifungals. These drugs, such as Lamisil (terbinafine), are prescribed if the infection has spread to your nails. They take weeks to begin working, and they have side effects.

Prevention

Watch your hygiene. Wear loose-fitting cotton socks and change them if they become wet. Wear flip-flops in public showers and locker rooms.

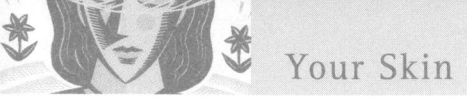

Bruises

Every time a part of your body meets a hard object, the impact smashes tiny blood vessels under your skin. Blood leaks out, pooling under your skin and leaving a black-and-blue mark. Eventually your body absorbs the blood and the bruise fades. As you age, your skin becomes thinner and your capillaries more fragile, and it takes less impact to create a bruise. Certain medications can intensify bruising, including blood thinners, birth control pills, diuretics, and aspirin.

Do This Now

Immediately after bumping into something you know will leave a bruise, follow these steps.

1. Apply a cold compress for 30 minutes.

2. Then apply a hot compress for three to five minutes.

3. Repeat Steps 1 and 2 at least twice over the next 24 hours for a mild injury, or every three or four waking hours over the next 48 hours for a more severe injury.

4. Apply arnica cream or ointment and repeat every one to two hours.

Why It Works

The cold compress reduces swelling and discoloration by shrinking blood vessels and sealing off leaking blood vessels. Conversely, the warm compress brings more blood and healing nutrients to the area, helping your body repair leaky blood vessels and reabsorb the blood quicker.

We love arnica for its ability to reduce pain and inflammation. It's the most common ingredient in homeopathic preparations for bruises.

Other Medicines
Herbs and Supplements

Bromelain. Studies find this enzyme, derived from pineapple stems, reduces swelling and bruising. It not only interferes with the inflammatory actions of chemicals called leukotrienes, but also disrupts the action of enzymes involved in inflammation. Take 500 milligrams two or three times a day. For a very large bruise, double the dose during the first 24 hours.

Other Approaches

Traumeel ointment or gel. This homeopathic product contains arnica, calendula, belladonna, and many other herbs known to reduce pain and swelling and speed healing. In one study, injured rats treated with the product had less swelling and healed more quickly than rats not treated with it. Rub a small amount into the bruise and reapply several times a day.

Prevention

Eat more brightly colored fruits and vegetables. They contain high amounts of flavonoids, antioxidant plant pigments that protect cell structures, enhance the action of vitamin C (see below), and reduce inflammation. Many high-flavonoid foods are also rich in vitamin K, which aids in blood clotting.

Take vitamin C with bioflavonoids. Vitamin C builds collagen around blood vessels and in the skin, preventing bruising. Take 1,000 milligrams twice a day for three weeks, then decrease to 500 milligrams twice a day.

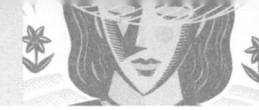

Burns

Heat has an amazing ability to breach the protective barrier of your skin and damage tissue. Burns can also result from chemicals, electricity, or radiation. We measure burns in degrees, from least severe (first degree) to most severe (third degree), based on which layer of skin the burn penetrates. If the burned skin feels leathery and doesn't hurt as much as you might expect given the seriousness of the injury, you likely have a third-degree burn and need immediate medical attention. Also seek immediate medical attention if the burn was caused by chemicals or electricity or if it covers an area larger than two hands put together. The advice here is geared toward less serious burns.

Do This Now

To treat a minor burn, do the following.

1. Run cool water over the area. If the burn was caused by a chemical, rinse the chemical off completely.

2. While you're at the sink, close your eyes, breathe deeply and picture a cooling blue breeze blowing on your burned skin.

3. Apply lavender oil.

4. Follow with an application of sap from an aloe vera plant if you have one. If you don't, use 100% aloe vera cream or lotion without fixatives. Then cover with a clean dressing that doesn't stick to the wound and keep dry.

5. Take 500 to 1,000 milligrams Tylenol or 400 milligrams ibuprofen.

Why It Works

The water cools the skin, and using your imagination to envision something cooling has been found to help relieve burn pain.

Lavender oil reduces inflammation and pain. It's also an antiseptic, so it helps prevent a secondary infection.

Aloe has long been used to soothe burns and speed healing. In one study of 27 patients with burns, patients treated with aloe healed faster than those treated with Vaseline-saturated gauze (often used in burn units). Don't use aloe vera gel, which can be drying.

The pain relievers, of course, help ease the pain.

Other Medicines

St. John's wort, calendula, or comfrey. You can buy salves, creams, or ointments containing these burn-soothing ingredients. For added benefit, mix one drop each of lavender and chamomile oil into the amount you plan to use, then apply and cover with a bandage or Telfa pad taped into place.

Other Approaches

Ripe papaya. Mash the pulp and apply. This is a common treatment in African and Central American hospitals. Papaya contains an enzyme that decreases inflammation and breaks down dead tissue. Alternatively, you can use a bromelain (pineapple enzyme) cream.

Homeopathy. *Urtica urens* and *Cantharis* are good for burns. Buy the 12C strength and take 1 to 2 tablets every 15 minutes for the first hour, then decrease the frequency as the burn heals.

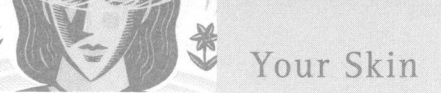

Cuts and Scrapes

Cuts and scrapes represent a breach of your body's most important protector—the skin. Once that barrier is compromised, all manner of germs can gain entry, potentially turning what once was a minor injury into a serious infection.

Do This Now

Treat your cut right by following these steps to prevent infection and speed healing.

1. Rinse the area thoroughly to clear any grit, dirt, or foreign material. Pick out any large bits that remain.

2. Clean the wound with an antiseptic (such as hydrogen peroxide) or tea tree soap, then rinse.

3. Put pressure on the wound with a clean cloth until the bleeding slows or stops.

4. Apply an antibacterial ointment like Bacitracin or Neosporin. Alternatively, you can use a calendula cream into which you've mixed a drop of lavender and tea tree oil.

5. Cover the wound with a clean, dry dressing such as a Telfa dressing and keep dry.

6. Begin taking 500 milligrams of vitamin C twice a day.

Why It Works

The rinsing removes particles you can't see. If you don't have a clean water source available (bottled water is ideal), cover the wound with a clean dressing and rinse it out as soon as possible.

The ointments provide a protective barrier until the skin grows back and help the injured tissue heal faster—often by several days.

Covering the cut is important to keep it clean. Telfa dressings, sold in drugstores, are cotton pads that won't stick to the wound and don't hurt when you take them off.

Numerous clinical studies find supplementing with vitamin C after an injury improves healing. The vitamin is a key component in collagen, the protein that makes up much of the connective tissue in skin.

Other Medicines

Anti-inflammatory supplements. Take 500 milligrams of the plant enzyme bromelain, 250 milligrams of rutin or quercetin, and 50 milligrams of grapeseed extract twice a day if you have a deep cut or large scraped area. These are the key ingredients, along with vitamin C, in a supplement called InflammEnz, which one study found significantly accelerated healing and reduced inflammation after injuries.

Pycnogenol gel. When researchers treated wounded rats with this antioxidant gel, their wounds healed about three days faster than those of rats not treated with it. The gel also reduced subsequent scarring. Rub a small amount into the injury and reapply several times a day.

Other Approaches

Liquid bandage. These products form a waterproof seal over your cut and also stop minor bleeding.

Arnica. This is a classic homeopathic treatment for injury. Take a 30X preparation every 15 to 30 minutes for the first one to two hours. Then decrease to one dose every hour for six to eight hours, then to three to four times a day for another day or two.

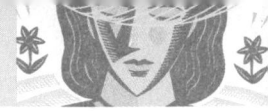

Dandruff

You know that scaly yellow stuff newborn babies get on their heads, called cradle cap? It's the same thing adults get, called dandruff. It can affect not only your scalp, but also your eyebrows. It's often triggered by an immune system overreaction to a yeastlike fungus called *Malassezia ovalis,* often present on our skin. Dandruff is like crabgrass—once you get it, it's all about keeping it from coming back.

Do This Now

To minimize flakes, follow these steps.

1. Wash your hair with a medicated shampoo containing ketoconazole (Nizoral). Leave the shampoo on your scalp for at least five minutes before rinsing.

2. Let your hair air-dry (skip the blow-dryer).

3. Several times a day, brush your hair firmly for 100 strokes with a natural bristle brush.

Why It Works

Although there are several different types of dandruff shampoos on the shelves, all with different ingredients, Nizoral is our recommendation. One of the few studies comparing several of the most common dandruff shampoos found that Nizoral, which contains the antifungal ingredient ketoconazole, was most effective at killing the fungus responsible for dandruff, particularly at the 2% prescription strength. Even the over-the-counter 1% strength was 10 times more effective than the other shampoos tested, which included Head & Shoulders and Selsun Blue.

Hair dryers not only dry the hair, but also the scalp, increasing flakiness.

Brushing distributes the oils from the top of the hair shaft down the length of the shaft, removing oil from the scalp and thereby decreasing irritation. Since *Malassezia ovalis* feeds on skin oil, this should also decrease the fungus on your scalp.

Other Medicines

Topical steroids. In severe cases of dandruff, your doctor may prescribe a topical steroid like triamcinolone solution or Luxíq (betamethasone valerate) once or twice daily to relieve itching and inflammation.

Other Approaches

Stress management. Stress definitely makes dandruff worse. See Part 2 for anti-stress tips.

Vinegar or lemon juice. Rinse your hair with 1/4 cup of either of these acidic liquids mixed with 1 cup water once a week after washing with dandruff shampoo to reduce flakes, improve your scalp's resistance to fungus, and ensure a neutral pH, which helps you resist fungal infection.

Essential oil therapy. Once a week, massage a solution of 2 to 3 drops each of lavender and rosemary essential oil mixed with 1 ounce carrier oil (almond or grapeseed) into your scalp and cover with a shower cap overnight. Wash with a medicated shampoo the next morning. These oils are antiseptic and anti-inflammatory.

Prevention

Follow an anti-inflammatory diet. For a detailed explanation, see page 38 (in Part 2).

Limit hair products. The less gel, spray, and mousse you add to your head, the better.

Eczema

Eczema, or atopic dermatitis, might sound benign—itchy skin. But it's really your body's way of telling you that your immune system has gone into overdrive, causing inflammation and itching. Eczema is closely related to asthma (page 76) or allergies (page 72). Outbreaks are often triggered by allergens such as dust mites, food allergens, and stress.

Although most common in children (who generally outgrow it), eczema can still be a significant problem for adults. Scratching just makes things worse, leading to swelling, cracking, and "oozing," and eventually resulting in crusty, scabby skin.

Do This Now

When a flare hits, start with these steps.

1. Begin using a prescribed corticosteroid treatment, or, if you don't have a prescription, use an over-the-counter hydrocortisone cream as directed.

2. Take a Claritin or a dose of Benadryl.

3. Fill the tub with lukewarm water and add 1 or 2 packages of Aveeno or 1 to 3 tablespoons oatmeal wrapped in a cheesecloth to the tub as it's filling. Take a soak.

Why It Works

Whether in a cream, lotion, ointment, gel, spray, foam, oil, or even impregnated tape, topical steroids are the first-line treatment for eczema. They work by suppressing the immune system, dampening inflammation. There are seven classes, ranging from weakest to strongest. Using the lowest effective dose is important because even topical steroids can lead to serious side effects, including thinning of the skin and possibly adrenal suppression.

To reduce the amount you use, ask your doctor if you can use it just once a day; there's some evidence that once-a-day application may be just as effective as the more commonly prescribed twice-a-day. Also ask your doctor about combining a topical steroid with a cream that contains retinoids, a form of vitamin A. A few studies have found that this combination is not only slightly better at reducing inflammation, but that retinoids, which are strong antioxidants, may reduce the risk of skin thinning.

Because eczema is an allergic reaction, we recommend antihistamines. They help quell the reaction by neutralizing inflammatory chemicals called histamines. Don't take a product that also contains a decongestant unless you also have significant nasal congestion; decongestants are drying and will make the itching worse.

The bath with oatmeal helps relieve itching and inflammation thanks to gelatin-like carbo-

❦ Helpful Hint

How Much Cream Is Enough?

Wondering how much cream or ointment to use to soothe your child's itchy skin? Try the fingertip unit (FTU) measurement. The tip of your index finger to the first joint is one FTU. It generally takes one FTU to cover the hand or groin; two for the face or foot; three for an arm; six for the leg; and 14 for the trunk. Always use the least amount possible.

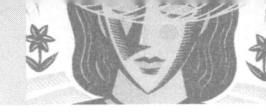

hydrates in oatmeal (which make it sticky) that moisten and soothe the skin.

Other Medicines
Herbs and Supplements

Licorice (*Glycyrrhiza glabra*) gel 2%. This anti-inflammatory gel, available in health food stores, is often used for skin conditions. Although there are few studies on its use for eczema, one study on 30 patients found that using it for two weeks improved redness, swelling, and itching.

Chamomile cream. Chamomile acts as an anti-inflammatory. Studies comparing the cream to topical hydrocortisone find it works just as well, if not better, in relieving symptoms. It is often used on a daily, long-term basis to prevent flares because it has no side effects (as long as you're not allergic to chamomile). One brand that's been studied in clinical trials is CamoCare.

St. John's wort cream. St. John's wort has both anti-inflammatory and antibacterial properties, which is why a group of German researchers decided to test its effects on eczema. Their study found that an extract standardized to 1.5% hyperforin was significantly better at treating the eczema of 21 patients than a placebo. The participants used the cream twice a day for four weeks. The skin treated with the cream also had less bacteria, which means less risk of secondary infection.

Probiotics. Several studies find these supplements can improve eczema symptoms in children, even infants. Researchers suspect they work by making the gut less "leaky," preventing large proteins that may trigger allergic reactions from leaking through. The usual dose is 1 or 2 capsules with meals for adults; half that for children 70 to 100 pounds, one-quarter the adult dose for children 50 to 70 pounds. Ask your doctor for the correct dosage for children under 50 pounds or less than six years old.

Ginkgo. Although there are no studies available on its use in treating eczema, the flavonoids in this herb block activation of a chemical that contributes to allergic responses. Take 120 milligrams twice a day. Use a standardized extract that contains 24% flavonoglycosides and 6% terpene lactones. You can take ginkgo on a daily basis or as needed to prevent flares.

Over-the-Counter Drugs

Coal tar. This old-fashioned therapy comes in many forms, including creams, gels, lotions, and salves. Although coal tar can be messy and smelly, it does work well for some people without the side effects of steroids. Follow package directions or your doctor's orders on dosage and frequency. Note that coal tar may stain the skin. The stain will disappear if you stop using the coal tar.

Prescription Drugs

Steroids. If your symptoms don't improve after treatment with a topical steroid, your doctor may prescribe an oral steroid such as prednisone. These drugs may have side effects if used long-term, however.

Immune modulators. These drugs, which include Elidel (pimecrolimus) and Protopic (tacrolimus), are the newest treatments for eczema. They work by suppressing the abnormal immune reaction in the skin. Because they're nonsteroidal, many doctors were quite excited when they first came on the market, thinking they could be used long-term to control flares with minimal side effects. But animal studies now find they increase the risk of cancer, so the FDA has placed strong warnings on them. They can be used for no more than six weeks, only in children older than two, and only after all other therapies have failed.

Other Approaches

Allergy shots. If your eczema flares are related to specific triggers, allergy shots, which slowly train your immune system to accept the allergen without reacting, might help.

Phototherapy. Ultraviolet (UV) therapy, in which you are exposed to bands of light, is being used more often to treat eczema, with studies finding good results. Don't try to self-treat by getting out in the sun, however; specific forms of light must be used, and you should be carefully monitored to avoid overexposure.

Mind-body therapies. The evidence is clear that stress can trigger eczema flares. One study found that about half of all cases of eczema are related to stress, and that people with eczema have higher levels of anxiety than those without. Various stress-reducing therapies, either used alone or with medical treatments, have been studied for eczema, including massage therapy, biofeedback, relaxation training, cognitive-behavioral therapy, and hypnosis, with varying benefits.

One well-designed clinical study compared four treatments—education about the condition, deep breathing, cognitive-behavioral therapy designed to help participants cope better with stress, and a combination of education and cognitive-behavioral therapy—with standard medical care. After a year, researchers found the psychological treatments—the cognitive-behavioral therapy and deep breathing—improved the skin condition significantly more than either the education alone or medical treatment.

Prevention

Supplement with omega-3 fatty acids. There's some thought that eczema may be the result of an inability to properly break down and use essential fatty acids, which are key to controlling inflammation. Some studies find that supplementing with high doses of omega-3 fatty acids can improve eczema. Start with 1 to 3 grams a day of fish oil or primrose oil. If you don't see an improvement in two to three months, talk to your health-care provider about increasing the dosage (up to 8 grams a day) or switching brands.

Reduce your exposure to allergens. Talk to an allergist about how to reduce your exposure to your allergy triggers.

Be careful about bathing. Stick with lukewarm water when bathing or showering. Very hot water is drying and will make the itching worse. Use soaps that don't contain perfumes or dyes.

Eczema and Food Allergies

Food allergies and eczema are strongly linked. In fact, more cases of eczema may be caused by food allergy than we previously thought. So try cutting out common food allergens one at a time through an elimination diet to see if your condition improves.

There are three types of elimination diets: eliminating one or several foods suspected of causing the symptoms, eliminating all but a defined group of "allowed" foods, and following a diet of liquid nutrients. Start with the first type. Eliminate one food at a time for at least two weeks. Start with wheat, including all gluten-containing grains such as oats, rye, and barley, then move on to dairy and nuts, followed by citrus, soy, eggs, and, finally, shellfish. If you have a flare during that time, add the food back and eliminate another.

If you go without a flare during that time, eliminate the food from your diet for at least several months. If you add the food back, do it slowly. If you have a severe reaction when you do, you should probably cut it out of your diet permanently.

Slather on the right moisturizer. After you get out of the shower or bath, pat, don't rub, your skin dry. Then apply a thick, rich moisturizing cream (Eucerin, Cetaphil, or Vanicream work well). Studies find this can reduce the risk of a flare. Buy the largest bottle you can find; you will be using a lot. You can even use vegetable shortening or petroleum jelly in a pinch if you have to, but these don't nourish the skin as well as some of the specially prepared products. They seem to work by preserving the outer skin layer, reducing susceptibility to irritants. Allow your skin to completely absorb the moisturizer before dressing. Avoid water-based lotions—look for a product that comes in a tub.

Topical corticosteroids. Although many patients (and their doctors) are loath to use corticosteroids on a daily basis to prevent eczema flares, there's a way to use significantly less and still get good results. Research shows that mixing a strong steroid like fluticasone propionate cream with bath oil (like baby oil) and applying twice a day to the areas that usually get the rash can significantly reduce the risk of flares with no negative side effects.

In one study, those using the cream had an average of 16 weeks until a relapse, compared to six weeks for those who used the placebo. You can mix the medicine into creams or lotions, too, such as Eucerin, Cetaphil, or Vanicream.

Hives

The red, itchy rash of hives occurs when histamine is released in response to an allergen (such as certain foods, penicillin, latex, or bee stings), an infection, parasites, or viral hepatitis. If you develop hives around your eyes or in your mouth, seek emergency medical help.

Do This Now

To soothe the itching and prevent infection, avoid the urge to scratch, and follow these steps.

1. Take 2 to 3 freeze-dried nettle capsules. Repeat with 1 to 3 capsules three to four times a day over the next 24 to 48 hours.

2. Take a cool bath in which you've sprinkled one or two packets of Aveeno and 2 cups concentrated chamomile tea. To make the tea, steep two handfuls of loose chamomile tea in 2 cups boiling water for 15 minutes. Strain.

3. If the hives are on a small part of your body, instead of the bath, add 20 to 30 drops of lavender oil to cold water, dip a clean cloth into it, and apply for up to 20 minutes.

4. Follow with an application of calamine or Eurax lotion.

5. Still itching? Take 50 milligrams of Benadryl and repeat in 30 minutes if necessary.

Why It Works

Nettle contains a compound called quercetin, which prevents the release of histamines and other inflammatory chemicals. The cool bath relieves itching and inflammation, thanks to the soothing oatmeal and the anti-inflammatory chamomile tea. Lavender also combats inflammation.

Calamine lotion, a zinc-based formula, soothes itching and has a mild antibacterial action. Eurax contains hydrocortisone, to reduce inflammation, and crotamiton, which relieves itching. Benadryl neutralizes histamines.

Other Medicines

Corticosteroids. These immune suppressors are sometimes used for a short time in severe cases.

Antihistamines. Zyrtec or Clarinex contain the same active ingredients as their over-the-counter cousins but last longer.

Epinephrine pen. These are used in cases of life-threatening allergies to reverse the reaction.

H_2 blockers. These drugs, including prescription and over-the-counter versions of Tagamet (cimetidine), Zantac (ranitidine), and Pepcid (famotidine), block a different form of histamine than Benadryl and other antihistamines do, so they're sometimes used for drug-resistant hives.

Other Approaches

Mind-body therapies. One study found listening to Mozart reduced hives in patients who were allergic to latex. Another study in young children found hypnosis relieved itching and reduced recurrences over the next 5 to 14 months.

Prevention

Avoid trigger foods. Hives are often related to a food allergy. Consider an allergy elimination diet as described in Eczema on page 200. Also watch out for spices and food additives (like tartrazine and sulfites), fermented cheeses, and cured meats.

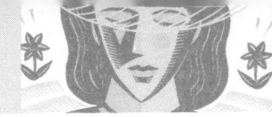

Poison Ivy

Between 50 and 70 percent of people are allergic to the plant oil urushiol, found in poison ivy, oak, and sumac. Brushing against any part of these plants can lead to a severe rash that can last for two or three weeks.

Do This Now

To reduce the allergic reaction and soothe the itch, follow this advice.

1. Immediately wash the affected area with Zanfel Poison Ivy Wash or Tecnu Extreme Poison Ivy Scrub. In a pinch, soap and water will do.

2. Apply cool compresses that have been soaked in 4 ounces water with 5 drops chamomile oil and 5 drops lavender oil.

3. For larger areas, soak in a cool bath in which you've sprinkled 1 or 2 packets of Aveeno. Also add 2 cups concentrated chamomile tea made with 2 handfuls loose chamomile tea steeped in 2 cups boiling water for 15 minutes, then strained and cooled.

4. After the bath, mix calamine and Benadryl lotions and spread on the itchy areas.

5. For severe itching, take an oral antihistamine like Claritin or Benadryl.

Why It Works

Zanfel and Tecnu are specially formulated to remove urushiol. Chamomile oil and lavender oil both have anti-inflammatory properties to soothe the itching.

The cool bath with oatmeal helps relieve itching and inflammation, thanks to gelatin-like carbohydrates in oatmeal that soothe the skin.

Calamine lotion is a zinc-based formula that soothes itching and has a mild antibacterial action to prevent infection. Benadryl, whether taken orally or used on the skin in gel form, works to block the action of inflammatory chemicals called histamines.

Other Medicines

Nettle. Take 2 to 3 freeze-dried nettle capsules immediately. Repeat with 1 to 3 capsules three to four times a day over the next 24 to 48 hours. Nettle leaves contain quercetin, and act as natural antihistamines.

Hydrocortisone 1%. Start with this low level of topical steroid to control the itching and rash. If that doesn't work, talk to your doctor about stronger prescription creams or, in severe cases, oral corticosteroids.

Other Approaches

Homeopathy. Use 12X or 6X preparations of *Rhus tox*, a homeopathic preparation made from the resin of poison ivy, every hour for two hours after exposure and then four times a day until symptoms respond. Stop if symptoms or rash gets worse.

Prevention

Wear long pants and a long-sleeved shirt anytime you may be near poisonous plants.

Apply IvyBlock. This cream contains a clay that blocks absorption of urushiol.

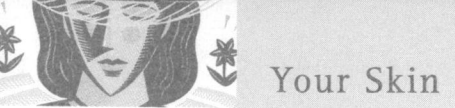

Psoriasis

Like eczema, psoriasis results from a problem with the immune system that leads to chronic inflammation. It often runs in families, which means your genes may be at least partly to blame. Unlike eczema, it's not related to an allergy. There are multiple forms of the disease, but the most common is plaque psoriasis, in which skin cells divide too quickly, building up into thick, scaly patches that cause pain and itching. Some people with psoriasis may have just a few scaly patches; others may have the scales on most of their body. Symptoms can persist for long stretches but can also disappear for long stretches.

As frustrating as the condition can be—and there's no cure—there is a wide variety of things you can do to reduce outbreaks and extend the length of remissions. Don't get discouraged if one thing doesn't work; go on and try another, or a combination of approaches. One important area to focus on is stress. It's clear that stress often triggers an outbreak, so pay special attention to the recommendations below, and revisit the section on stress in Part 2 on page 52.

Do This Now

Prescription topical or oral drugs, and possibly light therapy, might be required to treat the underlying condition. But for additional at-home relief:

1. Use your fingernail or tweezers to gently scrape away the heaviest scales on the plaque. Only take off the scales that come off easily—don't pull and damage the skin.

2. Once a day, soak in a warm bath to which you've added a handful of Dead Sea salt, available in health food stores and online. If you don't have Dead Sea salt, try Epsom salt.

3. After your bath, massage in just enough sesame or jojoba oil to cover the scales.

4. Apply an over-the-counter 1% hydrocortisone cream. Do this two to four times a day, applying more oil beforehand.

5. Find 15 minutes every day to sit in the sun with the affected area exposed.

Why It Works

Scraping away the scales (in other words, the dead skin) lets oils and creams penetrate the skin better. Soaking in the salty bath relieves itching and soothes inflammation (and, as a valuable side benefit, it also relaxes you). Dead Sea salts are a popular treatment for psoriasis. In fact, clinics along the Dead Sea specialize in treating psoriasis, and according to several studies, 75 percent or more of the people who go to one find significant relief after several weeks. You don't have to go to Israel for this therapy, though—your own bathtub will work.

The bathwater helps the sesame or jojoba oil penetrate the skin. In turn, the oils keep the skin moist and supple, making it easier for the hydrocortisone to penetrate. Hydrocortisone soothes the itching and flaking by dampening inflammation.

Dead Sea clinics combine soaks with plenty of sunlight exposure. We suggest sitting in the sun for 15 minutes because ultraviolet light destroys certain immune system cells in the plaques, slowing skin turnover. It's why you have fewer flares in the summer.

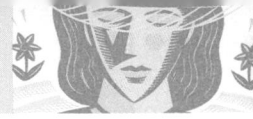

Other Medicines
Herbs and Supplements

Aloe vera cream. One study in 60 patients with mild-to-moderate psoriasis found applying a 0.05% cream three times a day five days a week for four weeks resulted in a complete remission in 85 percent of the patients, compared to just 6 percent of those using the placebo cream, with no side effects. (The patients weren't followed long-term, so there's no information on how long the remission lasted.)

Honey, beeswax, olive oil. Mix equal parts of honey, food-grade beeswax, and olive oil in a jar and smooth onto the affected area at night. Cover with plastic wrap, then hold in place with elastic bandages. One study found this mixture along with a topical corticosteroid enabled most participants to use less steroid medicine than people who used the steroid alone.

Over-the-Counter Drugs

Coal tar. This old-fashioned therapy comes in many forms, including creams, gels, lotions, and salves. Although it can be kind of messy and smelly, it works very well with no side effects. Follow package directions.

Salicylic acid cream. The cream is often used with steroids, tar, or other topical treatments because it dissolves the scales so the medicine can penetrate more deeply. A milder version of this is used on warts. You can find it in drugstores. Just smooth it on before you use the medicine.

Prescription Drugs

Topical drugs. Most cases of mild to moderate psoriasis respond to topical prescription drugs. Doctors often prescribe more than one at the same time because they target different underlying causes of the disease, enhance each other's effects, and reduce side effects. Prescription corticosteroids can lead to thinning of the skin and stretch marks, and the longer they're used, the more likely you'll become resistant to them.

- **Tazorac (tazarotene) gel and cream** is a form of vitamin A also known as a topical retinoid. It works by slowing the growth of skin cells.

- **Dovonex (calcipotriene)** is a synthetic form of vitamin D. It slows skin cell turnover, flattens lesions, and removes scales.

- **Drithocreme (anthralin)** is a synthetic form of chrysarobin, found in Goa powder from the bark of the araroba tree of South America, which has been used as a psoriasis treatment for more than 100 years. It slows the growth of skin cells, and is often prescribed with a steroid cream to reduce skin irritation.

Systemic drugs. If you have severe psoriasis, your doctor may prescribe methotrexate, Soriatane (acitretin), cyclosporine, or immune modulators (Amevive, Enbrel, or Raptiva) to suppress the immune system. These can have very serious side effects, however. Cyclosporine, for instance, may cause high blood pressure and kidney damage; while methotrexate (also used as a chemotherapy drug) can cause liver damage. Methotrexate is used only if no other drug works. Soriatane, similar to the acne drug Accutane, can raise cholesterol levels and may cause liver and bone problems. All of these drugs are reserved for only the most serious cases.

Other Approaches

Phototherapy. This treatment uses ultraviolet light to treat the disease, either in a doctor's office or with a special light at home. The light is directed just to the affected area, and other parts

WARNING

Certain medicines can make psoriasis worse or trigger a flare, including lithium, beta-blockers, and nonsteroidal anti-inflammatory drugs (NSAIDs), as well as some medications for malaria. Make sure your doctor knows you have psoriasis before filling any prescription.

of your body are protected during therapy. During medical phototherapy, you may need to take psoralen, a medication that enhances light's effects. While actual phototherapy can take weeks to have an effect, even a few minutes a day in the sun helps with less serious outbreaks.

Mind-body therapies. Studies find that one-third of psoriasis outbreaks are stress related, making this condition ideal for relaxation techniques. Specifically, studies show some benefits from individual and group psychotherapy, meditation, and hypnosis. One study found patients who used meditation-based relaxation tapes during phototherapy healed faster than those who didn't use the tapes. A study using hypnosis in 11 people found their skin improved more than those only taught to relax.

Prevention

Bathe in lukewarm water. Skip steaming showers and baths; they're too drying. Instead, soak in a lukewarm bath to which you've added 1 tablespoon jojoba or sesame oil to moisturize skin. Alternate soaks with Dead Sea salts. Use soaps that don't contain perfumes or dyes. Pat, don't rub, your skin dry after bathing.

Slather on a heavy-duty moisturizer. Buy a large jar of heavy moisturizer for sensitive skin (no additives or perfumes) and use after bathing and several times a day. Good brands include Eucerin and Cetaphil.

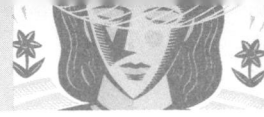

Rosacea

It might look a little like acne, but rosacea is a different condition altogether—one that usually strikes adults over 30, often those with fair skin. Symptoms include flushed, pimply, thickened facial skin, watery eyes, and visible blood vessels, and they typically get worse without treatment.

Although we don't know what causes rosacea, there's some evidence that food sensitivities, inflammatory disorders, and *H. pylori* (the bacterium that causes ulcers) may play a role. Anything that causes your face to flush—including menopausal hot flashes and humid weather—can also set off a flare.

There's no cure, but you and your doctor can do plenty to minimize symptoms and keep them from recurring.

Do This Now

When you're having a flare, take these steps to cool the heat and stop the sting.

1. Soak a washcloth in cool water to which you've added 5 drops rose, lavender, and chamomile oils. Place over your face for 10 minutes several times a day.

2. As you rest with the washcloth over your face, breathe deeply and slowly, filling your abdomen with each breath, and exhaling through your mouth.

Why It Works

The cool compress constricts blood vessels that cause flushing, reducing redness. The herbs, especially chamomile, are traditionally used to soothe skin inflammation and irritation.

Deep breathing reduces stress, a major trigger for rosacea. If you calm yourself down quickly enough, you might even be able to halt the flare.

Other Medicines
Herbs and Supplements

Digestive enzymes. For some reason, these enzymes appear to help with rosacea. When researchers gave 21 rosacea patients pancreatic enzymes—a type of digestive enzyme—with meals, their condition improved. This remedy seems to work best in people who experience stomach upset—gas, bloating, diarrhea, and/or constipation—along with the typical symptoms of rosacea.

There are several possible explanations for why these enzymes work; most are based on the idea that people with rosacea don't make enough stomach acid. This in turn can encourage the growth of *H. pylori* (which is suppressed by stomach acid) or perhaps allergic reactions triggered by the incomplete digestion of proteins (digestive enzymes break down food). We also know that digestive enzymes decrease inflammation, which is present with rosacea.

Hydrochloric acid. This supplement normalizes stomach acid levels. Take with meals if you have excessive gas, chronic diarrhea, and/or constipation along with rosacea symptoms. Follow the directions on the bottle.

Fish oil. Because rosacea is an inflammatory condition, fish oil supplements—which fight inflammation throughout the body—may help. Take 1,500 milligrams twice a day. Fish oil has multiple benefits—it will also help protect you against heart disease, for instance.

Prescription Drugs

MetroGel, MetroLotion (metronidazole). The first topical therapy approved for rosacea, this drug controls rosacea through its anti-inflammatory properties, not by killing germs, even though it's an antibacterial. One study of 90 patients found 76 of those using topical metronidazole for eight weeks had less redness and flushing than a control group.

Azelex (azelaic acid). If metronidazole doesn't work, azelaic acid may. Studies find it significantly reduces the number of skin lesions. Like metronidazole, it probably controls rosacea through its anti-inflammatory properties, but we don't know for sure. Because azelaic acid can cause mild stinging, burning, and dry skin, try metronidazole first.

Accutane or Roaccutane (isotretinoin). Studies show this oral retinoid—a form of vitamin A—can quickly bring rosacea under control, probably through its anti-inflammatory mechanisms. Because it poses side effects such as sun sensitivity and birth defects in women who are pregnant or may become pregnant, it shouldn't be used for more than two weeks.

Other Approaches

Lasers. A dermatologist or plastic surgeon uses lasers to target enlarged blood vessels just under the skin. The laser's heat builds in the blood vessel, causing it to disintegrate. You'll need at least three treatments to see results.

Makeup. Although it won't reduce rosacea, makeup—especially green-tinted foundation—can hide it. Keep in mind that the wrong type of makeup, however, can aggravate rosacea. Choose water-soluble makeup with few preservatives and no fragrances. If you're using topical medications, wait 10 minutes after using before applying makeup.

Gentle skin care. Gently cleanse your face each morning using a moisturizing, foaming cleanser that is not grainy or abrasive. Rinse your face with lukewarm water, then gently blot dry. Let your face totally air-dry before applying any topical medications. Don't use glycolic acid, alcohol, astringents, or exfoliant facial cleansers and toners, all of which further irritate skin.

Prevention

Avoid alcohol, spicy foods, and hot liquids. All of them can contribute to facial flushing.

Stay cool. Heat and humidity can make rosacea worse. Use air conditioning, avoid hot stoves (an excuse to order out!), and skip the hot tub and sauna.

Slather on the sunscreen. Wear UVA and UVB sunscreen with an SPF of 15 or higher (at least 30 if you're going to be outside for any length of time), and try a stronger sunblock with zinc oxide for your nose and ears. Also wear a hat that protects your face. Dry, cold, windy weather can lead to windburn and facial chapping, which aggravates rosacea, so wear sunscreen even during the winter.

Avoid stress. Anger, frustration, and embarrassment can literally make you "red in the face." Practice yoga, meditation, deep breathing, or some other form of relaxation regularly.

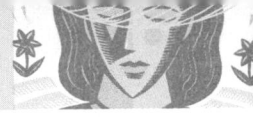

Shingles

If you've ever had chicken pox as a kid, you're susceptible to shingles as an adult. After a case of the chicken pox, the virus that causes it, called varicella zoster, hibernates in your nerve endings—usually forever. But sometimes the virus "reawakens" decades later, causing a painful, blistery condition called shingles.

While most adults harbor the varicella zoster virus, only about 500,000 people a year develop shingles, most of them elderly. Researchers are pretty sure the outbreaks are related to an immune system weakened by chronic disease, stress, major depression, or sleep problems, among other factors. Preventing recurrences, then, means addressing these aspects of health head-on to keep your immune system strong.

It's critical to treat the first sign of shingles with antiviral drugs to avoid the more serious condition called postherpetic neuralgia, which results from virus-damaged nerves.

Do This Now

At the first sign of shingles (an itching or tingling sensation followed by a rash), do the following.

1. See your doctor for an antiviral medication such as acyclovir or famciclovir.

2. Take 500 to 1,000 milligrams Tylenol along with 400 milligrams ibuprofen up to two to three times a day.

3. Soak in a warm (not hot) bath to which you've added 1/4 cup baking soda or one brimming handful of dried milk powder or Aveeno. Soak for 15 to 20 minutes, then shower off and pat—don't rub—skin dry.

4. Apply aloe vera ointment to the affected skin.

5. On top of the aloe, apply calamine lotion.

6. Cover any open sores with a clean sterile dressing such as a Telfa pad.

7. Once a day, remove the dressing and clean the area with water and gentle soap. Then repeat Steps 4 through 6.

8. Stay away from very young children and immune-compromised people.

Why It Works

Studies find that antiviral therapy can significantly reduce the severity of shingles and prevent postherpetic neuralgia, but fast action is key—you need to start the drugs within 72 hours of the outbreak. You can recognize a shingles rash because the blisters usually form a swath or band on one side of the body.

The Tylenol and ibuprofen help with pain; studies find that taking both at the same time provides more pain relief than taking either separately.

The warm bath with added skin-soothers immediately helps with itching and inflammation.

The aloe and calamine lotion hit shingles with a one-two punch: The aloe jump-starts the healing process; the calamine dries up the area and forms a barrier to seal off blisters from the air, which helps with the pain. Covering blisters with a sterile dressing helps prevent infection. Telfa pads are especially good because they don't stick to the wound when you change them.

Shingles itself isn't contagious, but kids and adults who've never had chicken pox can catch it from you when you have shingles.

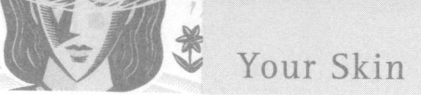

Other Medicines

Herbs and Supplements

St. John's wort cream. St. John's wort cream is a traditional treatment for nerve pain and burns. Since the blisters of shingles are similar to burn blisters, it also works well for this condition, and its antiviral properties may help keep the virus in check.

Lemon balm ointment. If you're having no success with the other creams mentioned here, try lemon balm ointment. Test tube studies suggest that this herb prevents the herpes virus from attaching to cells, thus blocking its ability to replicate. Although there haven't been any studies on its use for shingles, the virus that causes herpes and the one that causes shingles are very similar.

Over-the-Counter Drugs

Capsaicin cream/ointment 0.025% or 0.075%. Capsaicin is the chemical that gives hot peppers their heat. It works by depleting a chemical called substance P from the nerves in the skin, short-circuiting the transmission of pain signals from the nerves to the brain. Apply it at least three to four times a day. Initially, you may feel some burning, but that fades fairly quickly. Make sure you wash your hands well after using and don't use on broken skin or blisters. Use regularly for at least two weeks—it takes a while to begin working.

Prescription Drugs

In addition to antiviral drugs that inhibit the virus, these drugs can help with pain:

- **Lidocaine patch (5%).** Applying to the skin over the most painful area for two weeks significantly reduces the pain. But it can only be used on intact skin; if you have blisters or open sores, you'll need to try other options.

- **Anticonvulsants** such as Neurontin (gabapentin) and Depakote (divalproex) are often prescribed for the chronic nerve pain of postherpetic neuralgia, even though they're not officially approved for that purpose.

- **Tricyclic antidepressants** such as Elavil (amitriptyline) and nortriptyline are very effective at relieving the pain of postherpetic neuralgia. They're usually taken in much smaller doses than you'd take for depression.

Other Approaches

Hypnosis. Several published reports find that hypnosis can reduce the pain of shingles and postherpetic neuralgia.

Epidural infusions. For very severe pain, an anesthetic can be infused directly into the part of the spinal cord responsible for that particular nerve branch. As well as providing immediate relief, it also helps the pain go away faster.

Peppermint oil. If there are no open sores, mix 10 drops peppermint oil with 30 to 40 drops massage oil and rub into the affected area. The menthol in peppermint interferes with the ability of the nerves to transmit pain signals to the brain.

Prevention

Get sleep and manage stress. These steps will help keep your immune system strong.

Treat any chronic health conditions.

T'ai chi. This Eastern practice combines meditation and gentle exercise, both of which have been found to positively affect the immune system. One study of 36 elderly people at risk of developing shingles found those who took three 45-minute t'ai chi classes a week for 15 weeks showed a significant increase in immune system cells that keep the shingles virus in check compared to a control group.

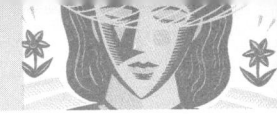

Sunburn

Who among us hasn't come in from a day at the beach bright red? Putting aside the fact that overexposure to the sun can increase your risk of skin cancer and age your skin, there's still the sting, burn, and eventual itch to contend with. The trick is to cool the heat, stop the inflammation that causes the itch—and remember to wear plenty of sunblock the next time.

Do This Now

When you're hot to the touch, follow these steps.

1. Soak in a cool bath to which you've added 2 cups calendula tea, black tea, or green tea (use two to four times the normal amount of tea leaves or bags to make a cup of tea), 15 drops lavender oil, and 3 tablespoons oatmeal tied up in muslin, or 1 to 2 packages of Aveeno. If the burn is on your face, add the same ingredients in one third or one quarter the amount to a large bowl of cool water, soak a cloth in the liquid, and apply the cloth for several minutes.

2. Apply undiluted lavender essential oil directly to the burned area.

3. Follow with an application of the sap from an aloe vera leaf. If you don't have an aloe plant, use 100% aloe vera cream or lotion without fixatives.

⁓ What About...

Ice?

Never ice a burn. The ice can further injure already damaged skin.

4. Take 500 to 1,000 milligrams Tylenol or 400 milligrams ibuprofen.

Why It Works

Cool water soothes raw, hot areas and rehydrates the skin. The ingredients you've added to your bath deliver extra benefits: lavender oil, calendula, and tea reduce inflammation that contributes to itching, and the oatmeal or Aveeno soothes itching and also reduces inflammation.

Dabbing on lavender oil after your bath provides a strong dose of this anti-inflammatory herb.

Aloe has long been used to soothe burns. It has ingredients that help with healing and pain relief and counter inflammation. Only use the salve or cream, not the gel, which can be drying.

Tylenol helps with the pain, as does the ibuprofen, which also counters inflammation.

Other Medicines

St. John's wort, calendula, and/or comfrey ointments. You can buy salves, creams or ointments containing these soothing ingredients. To boost the effect, mix 1 drop lavender and 1 drop chamomile oils into a small amount, then apply and cover with a bandage or Telfa pad.

Witch hazel 10% solution. Add 5 to 10 drops of lavender oil per ounce of witch hazel and apply. Cold witch hazel is even more soothing.

Other Approaches

Plain yogurt. Apply to the skin for 15 or 20 minutes of cooling relief, then rinse with cool water and apply an ointment as described earlier.

Varicose Veins

You know how an old, weak rubber band loses its snap? The same thing can happen to veins. In healthy veins, blood flows only one way—toward the heart. That means blood in the leg veins has to fight gravity to get where it needs to go. It does it thanks in part to tiny valves that close off the vein when blood tries to flow "backward." But in veins that have been weakened over time, these valves can give way, letting blood pool in the legs. This pooling results in bulging veins and painful swelling, itching, and leg heaviness. Eventually a buildup of pressure in the veins can cause fluid to leak out into the spaces between cells, triggering swelling of the leg and changes in skin pigmentation.

Varicose veins are not only unsightly and uncomfortable, they can lead to inflammation of the vein (phlebitis) or open sores (skin ulcers) on the leg, caused when the skin is deprived of blood. They can even increase the risk of a blood clot in the leg, which can break loose and travel to your lungs or brain.

Although you may have heard about surgical and other medical treatments for varicose veins, some of the simplest remedies, such as compression stockings, often work the best.

TIME TO WORRY

- If one leg swells or is painful when you walk or flex your foot—this could be a sign of a blood clot.
- If you have a lump in the leg, superficial redness, or heat—this could be a sign of phlebitis.
- If you have severe swelling in both legs at the same time—this could be a sign of heart or kidney disease.

Do This Now

If the varicose veins in your legs are painful and/or swollen, do the following now.

1. Put on elastic or compression stockings (available in medical supply stores). Make sure they fit properly and don't bind at the knee, which can make things worse. If your swelling is minor, you might be able to get away with support hose instead.

2. Sit or lie down and elevate your feet above your heart for about 20 minutes. If you can't get off your feet and you have to stand in one place, move your legs around as much as possible to keep the blood flowing.

3. After elevating your feet, go for a walk.

4. Mix 5 drops rosemary, peppermint, and juniper essential oil with 20 drops massage oil and massage into your legs.

Why It Works

Compression stockings force blood back to the heart and reduce fluid leakage from veins. Most people need stockings with a compression of 30 to 40 mm/Hg. Ask your doctor for a prescription; insurance usually covers the cost.

Elevating your feet uses gravity to return blood to the heart, reducing swelling and pain. Walking improves blood flow and pushes the blood in your legs back up to your heart. It's particularly important after a long airplane flight to prevent excess swelling and blood clots.

Rosemary and peppermint oil stimulate blood circulation, while the juniper oil helps relieve that feeling of heaviness.

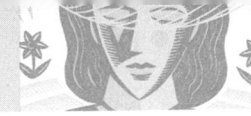

Other Medicines
Herbs and Supplements

Horse chestnut. If you only take one supplement for varicose veins, this is the one to take, hands-down. Numerous studies find that it can reduce swelling in the lower legs. It's thought to work by blocking inflammation and improving the strength of veins. Compounds in horse chestnut also thin blood so it can flow more easily out of veins into capillaries, preventing clots. Take 300 milligrams of horse chestnut extract standardized to 50 milligrams aescin twice a day. A good brand is Venastat.

Flavonoids. Flavonoids such as rutin or quercetin (sold as citrus flavonoids), pycnogenol, and grapeseed strengthen blood vessels, preventing fluid leakage. In numerous studies a flavonoid product called Daflon significantly improved the overall health of blood vessels in the legs and helped leg ulcers heal. Daflon isn't available in the United States, but you can get similar results by taking 500 milligrams citrus flavonoids, 50 milligrams pycnogenol, or 100 milligrams grapeseed extract twice a day.

Gotu kola. This tropical herb is well studied as a treatment for varicose veins. One study comparing it to placebo in 94 patients found it significantly improved symptoms, including heaviness in the lower limbs and swelling. It also improves vein strength and the veins' ability to stretch—important in preventing vein "sagging" that contributes to fluid leakage. Take 60 milligrams of a standardized extract once or twice a day.

Bilberry. This fruit, extremely high in antioxidants, improves the integrity of blood vessels and helps prevent fluid leakage. Take 160 to 480 milligrams a day of an extract standardized to 25% anthocyanidins in two or three divided doses.

Other Approaches

Sclerotherapy. This is one of the most common medical treatments for varicose veins. A substance such as salt water or a foaming agent is injected into the vein, ultimately destroying it. It works best in smaller veins.

Laser and pulsed light therapy. This is used primarily for small, more superficial veins when sclerotherapy isn't an option. The laser heats the hemoglobin in the blood vessel, injuring the blood vessel wall and destroying the vein. Several sessions are usually required.

Surgery. Many surgical techniques are available, including "stripping" the vein out of the leg, or destroying the path of blood to the vein so it dies.

Low-salt diet. Excess sodium leads to fluid retention, which makes swelling worse.

Prevention

Increase the amount of flavonoid-rich fruits and vegetables in your diet to strengthen blood vessel walls.

Don't just stand there. Sit instead. Standing on your feet all day significantly increases your risk of developing varicose veins.

Control your weight. Extra pounds put extra pressure on your legs and leg veins.

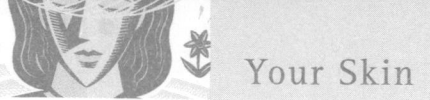

Warts

The same family of viruses responsible for cervical cancer also causes warts. Luckily, warts are much less dangerous. You don't *have* to treat them; studies find that about 20 percent disappear without treatment within six months, and 65 percent vanish within two years.

Of course, most people don't want to wait that long, so they often turn to some form of treatment, usually topical wart solutions that "burn" the wart away. These are fine, but our combination of essential oils and a common household product work just as well or better.

Because warts are linked so closely to the immune system (if it's weakened in any way, the virus can gain the upper hand), review our tips for strengthening the immune system (see Super Threat #5 on page 58).

Do This Now

Although nothing works quickly to remove a wart (except surgery), these remedies should eventually help and should be your first steps.

1. Soak the wart in warm water for 15 minutes before using any remedy.

2. Now apply 1 drop tea tree, lemon, clove, or thyme essential oil diluted with 1 drop carrier oil (like almond oil). Reapply every 24 hours.

3. Cut a piece of duct tape slightly bigger than the wart and cover the wart with it. Change the tape every day and reapply the essential oil before you put the tape over it. Make sure the piece of duct tape is large enough so it sticks to the non-oily skin.

Why It Works

Soaking the wart softens it so other remedies can work better. The essential oils contain compounds that fight viruses. As for the duct tape, it's surprisingly and amazingly effective. A study in 61 people with warts found that using duct tape for two months worked better than freezing the wart with liquid nitrogen every day for two to three weeks, with the wart disappearing in 85 percent of those who used duct tape (usually within a month) compared to 60 percent of those who used the liquid nitrogen. The duct tape might cause minor skin irritation, but trust us, that's nothing compared to the pain of liquid nitrogen therapy. In fact, the skin irritation may be why the duct tape treatment works—it triggers an immune-system reaction that finally rids the body of the wart.

Other Medicines
Herbs and Supplements

Garlic. Although the evidence is only anecdotal, garlic, which has strong antiviral properties, is a commonly used folk remedy. Don't

TIME TO WORRY

- If your warts are red, swollen, and filled with pus. They're likely infected and need medical attention.

- If warts suddenly appear in large numbers. This implies something is significantly wrong with your immune system.

- If you have warts on your feet or legs that require treatment and you have diabetes or a suppressed immune system.

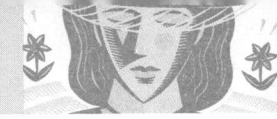

use on your face or genitals, however, because the juice can irritate or even burn sensitive skin. In fact, you should rub olive or massage oil on the skin around the wart to protect it from the garlic oil. There are several ways to use garlic on warts:

- Place a thin slice over the wart and cover with a bandage or duct tape for several hours (no longer than 24 hours).

- Rub a cut half on the wart, then cover.

- Apply a liquid extract of garlic.

Over-the-Counter Drugs

Salicylic acid. Over-the-counter preparations like Compound W that contain salicylic acid literally dissolve the wart. Make sure you soak the wart for 10 to 15 minutes before every application to soften it so the medicine can work. Every couple of days, carefully pare away the peeling tissue by rubbing it with a pumice stone or emery board. While it may take weeks or even months to totally remove the wart, it won't leave a scar and is very safe. If an over-the-counter approach doesn't work, see your doctor for prescription-strength solutions.

Tagamet (cimetidine). This medication, used for peptic ulcers, can turbocharge immune system cells that fight the wart virus. Anecdotal reports, as well as several studies in children and adults, find it can be quite effective. Take the recommended over-the-counter dose.

Other Approaches

Hypnosis. The mind has incredible powers to rid the body of warts. One study comparing hypnosis, placebo, and salicylic acid treatments

WARNING

Warts can spread, so cover existing warts with a bandage or tape. And don't share towels, razors, or fingernail clippers with people who have warts. If you're prone to warts, clean such equipment regularly.

found that people who underwent hypnosis lost more warts than those who used salicylic acid or a placebo. It appears that hypnosis and the closely related therapy of guided imagery help spur the immune system to better fight off the virus. You can find a practitioner who is trained in medical hypnosis online at the American Psychotherapy and Medical Hypnosis Association at http://apmha.com/page2.htm.

Cryotherapy. In this procedure, the physician "burns off" the wart by freezing it with liquid nitrogen. However, several sessions may be required, and it is fairly painful (which is why it usually isn't used on children). An over-the-counter product, Wartner, also freezes warts, which are supposed to fall off about 10 days after treatment. There may still be pain or stinging.

Burning. The doctor burns the wart off using a laser or electrical cauterizing instrument. It is painful and may leave a scar.

Surgery. If your wart doesn't respond to other treatments, the doctor can scrape it away surgically. However, this often leaves scars and may spread the virus.

Immunotherapy. The wart is injected several times with candida or mumps proteins (common agents everyone has been exposed to) to stimulate a local immune response to help eliminate the wart. One study found injecting the proteins into just one wart helped eliminate others.

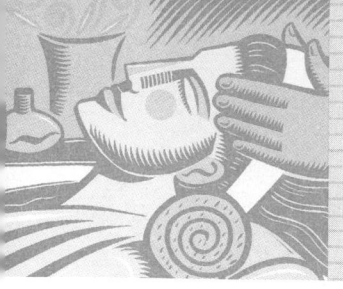

Anxiety

Our bodies have a built-in survival mechanism that swings into action when we're faced with a threat, real or perceived. That mechanism dilates our pupils, speeds our heart rate, induces sweating, and shunts blood away from our stomach to our muscles. This so-called fight-or-flight response comes in handy when we have to run away from a mugger or steer the car around a four-car pileup. It's not so handy, however, when it kicks in during the normal course of the day.

You might know this as stress, but taken to the extreme, stress becomes anxiety. If that anxiety affects your life, including work, relationships, etc., then you have an anxiety disorder. Anxiety disorders (see "Anxiety in Excess" on page 219) affect nearly one out of five people in the United States. If you have some of the symptoms, see your family doctor, who should rule out medical conditions such as thyroid and cardiac abnormalities that can mimic the signs and symptoms of a panic attack.

Do This Now

When the rapid heartbeat, shallow breathing, and claustrophobia of an anxiety attack hit, try this.

1. Place 5 to 20 drops of a tincture extract of Bach's Rescue Remedy (available in most drugstores) under your tongue several times a day, or apply 1 to 3 drops to pulse points along your wrist and throat.

2. Spend 15 minutes playing with or petting a dog or cat (if you have one or have access to one).

3. Set a timer for 5 minutes and give yourself a time-out. During that time, sit up straight and listen to the most relaxing music in your collection.

4. Place a couple of drops of lavender, jasmine, sweet orange, or geranium essential oil on a Kleenex and inhale deeply. While inhaling, breathe slowly and evenly, bringing the air into your belly, and count the length of each breath, trying to maintain an even rhythm.

Why It Works

The Bach Rescue Remedy contains a variety of flower extracts, including star-of-Bethlehem, clematis, cherry plum, impatiens, and rockrose. While the evidence in favor of it is purely anecdotal, we find it works well at soothing episodic anxiety, and it has no side effects.

Playing with a pet is amazingly soothing because pets offer the ultimate form of unconditional love. It's no surprise that studies have linked petting animals with reduced fear and anxiety.

If you don't have access to a pet, a short time-out will also work. Setting the timer helps you mentally put aside your to-do list. During this time-out, sit up straight with your shoulders back and your sternum lifted. At least one study links

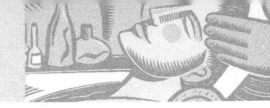

this posture with positive thinking. The posture also enables deep, relaxed breathing, which triggers the relaxation response (just the opposite of the fight-or-flight response).

Studies prove that music—particularly soft music such as classical, New Age, or nature sounds—triggers relaxation. In one study of 143 women undergoing breast biopsies, women who listened to classical music during the procedure found their anxiety levels dropped as much as women who took a prescription anti-anxiety medication.

As for the aromatherapy, your sense of smell resides in the most primitive part of your brain, the part that processes emotion. Teach yourself to associate the scent of one of these oils with your relaxing time-out and to reinforce the relaxation response.

Finally, counting your breaths helps focus your mind away from anxiety-producing worries.

Other Medicines

Herbs and Supplements

Kava. This pepper plant from the Pacific islands has been used for centuries to induce sleep and soothe anxiety. It works by affecting levels of calming chemicals in the brain. However, high doses can cause liver damage, so we don't recommend kava if you have an increased risk for liver disease (if, for example, you drink heavily or take medications that also stress the liver). Also, talk to your doctor before taking the herb, as it can interact with other herbs and prescription medication. You'll also need your doctor to monitor your liver function. The herb is not without risks, but it's less risky than most anti-anxiety drugs, which also carry a threat of liver toxicity—and addiction too.

Valerian. Various studies link use of this herb with improved sleep, often a problem when you're anxious. Take 300 to 400 milligrams of a product standardized to 0.4% valerinic acids. You'll need to take it for a couple of weeks to get the best effect.

St. John's wort. This herb is typically used for depression, but a few studies and case reports indicate it may also help reduce symptoms of obsessive-compulsive disorder and generalized anxiety disorder. For best results, take it along with the herb valerian. But talk to your doctor first because St. John's wort can interact with some prescription drugs. Take 300 milligrams of a product standardized to 0.3% hypericin or 2% to 5% hyperforin three times a day.

L-theanine. Although clinical trials have yet to find a definitive link between this amino acid and reduced anxiety, many patients report good results after taking it. As a result, L-theanine has made its way into many "calming" herbal preparations on the market. Take 200 milligrams daily.

Passionflower. In one study of 36 people with generalized anxiety disorder, those who took passionflower extract for four weeks found their anxiety improved as much as those who took the prescription medication Serax (oxazepam). Although the drug worked faster, it also had more side effects, including impaired job performance. Take 1 to 2 droppersful of a passionflower tincture three or four times a day. You can drop the tincture right in your mouth or put it in a bit of hot water and swallow.

Magnesium. When you feel anxious and your body heads into fight-or-flight mode, you use up the magnesium in your body. This can create a vicious cycle, since low magnesium levels can contribute to anxiety. Take 100 to 200 milligrams magnesium two to three times a day.

Prescription Drugs

Anxiolytics. These drugs reduce anxiety, but they also cause bothersome side effects such as memory loss, balance problems, and diminished

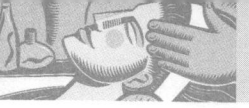

alertness in drivers. They can also lead to rebound insomnia and anxiety once you stop using them. If your doctor recommends one of these drugs, ask about starting with BuSpar (buspirone hydrochloride), which isn't as habit-forming as more well-known anxiolytics like Ativan (lorazepam), Xanax (alprazolam), and Valium (diazepam).

Antidepressants. In addition to depression, selective serotonin reuptake inhibitors (SSRIs) such as Lexapro (escitalopram) can also treat anxiety. Studies show they help up to two-thirds of people taking them for that reason.

Beta-blockers. These drugs treat heart disease by slowing the heart rate, which, of course, also helps soothe anxiety.

Other Approaches

Cognitive-behavioral therapy. This practical form of psychotherapy helps you resolve issues that make you feel anxious. You also learn how to change thoughts and beliefs that trigger anxiety and choose new ways of responding when anxiety hits. Considered one of the best treatments for generalized anxiety disorder, cognitive therapy helps more than half of people who try it.

Progressive muscle relaxation. Many studies show this simple relaxation technique—which involves systematically tensing and then relaxing your muscles, starting from your feet and working your way up to your head—reduces just about any type of anxiety, including dental phobia, test anxiety, and panic disorder. Practice it for 15 minutes twice a day for best results.

Meditation. Several studies show that various types of meditation can bring about a deeply relaxed state.

Neurofeedback. Using an EEG machine to provide feedback, this therapy teaches you to alter your brain wave patterns to reduce anxiety. During training, which can take 12 weeks or more, sensors are attached to your head. They feed information to a machine that visually depicts your brain waves. You learn what they look like when you're agitated, and what they look like when you're calm, then learn how to return to the "calm" state when you feel anxious.

Hypnosis. During hypnosis, you enter a state of deep relaxation in which you're open to affirmations and suggestions. It's especially helpful when combined with other mind-body therapies, such as cognitive-behavioral therapy. Hypnosis may also be helpful for children undergoing uncomfortable medical procedures.

Autogenic therapy. In this mind-body therapy, you enter a deeply relaxed state by focusing on creating sensations of warmth and heaviness in your arms and legs in order to reverse the blood vessel constriction and coolness in the extremities that anxiety can cause. In a study of 31 women undergoing breast lumpectomies, those practicing autogenic therapy had less anxiety and depression during and after the procedure than women who didn't. You can see a medical hypnotherapist, a stress reduction counselor, or a biofeedback therapist for this treatment.

Exercise. Aerobic exercise lifts your mood and blasts away stress, but it's best to get your workout all at once. In one study of 40 men and women, participants who walked 30 minutes a day at one time reduced their anxiety levels more than those who walked 10 minutes three times a day.

Yoga. Studies show that yoga's unique combination of stretching, strengthening, breathing, and relaxation works better than prescription drugs at reducing generalized anxiety.

T'ai chi. Participants in one study who practiced t'ai chi for 40 minutes three times a week for 12 weeks significantly reduced their blood pressure, cholesterol, and anxiety compared to study participants who didn't practice the mind-body exercise.

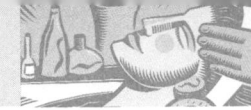

Anxiety in Excess

Everyone is anxious now and then, but some people have actual anxiety disorders. These disorders include the four below. If any of these symptoms sound familiar, make an appointment with your doctor. And take heart: The National Institute of Mental Health estimates that more than 90 percent of people with an anxiety disorder can recover.

• **Generalized anxiety disorder.** You may have this if you have excessive, uncontrollable worry about everyday things.

• **Panic disorder.** If you've had at least two panic attacks, you may have panic disorder. During a panic attack you feel intense fear along with at least four of the following symptoms: a feeling of imminent danger or doom, the need to escape, palpitations, sweating, trembling, shortness of breath or a smothering feeling, a feeling of choking, chest pain or discomfort, nausea or abdominal discomfort, dizziness or lightheaded- ness, a sense of things being unreal, a fear of losing control, a fear of dying, tingling sensations, chills or hot flushes.

• **Post-traumatic stress disorder (PTSD).** Exposure to traumas such as a serious accident, a violent crime, or natural disaster can bring on intense anxiety. You may have PTSD if you've had the following symptoms for more than one month: re-experiencing the event in the form of intrusive thoughts or dreams; avoiding activities, situations, people, and/or conversations that you associate with the trauma; a general feeling of numbness and loss of interest in your surroundings; insomnia, anxious feelings, an overactive startle response, and irritability.

• **Phobias.** You have a phobia when you have an excessive and unreasonable fear of an object or a situation. Exposure to the feared object or situation can result in a panic attack.

Acupuncture. Acupuncture increases levels of mood-boosting endorphins as well as bumping up nighttime levels of melatonin to induce sleep. In one study of 18 anxious adults, five weeks of acupuncture treatments improved sleep and significantly reduced anxiety.

Massage. The touch of another human being can be remarkably calming. For best results, ask your therapist or partner to add 15 to 20 drops of the relaxing essential oils lavender, geranium, rose, or chamomile to the massage oil.

Prevention

Limit caffeine. For the same reason it gives you energy, caffeine also makes you jumpy.

Stop drinking alcohol. Alcohol affects the brain similarly to anti-anxiety medication, inducing an initial state of calmness. But chronic alcohol consumption leads to rebound anxiety. Heavy drinking can also cause life problems (financial or relationship difficulties, for example) that create anxiety.

Stop smoking. As with alcohol, nicotine can help calm anxiety. However, it's addictive, and you'll eventually need more and more nicotine to keep anxiety levels low. Although quitting will temporally trigger anxiety, these symptoms will subside within four weeks. For more on quitting smoking, see Nicotine Addiction (page 251).

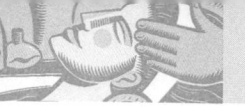

Bee Stings

Without bees we wouldn't have flowers, but a bee sting sure can put a damper on a picnic. Bees sting with a hollow stinger, through which they inject venom—the real culprit behind all the swelling and itching. For most people, a sting is just a temporary annoyance. But if you're allergic to the venom, it could turn into a life-threatening situation. People can also be allergic to hornets, wasps, and yellow jackets.

Remember, bees only sting when they feel threatened, so the best way to avoid bee stings is to leave the bees alone (and wear shoes so you don't accidentally step on one).

Do This Now

Immediately after a sting, do the following to minimize the allergic reaction and discomfort.

1. Remove the stinger as soon as possible, any way you can—scrape it away with the edge of a knife or credit card or pluck it out with your fingernail or tweezers. Just get it out fast.

2. Use your EpiPen if you've had a previous allergic reaction.

3. Take 25 to 50 milligrams oral Benadryl.

4. Apply a paste of ice water and meat tenderizer to the sting area for 10 minutes.

5. Elevate and ice the sting area for 20 minutes at a time throughout the first 24 to 48 hours.

Why It Works

The faster you remove the stinger, the less venom is released. One study (in which researchers were stung themselves) found the longer it took to remove the stinger, the larger the area of irritation, no matter how the stinger was removed. (The old advice not to pinch the stinger was based on a misconception of the anatomy of the stingers, according to the researchers.)

Only use the EpiPen if you have previously experienced a severe reaction to a sting. This shot of synthetic adrenaline (epinephrine) prevents a life-threatening allergic reaction, buying you time to get to a hospital.

For less severe allergic reactions (i.e., your arm swells but you have no trouble breathing), Benadryl stems the reaction and is the fastest-working antihistamine available. If you have a history of allergic reactions (non-life-threatening) to bee stings, take a 10-milligram Claritin with the Benadryl to provide longer coverage.

The meat tenderizer is actually papain, a plant enzyme, which helps break down the venom. If you don't have meat tenderizer but you happen to have a papaya, lay a slice over the area. If you don't have either one, apply a paste of baking soda and water to soothe the itching.

Icing and elevation reduce swelling, which causes the itching.

Other Medicines
Herbs and Supplements

Bromelain. Bromelain is plant-based enzyme like papain, and, like papain, it's an excellent anti-inflammatory. Take 500 milligrams three times a day for the first 24 to 48 hours after a sting. Look for products that contain at least 3,000 MCU/500 milligrams.

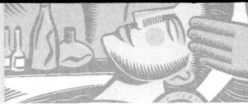

Other Approaches

Echinacea tincture. Put 1 to 2 drops directly on the sting. Most people don't realize it, but the tincture contains compounds that act as topical painkillers. Echinacea also has antiseptic and anti-inflammatory properties, so it's a great choice for bee stings.

Soothing gels. To soothe the itchy skin, smooth on some aloe vera gel or calendula, chamomile, or plantain cream. For a stronger effect, mix 10 to 20 drops of a combination of lavender, tea tree, chamomile and/or eucalyptus essential oils into 1 ounce of ointment. These oils have antiseptic and anti-inflammatory properties.

Lavender oil or tea tree oil. You can add these to the gels mentioned above, or use them on their own. Apply liberally to the sting to reduce pain and itching.

Apis Mellifica. This homeopathic remedy is made from the venom of the honeybee. Using a 12C or 30C concentration, put two tablets under your tongue three to four times a day for the first 24 to 48 hours.

Prevention

Start allergy shots to desensitize you to the venom if you're allergic to bees. One study found the benefits in children may last up to 20 years after the final shot. And take an antihistamine before each shot; it might increase the safety and efficacy of the therapy. If you're squeamish about shots, consider this: One study found the treatment significantly improved the quality of life of people who were allergic to yellow jackets.

Keep food, drink, and garbage covered outside so you don't attract bees.

Wear light-colored clothing and cover your arms, legs, and feet when you're outside.

Use unscented products, including shampoo, hair spray, and deodorant if you're planning to be outside.

Back away slowly from flying insects instead of swatting at them. Swatting can agitate the insect and encourage stinging. Plus, although bees die after the first sting, wasps, hornets, and yellow jackets don't. And bees can recruit other bees before they die.

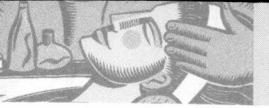

Fatigue

Chances are, if you go to your primary care doctor and tell her you're tired, she'll run a few tests but will ultimately tell you you're just slowing down as you get older. Don't accept that answer. It's important to get to the bottom of what's causing your fatigue (defined as a pervasive sense of tiredness and lack of energy that doesn't go away with rest). Although fatigue can exist on its own, it's more likely to be caused by a condition such as low thyroid, iron deficiency anemia, depression, sleep disorders, heart disease, or kidney failure. Stress, poor physical condition, and even your diet can also lead to fatigue, so there's also plenty you can do on your own to get your pep back by tweaking your daily habits.

Fatigue is particularly devastating for cancer patients. Not only is it the most common symptom they experience, it's the one most distressing and the most likely to interfere with daily life. See Integrative Cancer Care (page 337) for more approaches that can help. If you have lingering exhaustion as well as other symptoms such as muscle and joint pain, it's possible you have chronic fatigue syndrome (page 320).

Don't confuse fatigue with daytime sleepiness. If you're falling asleep easily while doing other activities (watching TV, reading, working), you may have narcolepsy or some other sleep disorder—or you may simply need more sleep.

Do This Now

The following steps won't make your fatigue go away, but they may give you enough of a pick-me-up to get dinner on the table or finish that report at work. Read on for longer-term treatments.

1. Put a drop or two of peppermint and/or rosemary essential oil on a tissue. Inhale deeply and evenly for 5 minutes.

2. If possible, take a short nap—no more than 20 minutes.

3. When you wake up, turn on all the lights in the room, drink a cup of caffeinated tea, and rinse your face with cold water.

4. Eat a small snack that contains both protein and carbohydrate, like yogurt, crackers with cheese, or a piece of apple spread with peanut butter.

5. Go for a 10-minute walk.

Why It Works

Peppermint and rosemary, along with pine and citrus scents, are stimulating and energizing. In addition to using them as described, you can make a cold compress by adding 1 to 2 drops to a cup of very cold water. Mix well, then thoroughly wet and wring out a washcloth with the mixture and use it to massage the back of your neck, face, and arms. Keep it away from your eyes.

Several studies find significant improvement in people's performance and energy level after brief naps, often no longer than 10 minutes. A short nap followed by exposure to bright light, a caffeinated drink, or washing your face with cold water provides more energy than the nap alone.

Eating something gives you a temporary boost of energy by raising your blood sugar level. Just don't eat anything that's pure sugar or low-fiber carbohydrate (e.g., a doughnut or cookie); it

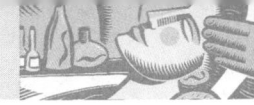

could raise your blood sugar level very quickly. That backfires when blood sugar comes crashing down, leaving you feeling even more wiped out.

Walking increases your heart rate, getting more oxygenated blood to cells, which boosts energy. It also stimulates the release of endorphins, feel-good hormones that improve mood, making you forget you're tired.

Other Medicines
Herbs and Supplements

Adaptogenic herbs. These herbs improve your body's ability to respond to stress by reducing the release of stress hormones. They may also increase stamina. They are not stimulants—they aren't going to give you a "burst" of energy. Rather, they support your body so that it can cope better with whatever's causing your fatigue. Some of the herbs also have positive effects on the immune system.

Talk with your health-care provider about which herb to try. Your choice depends in part on what other health conditions you have. For instance, if you have diabetes or high blood pressure, stay away from ginseng.

- **Goldenroot (*Rhodiola rosea*).** Studies on this herb find it can counter fatigue from several causes, including shift work and stress. One study tested its effects on the mental performance of young physicians during night shifts and found a significant improvement in the doctors' cognitive abilities. Take 50 to 100 milligrams two to three times per day.

- **Siberian ginseng (*Eleutherococcus senticosus*).** Although there are no clinical trials showing it is effective for fatigue, clinical experience finds it helps, and we recommend it to combat that run-down feeling.

GETTING TESTED

If you are suffering regularly from fatigue, talk to your doctor about the following tests:

- **Morning and afternoon temperature.** If you have a fever during these times of the day, it could indicate an infection or even some forms of cancer. If your morning temperature is low, it could indicate an underactive thyroid.

- **Basic metabolic panel.** Includes tests for glucose, electrolytes, kidney and liver enzyme levels, calcium, phosphorus, and other hormones and minerals.

- **Urinalysis.** Tests for renal disease and protein in your urine (could be a sign of diabetes or high blood pressure).

- **Complete blood count (CBC).** Helps determine your general health status and screens for a variety of fatigue-related disorders, such as anemia and infection.

- **Erythrocyte sedimentation rate (sed rate).** Measures inflammation in the body, a sign of infection, stress, or certain medical conditions.

The method of preparation varies among brands, so check the box for the exact dose. Don't take it after 3 p.m., or it could interfere with your sleep.

- **Schisandra/Schizandra (*Schisandra chinensis*).** This preparation, extracted from a woody vine commonly found in northern China, Russia, and Korea, has antioxidant and anti-inflammatory properties. Take 500 to 1,000 milligrams of the extract twice daily.

- **Ginseng (Panax and American).** You can use either species, as both seem to work equally well. Take 100 to 200 milligrams once or twice a day, but check with your doctor first if you have diabetes or low

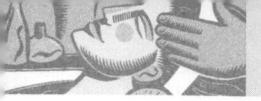

blood sugar (they can lower blood sugar) or high blood pressure.

• **_Cordyceps sinensis._** This fungus is sold in pill form as CordyMax. Although there are few studies on its effectiveness (except one on mice, which showed it reduced the effect of stress on their body and improved their energy), clinical experience suggests it works well. Take one to two pills twice a day.

Vitamin B$_{12}$. Shots of this vitamin are a classic treatment for unexplained fatigue, but self-treating with B$_{12}$ pills is worth a try too. Take 300 micrograms a day for two weeks; if you don't feel any effect, increase the dose to 1,000 micrograms daily for another two weeks. If you see a benefit, then decrease the amount 100 micrograms or less per day until you're taking the lowest possible dose that still has an effect.

Iron. Even if your blood tests show you're not anemic, you may still benefit from a trial of iron supplements. In one study, 144 women with unexplained fatigue took 80 milligrams of elemental iron a day or a placebo. While the iron group's fatigue improved more than that of the placebo group, the greatest improvement came in women whose blood iron levels were low or borderline but not low enough to be considered anemic. Iron is generally safe to take unless you have liver disease or already high blood levels of iron, but check with your doctor first. If you _are_ anemic, you may need a prescription-strength supplement. If you do take iron, take with 500 milligrams vitamin C, which aids in digestion.

Prescription Drugs

Antidepressants. Because fatigue is so often related to depression, antidepressants that improve your mood could also improve your energy level. See the entry on Depression (page 272) for more information.

Testosterone. While supplemental testosterone doesn't seem to have much effect on men's energy levels, it can help women have more energy, feel better overall, and, as a side benefit, increase libido and reduce bone loss. It's usually prescribed as a patch. Talk to your doctor about potential side effects.

Other Approaches

Exercise. You'd think that exercise would tire you out, but in fact it raises your energy level. Studies find it is one of the most effective treatments for unexplained fatigue and cancer-related fatigue. In cancer patients, for instance, it helps maintain muscle strength and endurance, thus reducing the fatiguing effects of performing everyday tasks. Studies also find that exercise can enhance the effects of certain antidepressants, such as Wellbutrin (bupropion), and it's a well-known antidote for depression, a common cause of fatigue. No need to take up running—brisk walking will do nicely. Don't overdo, however. Start slowly and gradually pump up your efforts.

Inversion. Getting more blood to the head is a great way to temporarily crank up your energy level. Obviously, you're not going to stand on your head in the middle of the work day, so do the next best thing: Stand with your legs a little wider than shoulder-width apart. Slightly bend your knees and then lean as far forward from your waist as you can. Let your head, neck, shoulders, and arms hang freely and feel all the tension from these muscles drop away. Breathe slowly and deeply for a minute, then slowly straighten up.

Green drinks. With names like Emerald Green, Pure Synergy, Green Magma, and Barley Green (available online or in health food stores), these drinks contain ingredients such as wheat germ, chlorella, and tonic herbs (herbs that improve energy), and are a great source of

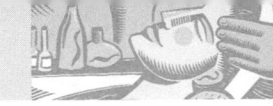

vitamin B_{12}. Although there are no published studies on their use for fatigue, experience shows they work well to combat short-term fatigue.

Energy drinks. These products, including Venom, Whoopass, Red Bull, and Adrenaline Rush, combine sugar, amino acids, caffeine, and, sometimes, herbal extracts to provide a quick pick-me-up. In one study of 20 people who fasted overnight, such a drink significantly improved attention, alertness, and memory. They're not recommended for daily use, however, because they contain such large amounts of caffeine.

Tea. If you need a caffeinated pick-you-up, choose tea over coffee. One study found that drinking tea all day improved alertness and performance just as well as coffee, but was less likely to disrupt sleep.

Traditional Chinese Medicine. The Chinese have thousands of years of history in treating "vague" diseases like fatigue. Rather than recommending specific herbs, we recommend you visit a naturopath or acupuncturist who can complete an evaluation and recommend the proper treatment regimen for you, whether it's herbs, acupuncture, and/or other lifestyle changes.

Prevention

Manage your schedule. Whether your fatigue is related to an underlying disease, cancer treatment, or stress, it's important that you take it seriously and don't try to ignore it. That means taking naps when you're tired, going to bed earlier, saying no to extra commitments, and conserving your energy for those things you absolutely *must* do.

Eat a high-fiber breakfast every morning and don't go more than three or four hours between meals. This helps you maintain steady blood sugar levels and avoid the highs and lows associated with fatigue.

Eat a high-protein lunch. It won't leave you feeling sluggish, unlike a bowl of pasta or other high-carb meal.

Make sure you're getting enough protein in general. Protein is an important source of vitamin B_{12}. Vegetarians who don't eat eggs or dairy could find themselves deficient in this vitamin. Get at least 0.5 to 0.6 grams of protein per pound of body weight. If you weight 150 pounds, that's 7.5 grams. A half-cup of canned kidney beans contains 6.6 grams; a cup of spinach contains 1.62 grams. Of course, if you're not a vegetarian, you can get plenty of protein from meat, poultry, and dairy products.

Drink 8 ounces of water every hour during the day. One of the first signs of dehydration is fatigue, so drink up.

Practice good sleep hygiene. That means going to bed and getting up at the same time every day, for instance. See more details in the Insomnia entry (page 235).

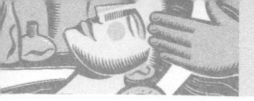

Hangover

You got a little carried away last night and now you're paying the price: a sandpapery mouth, a pounding headache, swollen eyes, sweaty skin, and a queasy stomach.

Although you probably didn't notice the ill effects of your drinking until this morning, your hangover actually hit soon after you downed your last glass. The alcohol bathed your brain in ethanol. When you stopped drinking, your blood and brain alcohol levels dropped and your brain cells went into alcohol withdrawal. Enter the hangover, which peaks when blood alcohol levels reach zero.

On top of alcohol withdrawal, you're also suffering from dehydration. (Alcohol is a diuretic, which explains all those trips to the bathroom.) Dehydration often triggers a headache. Last night's frequent urination also drained important nutrients from your body, including sodium and potassium, minerals needed for maintaining fluid balance and for proper cell functioning. Lack of these electrolytes can lead to headache, fatigue, and nausea. Finally, when your body metabolizes alcohol, your blood becomes slightly more acidic, inducing sweating and nausea.

Our remedies to the rescue!

Do This Now

When you wake up after a night of indulgence feeling worse than death warmed over, take the following five steps.

1. Drink two 8-ounce glasses of 100 percent fruit juice mixed with a spoonful of honey and a dash of salt, or the same amount of a sports drink like Gatorade.

2. Drink a cup of coffee or tea.

3. Draw a warm bath, adding a handful of sea salt or Epsom salt and 10 drops peppermint essential oils. Start soaking.

4. Eat a piece of toast.

5. Take two aspirin or ibuprofen.

Why It Works

Here's why we want you to drink the beverages in Steps 1 and 2: The fruit juice helps rehydrate your parched system and replace essential nutrients like sugar, minerals and other electrolytes, while the salt and potassium (from the fruit juice or sports drink) help your body absorb and hold on to the fluid. The fruit juice and honey also contain fructose, which some studies suggest may help your body burn any remaining alcohol faster. Fruit juice also helps normalize your blood pH, making the blood less acidic because of the way the juice is metabolized. The caffeine in the coffee shrinks swollen blood vessels, easing that pounding in your head. (Use whatever form of caffeine is least likely to upset your stomach.)

As for the bath, the Epsom salt helps clear out the toxic remnants of the alcohol your body has broken down, while peppermint oil helps fight nausea as you breathe it in.

The aspirin and ibuprofen can help ease your pain and reduce tissue swelling, but eat something innocuous first, like dry toast, to line your stomach, because the medicine can irritate the stomach lining, which has already been irritated by the alcohol.

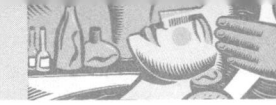

Other Medicines

B$_6$ **vitamins.** Alcohol drains the body of B vitamins—especially B$_6$. Studies find that quickly replacing it may reduce a hangover. Take 400 milligrams of B$_6$ when you wake up. (If you know you're going to indulge, take 400 milligrams before your first drink, 400 milligrams after three hours of drinking, and 400 milligrams at the end of the party to halve your risk of hangover.)

Other Approaches

Nux vomica 6C or 12C. This homeopathic remedy, from the bitter-tasting seeds of the poison nut plant, helps quell nausea and soothe an upset stomach. Take three tablets every 30 minutes for 4 to 6 hours until your symptoms subside.

Lime and baking soda. Ayurvedic medicine holds that hangovers are caused by an excess of pitta, one of three "doshas" that govern bodily processes. The following drink helps balance pitta (plus, it contains sugar, potassium, and salt for fast rehydration along with lime juice to reduce blood acidity). Mix 2 teaspoons fresh lime juice, 1/4 teaspoon sugar, a pinch of salt, and 1/2 teaspoon baking soda into 8 ounces water and drink.

Prevention

Know when to stop. For most men, that means no more than one drink an hour; for women, no more than half a drink per hour (a "drink" is 1 ounce of liquor, 5 ounces of wine, or 12 ounces of beer). Stop drinking after four hours.

Steer clear of sugary tropical mixed drinks such as piña coladas. You're more likely to drink them too fast.

Drink one glass of sparkling water, seltzer, or sports drink for every alcoholic drink. It slows your drinking and prevents dehydration and electrolyte depletion.

❧ What About...

The Hair of the Dog?

Is "the hair of the dog that bit you"—in other words, another drink—a way to counteract a hangover? Although we don't recommend this remedy (it's a sign of an alcohol problem), there is some logic behind it. A hangover is caused primarily by alcohol withdrawal, and having another drink bathes your brain cells in alcohol, reducing hangover symptoms. The traditional post-party Bloody Mary also contains valuable vitamins and electrolytes. But the benefits are temporary. Unless you plan to continue drinking indefinitely, your brain will eventually go through alcohol withdrawal again and your hangover will return.

Nibble some cheese or crackers to coat your stomach before you start drinking. This slows the entrance of alcohol into your bloodstream.

Drink purer forms of alcohol. Certain types of alcohol, including bourbon, whisky, brandy, and other colored hard liquors, contain congeners, impurities that trigger hangovers. So stick with clear liquors, such as vodka. Also limit your consumption of red wine, which contains tyramine, a histamine-like substance that triggers headaches.

Take 175 milligrams milk thistle standardized extract (such as the brand Legalon) three times daily for three days leading up to a big event. It raises levels of detoxifying enzymes in the liver and improves liver function, helping your body process alcohol more quickly.

Take 800-1600 IU prickly pear 2 to 5 hours before drinking. One study of 64 people who took this supplement before drinking found they had less nausea, dry mouth, and other hangover symptoms than a control group. Overall, they slashed their risk of a severe hangover in half. The supplement is thought to work by reducing levels of inflammation.

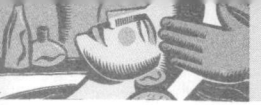

Headache

They say there are only two things in life you can count on: death and taxes. But most of us can also count on an occasional headache. Of course, you can pop an aspirin or two and you'll usually get relief (unless you reach for aspirin too often, in which case, you can expect a rebound headache when it wears off). But it's also worth trying other, natural ways to assuage the pounding because they're quite effective, especially when combined with your headache medicine.

Garden-variety tension headaches are thought to be caused by chemical changes in the brain that contract and then dilate blood vessels in the head. (Muscle tension in the face and neck certainly doesn't help, though.) Headaches can also be caused by sinusitis (page 88), allergies (page 72), PMS (page 154), and temporomandibular joint syndrome or TMJ (page 185). It's a wonder more of us aren't walking around holding our aching heads in our hands! More serious causes include glaucoma (page 178) and depression (page 272). If migraines are the type of headache you get, see page 245.

Do This Now

To put an end to the classic tension headache, take these steps.

1. Take Aleve (225 milligrams) or a product combining acetaminophen, aspirin, and caffeine, such as Excedrin. Take one Aleve or two Excedrin every four hours for up to two days. Wash it down with a caffeinated beverage like tea, coffee, or cola.

2. Mix 1 drop peppermint oil in 9 drops massage oil and massage it into your temples,

hairline, and along the base of your skull. Wash your hands thoroughly afterward.

3. Rub the fleshy area between your thumb and index finger very firmly and rhythmically while sitting quietly with your eyes closed and breathing deeply for 5 to 10 minutes. As you breathe out, ease up on the pressure on your hand and imagine all the tension and pain in your head draining out as your breath relaxes.

4. If you still have a headache, put an ice pack on your forehead and the back of your head for 15 minutes while lying in a quiet place and breathing in and out slowly and deeply.

5. If neck tension is contributing to your headache, do these neck stretches. Sit up straight in an armless chair. Grab the edge of the chair with your right hand and lean your neck over to the left, trying to place your left ear onto your left shoulder. Hold for 10 seconds, then repeat on the other side. Moving your hand back on the chair seat stretches muscles in the back of the neck; moving it forward stretches muscles in the front.

6. Finally, eat a small snack that combines carbohydrates and protein, like cheese and crackers, or a container of yogurt, or a piece of fruit and a slice of deli meat.

Why It Works

Unless you're suffering from a rebound headache caused by overuse of pain relievers, aspirin and other NSAIDs still provide the fastest, best relief. They work by blocking production of inflammatory chemicals that cause the swelling of blood

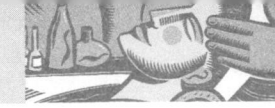

vessels in the head. Taking them with caffeine helps them work better because caffeine constricts blood vessels. Don't overdo the caffeine, though—more than 3 to 5 cups of coffee a day (less if you're sensitive to the stimulant) can backfire, leading to headaches as the caffeine "hit" wears off.

The menthol in peppermint oil is a topical pain reliever that also relaxes muscles; the scent also helps with nausea that sometimes accompanies bad headaches. These effects are enhanced by the gentle massaging motion you use as you apply the oil. Keep the oil away from your eyes, and don't use it on very small children or if you have asthma. You can also find peppermint essential oil in rub-on stick form.

Pressing the web of your hand as described above is an effective acupressure technique for tension headaches.

The ice decreases the inflammation of throbbing blood vessels, and the deep breathing eases muscle tension, as do the stretches.

Finally, we want you to eat something, because low blood sugar can cause a headache. A snack that contains some protein is best because it won't cause a blood sugar crash later, unlike a candy bar.

Other Medicines
Herbs and Supplements

Magnesium. For migraine (page 245) we recommend magnesium. It is also effective for tension and cluster headaches. Take 300 to 500 milligrams at the first sign of a headache. One caution: It may lead to some temporary diarrhea.

Prevention

Book appointments for acupuncture. Numerous studies attest to acupuncture's benefits in treating and preventing chronic headaches. For instance, in one well-designed study, German researchers divided 270 tension headache patients into three groups, giving one group acupuncture, one group sham acupuncture (using needles on sites that are not true acupuncture points), and one group no treatment over eight weeks. Those who received the real acupuncture and sham acupuncture saw their headache rates drop by almost half, while the control group saw little change. Plus, those who received the real acupuncture treatment found they had fewer headaches for months after the treatment ended. Start with a series of six to eight treatments once or twice a week, depending on the severity of your symptoms.

Have your feet rubbed. Reflexology—which involves massaging or pressing specific points on the feet—improved headaches in 81 percent of 220 chronic headache patients who participated in a clinical trial testing it. However, there was no control group in this study, so we can't be sure how much of the benefit was due to the placebo effect. If it gets rid of your headache, though, does it matter?

See a chiropractor. One review of eight clinical trials found that spinal manipulation improved chronic tension and migraine headaches as well as, or better than, aspirin or placebo. Other studies find chiropractic combined with exercise is even more effective. However, if you have osteoarthritis of the neck, rheumatoid arthritis, cerebral vascular disease, or heart disease, skip the chiropractic, since it could increase your risk of stroke.

Give biofeedback a try. There's good evidence that biofeedback can help relieve and prevent chronic tension headaches. In one study, young headache sufferers who learned biofeedback had fewer headaches in the 6 to 12 months after their treatment than those in a control group. You'll need to see a biofeedback professional for training; afterward you can practice the techniques yourself without the sensors that give the "feedback."

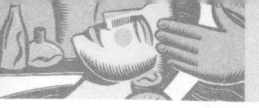

Try 5-HTP. Studies find that taking 150 milligrams twice a day of this amino acid (5-hydroxytryptophan) for two weeks can reduce the intensity of chronic tension headaches, as well as the use of pain relievers, probably by raising levels of serotonin, a neurotransmitter that helps nerves communicate and plays a role in pain perception. Try it if your headaches are related to overuse of pain relievers and you're trying to wean yourself off daily use. Don't use it for more than three or four weeks without your doctor's okay.

Decline that drink. Alcohol is a known headache trigger. Just half an hour after that first sip of wine, you could wind up with a throbbing noggin.

Cut out any food triggers. Some foods can provoke headaches, including citrus fruits, chocolate, dairy, and foods that contain tyramine, like aged cheese and cured meats. So can some food additives, including sodium chloride, sodium nitrate, monosodium glutamate, and the sweetener aspartame.

Improve your posture. If you sit in front of a computer all day, eye and neck strain can lead to headaches. Have an ergonomics expert evaluate your workstation. Hint: Your legs and arms should be bent at right angles, and your head shouldn't tilt up or down.

Get a good night's sleep. Insomnia or restless sleep can land you with a headache the next day. See Insomnia (page 235) for our advice.

Talk with your doctor about antidepressants. Research shows that regular use of tricyclic antidepressants such as Elavil (amitriptyline) or selective serotonin reuptake inhibitors (SSRIs), such as Prozac (fluoxetine) can prevent chronic headaches, whether migraine or other types. They probably work by affecting the release of certain brain chemicals that lead to headaches, and studies suggest they work twice as well when combined with stress-reducing therapies like biofeedback.

Swallow fish oil supplements. Because inflammation contributes to headaches and fish oil counters inflammation, try taking 3 grams fish oil a day to relieve frequent headaches. It's good for your heart and the rest of your body too.

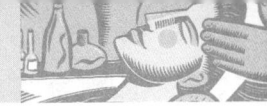

Hemorrhoids

Think of hemorrhoids as the varicose veins of your bottom. Like varicose veins (see page 212), they are swollen veins that can cause itching and pain—in this case, especially when you've been sitting for a while. Since the veins of the anus are more delicate than other veins, they can easily bleed, leaving bright red blood in your feces, in the toilet, or on toilet paper, scaring the heck out of you. It's a good thing to be scared, however. Other, more serious conditions—such as colon polyps—also cause bleeding. So never assume you have a hemorrhoid when you see red. Make an appointment with your doctor to rule out other possible problems.

Although most hemorrhoidal flare-ups resolve on their own in just a few days, the swelling will return—and more hemorrhoids may form—unless you get at the original cause.

Do This Now

To quickly soothe the itchiness and pain of a hemorrhoid, follow these steps.

1. Draw a hot bath and add a handful of Epsom or sea salt. Get in and sit down with your knees raised for 10 minutes. Repeat several times a day.

2. Apply an over-the-counter hemorrhoidal cream such as Preparation H after each bath.

Why It Works

The warm water brings more blood to the affected area, reducing pain. It also relaxes your anus and rectum, which reduces pressure on the hemor-

rhoid. The salt helps shrink the blood vessels. In one study, 28 people with hemorrhoids sat in warm baths of varying temperatures for 10 minutes. The hottest temperature used in the study, 122°F, reduced pain for the longest time—as long as 70 minutes.

As for the cream, although it won't cure your hemorrhoid, the witch hazel it contains cools the burning and itching and shrinks swelling.

Other Medicines
Herbs and Supplements

Flavonoids. Flavonoids such as rutin or quercetin (sold as citrus flavonoids), pycnogenol, or grapeseed strengthen blood vessels and also reduce swelling through their anti-inflammatory action. Take 500 milligrams citrus flavonoids, 50 milligrams pycnogenol, or 100 milligrams grapeseed extract twice a day.

Ginkgo. Supplements made from this large shade tree increase blood flow and improve blood vessel function throughout the body. In one study, 22 people with hemorrhoids who took ginkgo supplements for a week experienced less bleeding, pain, and discharge than before taking the supplement. Take 2 capsules of standardized extract (24% flavonoids, 7.5% terpenoids) twice daily.

Witch hazel. This natural anti-inflammatory shrinks swollen veins, bringing immediate relief. Chill the witch hazel for 15 minutes, then soak a wad of cotton in it and place the cotton ball near the hemorrhoid. This remedy works particularly well at night, helping to relieve pain and itching so you can sleep.

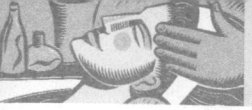

Prescription Drugs

Doxium (calcium dobesilate). Used to treat diabetes and various blood disorders, this medication can provide efficient, fast, and safe relief from your symptoms by strengthening your blood vessels. In a study of 29 patients, hemorrhoid symptoms improved within two weeks in 86 percent of those taking the drug.

Other Approaches

Fiber. Straining during a bowel movement is a major cause of hemorrhoids. To stay regular and pass soft stool, you need to eat 25 to 30 grams of fiber a day, but the average American consumes only 8 to 15 grams. A daily fiber supplement, along with a fiber-rich diet that includes whole grains, legumes, and fruits and vegetables, will get you to that goal.

Psyllium and other over-the-counter soluble fiber supplements also help soften stool, making it less painful to pass (and less likely to irritate your hemorrhoid). Studies find these fiber supplements reduce the bleeding and pain associated with hemorrhoids, while increasing the effectiveness of other therapies, such as surgery, possibly by reducing future flare-ups. The best fiber supplement for you is the one you'll most likely take. Choose one that tastes good and dissolves easily in water or food and follow package directions.

Careful hygiene. You can easily nick a hemorrhoid, making it bleed. So use baby wipes or Tucks pads instead of toilet paper to wipe carefully and gently after bowel movements. When showering, avoid perfumed soaps, which can irritate hemorrhoids.

Guided imagery. Hemorrhoids can cause insane itching, but giving in and scratching may irritate your hemorrhoid further, prolonging and intensifying your symptoms. Most people can ignore the itching during the day, but find it drives them crazy at night. The good news: The relaxation technique called guided imagery can teach you to use mind over matter to ignore the itching and pain. In a study of 86 people recovering from hemorrhoid surgery, participants who listened to a guided imagery CD reported less pain and improved sleep compared to patients who did not listen to the tape. For more on guided imagery, see page 24.

Rubber band ligation. In this procedure, a physician places a rubber band around the base of the hemorrhoid inside the rectum. The band cuts off circulation, and the hemorrhoid withers away within a few days.

Sclerotherapy. In this procedure, a physician injects a chemical solution around the blood vessel to shrink the hemorrhoid.

Surgery. As a last resort, a surgeon can remove your hemorrhoid via a hemorrhoidectomy. Consider this method only after more conservative treatments, including rubber band ligation, fail. Although hemorrhoidectomy has a better success rate than other surgical procedures, its potential risks include postoperative bleeding, infection, and incontinence.

Prevention

Drink 8 to 10 glasses of water daily. In addition to helping your body to process the extra fiber, the water softens stools.

Eat a high-fiber breakfast. In a study of 47 people, those who ate breakfast were seven times less likely to have hemorrhoids than people who didn't, possibly because many breakfast foods—such as bran cereals—are high in fiber.

Take a 30-minute walk every day. Regular exercise helps you have regular bowel movements.

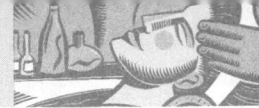

Insect Bites

A mosquito bite used to be nothing more than an itchy annoyance. Now it brings a small risk of the dangerous West Nile virus, carried by infected female mosquitoes, so wearing insect repellent is smart. If you do get bitten (and who can avoid a few mosquito bites now and again?), we have strategies to stop the itch before you scratch yourself silly. Remember that welts from insect bites are the result of an immune system reaction to the insect's venom that causes inflammation. Stopping the inflammation is key to soothing symptoms.

Do This Now

If last night's cookout left you with more bumps than a braille encyclopedia, follow this advice to soothe the itch.

1. Resist the urge to scratch.

2. Wash bitten areas with chilled chamomile tea.

3. Next, apply an anti-itch lotion like Benadryl or hydrocortisone, or, if you don't have one, smooth on aloe vera gel.

4. If you're still itching, bring in the big gun: Take 25 milligrams Benadryl.

Why It Works

Scratching just spreads the venom deeper under your skin, and can open the skin, risking a secondary infection. The chilled liquid reduces inflammation, helped along by the anti-inflammatory benefits of chamomile.

Benadryl and hydrocortisone subdue the immune response that results in the itching and redness. Aloe won't stop the immune response, but it does have anti-inflammatory properties.

If you have a significant response to the bite—common in children in particular, and marked by a huge red bump—you may need an oral antihistamine like Benadryl to stop the reaction from inside your body.

Other Medicines
Herbs and Supplements

Echinacea angustifolia or purpurea alcohol extract. Put 1 to 2 drops of either extract directly on the sting. These species of echinacea contain topical pain relievers.

Soothing gels. Apply calendula, chamomile, or plantain cream, all of which have anti-inflammatory properties. For a stronger result, mix 10 to 20 drops of a combination of lavender, chamomile, or peppermint essential oils into 1 ounce of ointment.

Over-the-Counter Drugs

Burow's solution. Also sold under the name Domeboro, this remedy soothes itchiness because the main ingredient, aluminum sulfate, is astringent. Pour two packets under cool running bathwater and soak for at least 10 minutes. You can also soak a cloth in the solution and apply.

> ❧ What About...
>
> ### Bug Zappers?
> Save your money. Studies find they don't work.

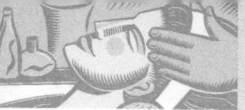

The Right Repellent

Insect repellent is your best defense against mosquitoes. Look for one of these ingredients:

• **DEET.** DEET is so common in insect repellents because it works so well. The minimum dose is a 10 percent concentration, with a maximum dose of 50 percent. Doses higher than that don't provide any additional protection. Use the lowest effective DEET concentration you can based on how buggy the environment is and how long you'll be outside. According to a 2002 study, a product containing 23.8% DEET provided five hours of protection from mosquito bites; 20% DEET provided almost four hours of protection. DEET may be used on children who are older than 2 months, but don't let children under 10 apply it themselves, and don't apply to young children's hands or around their eyes and mouth. Don't apply DEET at the same time as you apply sunscreen. It could result in a toxic buildup of DEET.

• **Picardin.** The newest insect repellent ingredient, picardin has been used in Europe for years. Studies suggest it is as effective as DEET, with less risk of skin irritation. This odorless repellent is available in the U.S. as Cutter Advanced Insect Repellent and is safe for infants and children.

• **Oil of lemon eucalyptus.** This strong-smelling, natural repellent protects against mosquitoes, midges, and ticks as well as repellents containing low concentrations of DEET, according to recent studies, but its effects last only about half as long, so you'll need to reapply often.

• **Permethrin.** Spray this product on your clothes, netting, and bedding. Although it's ineffective on skin, this plant-based repellent binds with fabric fibers to repel numerous insects, including ticks and mosquitoes. One application lasts weeks. Using it together with a DEET repellent provides near 100 percent protection against insect bites.

You can also make your own repellent by mixing 15 to 20 drops lemon eucalyptus, lemongrass, and citronella essential oils into 1 ounce carrier oil. Reapply often.

Prevention

Apply insect repellent to your skin and clothes before going outside (see "The Right Repellent" above). Don't apply to any abraded or broken skin.

Cover your arms and legs if you're outside at dawn and dusk, when mosquitoes are most active.

Sleep in mosquito netting or a zipped tent when sleeping outdoors.

Remove all standing water from your property. If you have any you can't get rid of, add tadpoles or fish to the water to eat mosquito larvae. You can often get them at the mosquito control division of your local health department.

Repair any torn window screens to keep flying insects out.

Light citronella candles and incense when you're outside. One study found they reduced the number of mosquito bites by 42 and 24 percent respectively when compared to no candles or unscented candles.

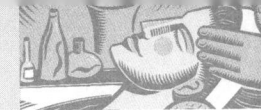

Insomnia

There's more to insomnia than just trouble falling asleep. Some people fall asleep just fine but wake up in the middle of the night and can't get back to sleep. Others sleep through the night but wake too early in the morning. And still others appear to sleep through the night with no problem, but never wake rested.

While it's normal to experience an occasional bad night of sleep, if your sleep problems become chronic, it's time to do something about them. Remember from Part 2 in this book that lack of sleep interferes with immune function and increases your risk of insulin resistance. Then there are the dangers of trying to get through the day (especially if you have to drive) when you're overtired.

Various health issues may contribute to sleep problems, including menopause, depression (early morning awakening is a common sign of depression), and just about any condition that causes pain. Other culprits include restless legs syndrome (see page 253) and sleep apnea, in which you slightly awaken dozens of times a night because your breathing stops.

Just as important as the ability to fall asleep and stay asleep is the ability to cycle in an orderly fashion through the five stages of sleep several times a night. This is critical to cell growth and repair and a strong immune system. If something (for instance, alcohol, heavy smoking, or abnormally hot or cold bedroom temperatures) interrupts the progression of these sleep stages, you won't feel well rested and your immune system, mood, and memory may suffer.

Not being able to sleep can be extremely frustrating. But before you turn to sleeping pills, there are plenty of natural approaches to try.

Do This Now

Getting rid of chronic insomnia will probably involve making some long-term changes to your habits. See the rest of the entry for advice. Meanwhile, on a week when you can't sleep, take these steps.

1. Go for a brisk 20-minute walk outside in the afternoon.

2. About two hours before bed, take a warm bath into which you've mixed 15 drops lavender essential oil.

3. If it's hot in your bedroom, turn down the thermostat or turn on the air conditioner.

4. Take 600 to 900 milligrams of valerian extract standardized to 0.4% valerinic acids.

5. Before you climb into bed, spend 20 minutes on some form of relaxation therapy, such as progressive muscle relaxation or meditation (described on pages 24-25), or write in your journal.

6. If you don't fall asleep within 30 minutes, get out of bed. Do something low key like reading or folding laundry until you feel tired. Then go back to bed.

7. If you still can't fall sleep, take a sleeping pill (if you have them) or an over-the-counter antihistamine such as Benadryl.

Why It Works

Few scientific studies show exercise has much benefit for insomnia, but those studies were conducted in labs, primarily on people who didn't

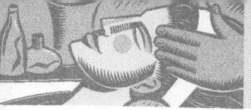

Habits for Better Sleep

"Sleep hygiene," a term doctors use, doesn't refer to how clean you are when you go to bed, but to sleep-promoting behaviors. The idea is to avoid habits that interfere with a good night's sleep and to follow habits that promote it. Studies find that 70 to 80 percent of people with chronic insomnia benefit from non-drug approaches like these.

• **Stop drinking caffeinated beverages** and eating caffeinated foods (including chocolate), even if you're sleepy during the day. Don't forget that some medications, like Excedrin, contain large doses of caffeine.

• **Go to bed and wake up at the same time** every day, even on weekends.

• **Hide the bedside clock.** That way, you won't see it when you wake up in the middle of the night and obsess over how little time you have left to sleep.

• **Prepare your room for sleep** by buying room-darkening shades or using a sleeping mask (available in drugstores) to block light, placing your bed against an inside wall to limit your exposure to noise, and using a white-noise machine to drown out any racket. And keep your bedroom cool.

• **Use the bedroom only for sleep** and sex. That way, when you get into bed, your body will know it's time to nod off.

bedtime because it could increase your metabolism and mental alertness.

The bath and the relaxation technique do several things for you. First, they relax tense muscles. And if you do them regularly, they form a nighttime ritual that signals to your brain that it's time to sleep. Stick to your ritual like glue every night and it will work like a charm.

After you get out of the bath, your body temperature will slowly start to drop—a precursor to sleep. (A cool bedroom also helps induce sleep, which is why we suggest adjusting the temperature.) We recommend adding lavender oil to the bath because lavender promotes relaxation and possibly sleep (see also lavender aromatherapy, under "Other Approaches," below).

Valerian is the core of our herbal treatment for chronic insomnia. It doesn't work like a sleeping pill—that is, it won't "knock you out." Rather, it works to stabilize sleep cycles, making it ideal for people who wake up still feeling tired or wake in the middle of the night. One study comparing valerian to a prescription sedative found both worked just as well at relieving sleep disturbances, although the valerian had fewer side effects. Be patient—it may take two to four weeks before you see any benefits from the herb. But it's very safe, with no risk of addiction as with the benzodiazepines, and with no morning "hangover."

Antihistamines are not a long-term solution to insomnia, but for a night or two they'll probably help you sleep, since they are sedating.

Other Medicines
Herbs and Supplements

Relaxant herbs. In addition to valerian, other relaxing herbs that are excellent for sleep problems include chamomile, hops, passionflower, lemon balm, and skullcap. We don't have a preference as to which you take, and you may even find all included in some herbal sleeping formulas

have sleep problems. In real life with real people suffering from insomnia, we find regular exercise to be critical to people's ability to get a good night's sleep. It doesn't need to be an intense workout—a walk is just fine. We want you to walk outside if possible because natural light helps regulate your body's sleep-wake cycle. Just don't exercise within three or four hours of

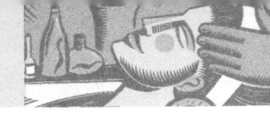

or teas. We often recommend such teas because the act of sipping a warm drink before bed is, in itself, relaxing (make it part of your nightly ritual, if you enjoy it). Follow the package directions, or make your own tea. Mix 1/2 teaspoon each of passionflower, lemon balm, skullcap, and chamomile tea leaves, and steep in 6 ounces boiling water for 8 to 10 minutes. Strain and sweeten with honey if desired. Sip a cup an hour or so before bed as part of your preparing-for-bedtime routine.

Melatonin. This supplement is most useful for sleep problems related to shift work or jet lag, but some people find it very helpful for insomnia. Start with the lowest dose available, increasing it by 0.5 milligrams a night until you reach the most effective dose (but no higher than 3 milligrams).

5-hydroxytryptophan (5-HTP). This amino acid is a building block for serotonin, a neurotransmitter that plays a major role in sleep. Take 100 milligrams before bed with a piece of fruit, glass of juice, or cracker (it works best when taken with a carbohydrate), but not protein. Or take 50 milligrams a half-hour before dinner and 50 milligrams with your bedtime snack. This supplement shouldn't be used for more than three or four weeks except under a doctor's supervision.

Over-the-Counter Drugs

Sleeping aids. Most over-the-counter sleeping pills contain antihistamines, which make you sleepy. But they're also very drying. If they work for you for occasional insomnia, just take a generic antihistamine instead of a sleeping pill; they're less expensive and just as effective.

Prescription Drugs

Benzodiazepines. These medications include Ativan (lorazepam) Valium (diazepam) and Restoril (temazepam). They're okay for a once-in-a-while use, but they interfere with the restorative phase of sleep called REM sleep and can be habit forming.

Non-benzodiazepine hypnotics. This newer class of sleep aids includes Ambien (zolpidem), Sonata (zaleplon), and Lunesta (eszopiclone). They work similarly to benzodiazepines, but have fewer side effects because they don't stay in your system very long.

Tricyclic or atypical antidepressants. These antidepressants, which include Elavil (amitriptyline), Sinequan (doxepin), and Desyrel (trazodone) have sleepiness as one of their side effects. If you have chronic insomnia, your doctor may prescribe low doses to be taken just before bed. They're especially helpful if you have sleep disturbances (i.e., waking in the middle of the night or early morning) or sleep problems related to chronic pain.

Rozerem (ramelteon). This is the newest drug approved for insomnia and the only one not considered a controlled substance. It works by mimicking melatonin in the brain, dimming signals that might keep you alert and prevent you from falling asleep.

Other Approaches

Warm milk. It's a cliché, but it has science behind it. Milk is a good source of tryptophan, the same amino acid found in turkey and other food sources, which contributes to the production of sleep-inducing serotonin. Plus, the warmth itself is relaxing. Other foods high in tryptophan include chicken, tuna, soy, yogurt, and whole grain crackers. Try a little snack before beginning your pre-bedtime routine.

Cognitive-behavioral therapy. Most people get panicky when they can't fall asleep, or wake up in the middle of the night and start to focus on how little time they have left to sleep, making it even harder to sleep. Cognitive-behavioral therapy

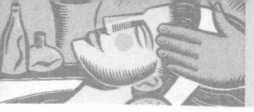

helps you change this thought pattern so you can relax and fall asleep. Look for a psychologist or counselor who's trained in CBT for sleep problems.

Acupuncture. Several studies find acupuncture can relieve various types of insomnia in all types of people (including pregnant women and anxious people). One study found five weeks of acupuncture increased participants' own melatonin secretion as well as significantly improved their ability to fall asleep, stay asleep, and sleep well.

Calms Forté. This homeopathic remedy from Hyland's is one of our favorite homeopathic patent remedies. It contains minute amounts of several herbs, including passionflower, oats, hops, and chamomile. It works well for children with occasional sleep problems, for elderly people (for whom benzodiazepines may be too sedating), and for people who wake up early in the morning.

Lavender aromatherapy. Spritz lavender spray on your pillow and sheets, put a few drops of lavender essential oil on a tissue and sniff it as you're trying to fall asleep, dab some on your pulse points before you get into bed, or use a plug-in diffuser. One small preliminary study found lavender improved mild insomnia in participants; other studies find it calms people with dementia, attesting to its relaxing effects.

Prevention

Maintain a normal weight. Studies find that obesity can make sleep problems like sleep apnea worse. It can also affect important sleep-related hormone levels in the body, increasing levels of the stress hormone cortisol while decreasing levels of sleep-inducing melatonin.

Manage stress. Do it however you can, whether it's yoga classes or meditation.

Check your medications. Many prescription and over-the-counter medications can interfere with sleep, including beta-blockers, thyroid medication, certain antidepressants like the selective serotonin reuptake inhibitors (SSRIs), decongestants, corticosteroids, and medications with caffeine. Talk to your doctor about changing dosages or medication if you're taking any of these drugs.

Avoid alcohol. Although many people think a glass of wine before bed can help with insomnia, the opposite is actually true. While alcohol might help you fall asleep, it's often the culprit behind middle-of-the-night awakenings as your body experiences alcohol withdrawal. It also interferes with your sleep cycle, so even if you do sleep through the night, you'll wake up tired.

Stop smoking. Yet another reason to quit: Nicotine is a stimulant. If you're still smoking, try not to smoke for at least two hours before bedtime (brush your teeth so you won't be tempted).

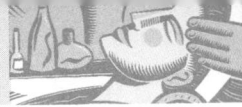

Jet Lag

You don't have to travel to Beijing to get jet-lagged. Fly from New York to Denver and back in three days and see how you feel over the next week. The truth is, for every time zone change, you need one day to recover. So flying from New York to London can put you off base for six days (every hour of flying time approximates one time zone).

You may not be able to completely avoid jet lag, but you can be one of those people who more or less breeze through it.

Do This Now

The best way to deal with jet lag is to prevent it.

1. Take 5 milligrams melatonin the day before your travel at a time that equals 5 p.m. in the new time zone, and take again on the plane if you're traveling eastward. Continue taking 1 to 3 milligrams melatonin at bedtime in your new time zone to continue your body clock's adjustment.

2. Avoid alcohol or caffeinated drinks while traveling, and skip the caffeine upon arrival, especially the first day.

3. If you arrive at your destination in the morning or afternoon, get settled and then take a brief (30-minute) nap.

4. Now go for a 30-minute walk outside.

Why It Works

Melatonin, also known as the sleep hormone, rises throughout the day, peaking in the evening and signaling your brain and body that it's time for bed. Supplementing with it when traveling can trick your body into thinking it's later than it is.

Even though a little caffeinated pick-me-up may be tempting, we want you to avoid caffeine as well as alcohol because both can interfere with sleep the first night in your new time zone.

A short nap upon arrival is refreshing—but don't sleep too long or you may have trouble falling asleep that night. Finally, exercise gets the blood moving and increases your heartbeat after hours of travel, providing a boost of energy that may see you through until bedtime. The sunlight helps reset your body clock to the new time zone.

Other Medicines

Valerian. Take 600 to 900 milligrams valerian extract standardized to 0.4% valerinic acids every night of your trip to help normalize your sleep cycles and provide a good night's sleep.

Other Approaches

Progressive muscle relaxation. When you get into bed that first night, you may feel wide-awake. Practice progressive muscle relaxation, in which you alternately tense and then relax every muscle in your body, starting at your toes and working up to your head.

Prevention

Try the Argonne diet. Also known as the Anti-Jet-Lag Diet, this diet uses a feast-or-famine regimen to adjust your body clock to the time zone of your destination. Find details at www.antijetlagdiet.com.

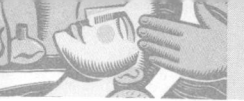

Lyme Disease

Lyme disease may seem like a recent phenomenon, but the bacterium that causes it (*Borrelia burgdorferi*) has been around for centuries. It's carried in the stomachs of deer ticks. When this country was first populated, deer were hunted nearly to extinction. Now they roam our backyards—and Lyme disease has become a force to be reckoned with. Today it's the most common insect-borne disease in the United States, and one of the most complicated bacterial diseases to treat.

The disease occurs in three stages. The first is often accompanied by a ringlike rash, sometimes with flulike symptoms, that hits days or even weeks after infection. This rash—when it occurs—is the only physical sign of infection with which doctors can make a reliable diagnosis, and the early stage the only time when a lab test for the bacterium is likely to identify it. This first stage is also the time when antibiotic treatment is most likely to result in a complete cure.

The latter two stages can arise weeks, months, or even years after the initial infection and may involve nearly every part of the body, from pain and swelling in the joints to excruciating headaches to heart arrhythmias.

To make matters worse, Lyme disease doesn't simply start and continuously get worse; it may get worse, then better, then worse again. Plus, not all people start at Stage 1 and move through Stage 3, and not all exhibit the same symptoms at each stage. Add to that the fact that many of the symptoms mimic other diseases, like fibromyalgia, arthritis, myocarditis, and facial palsy, and you can see why it can be difficult to diagnose and treat. It's much better to prevent a tick bite in the first place.

Do This Now

1. If you discover a tick attached to your body, remove it. Forget matches. To remove a tick, use thin-tipped tweezers to remove the whole tick, making sure you get the mandible, or mouth, to prevent transfer of the bacterium. Grasp the tick in the tweezers and pull straight back. Don't twist.

2. Save the tick in a plastic bag to show your doctor so the tick can be identified and tested for the *Borrelia* bacterium.

3. If you've discovered a tick on your body, or you live in an area with deer ticks and/or have been outside in recent days and experience any of the symptoms under "Lyme Disease Symptoms" (below) see your doctor immediately for an antibiotic, especially if you haven't discovered and removed the tick right away.

Why It Works

Removing the tick promptly enough can prevent Lyme disease. That's because the tick needs to be attached for more than 24 hours to transmit the bacterium. So if you've been hiking for two hours,

---

Lyme Disease Symptoms

Early symptoms:
- A ringlike red rash
- Flulike symptoms and headaches

Later symptoms:
- Swollen or painful joints
- Irregular heartbeats or chest pain

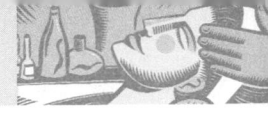

and an hour later see the tick and cleanly remove it, you probably don't need antibiotics.

Treatment within 72 hours of a tick bite with just one dose of the antibiotic doxycycline can prevent Lyme disease in 87 percent of people.

Other Medicines
Herbs and Supplements

Fish oil. If your Lyme disease has progressed to one of the later stages that involves inflammation, take 3 to 6 grams of fish oil a day in two or three divided doses.

Probiotics. Use these tablets while you're taking an antibiotic. Antibiotics reduce amounts of all bacteria in the body—friendly or otherwise—allowing unfriendly organisms such as yeast to get a foothold, causing diarrhea and other side effects. Probiotic preparations contain healthful bacteria, alleviating these side effects. Take 1 or 2 tablets with each meal and at bedtime.

Over-the-Counter Drugs

Analgesics. For flulike aches and headaches, take up to 1.5 grams aspirin, 4,800 milligrams ibuprofen, or 550 milligrams naproxen a day for a day or two.

Prescription Drugs

Antibiotics. These are the first-line treatment. The most commonly used antibiotic is doxycycline, primarily because you can take fewer pills for a shorter time than other antibiotics.

Unfortunately, once you've progressed to the later stages of Lyme, even aggressive use of antibiotics is not always effective. This may be because what started as an infectious disease has been transformed by the body into an autoimmune condition. One study found that penicillin improved arthritis in just 55 percent of those whose condition had progressed to this stage.

Other studies find that even if you initially get better, arthritis and other symptoms often worsen later. And antibiotics don't necessarily improve other Lyme symptoms.

There's no real consensus on the best antibiotic treatment for later-stage disease, either the type or the number of treatments. Get in to see a good specialist in infectious diseases or a rheumatologist who has experience in treating late-stage Lyme disease.

Other Approaches

Anti-inflammation diet. For Lyme-related joint pain, follow the anti-inflammation diet on page 42. Also follow our recommendations for rheumatoid arthritis on page 306.

Physical therapy. If your joints are affected, talk to your doctor about a prescription for physical therapy, which could help reduce pain and improve movement.

Prevention

Do a thorough inspection for ticks when you come in from a tick-infested area. First take a shower and wash your hair. Then look over your skin carefully. Ask someone else to check areas you can't see. Remember that most ticks that carry the Lyme disease bacterium are tiny and can look like freckles.

Use an insect repellent containing DEET to prevent tick bites. Also spray a commercial product containing permethrin on your clothes, netting, and bedding. Permethrin binds with fabric fibers to repel ticks and mosquitoes. Applying it with DEET products provides nearly 100 percent protection against insects.

Dress to repel ticks. This means wearing light-colored long pants and long-sleeved shirts, tucking pants into socks, and keeping your feet (including your ankles) completely covered.

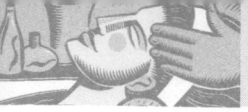

Memory Problems

The more we learn about the brain, the more we understand that it is a pliable organ, capable of growing and changing throughout life. And if you treat it right, it will serve you well into old age. That said, like the rest of the body, the brain does age. Brain cells, or neurons, shrink, accumulate extra gunk around them, and lose some of the fatty material called myelin that enables them to efficiently send electrical signals to other neurons. They also churn out fewer neurotransmitters like acetylcholine, chemicals that help act like a kind of cerebral FedEx, carrying messages instead of packages from one neuron to the next.

The good news? Many of the same steps that reduce your risk of chronic diseases, like heart disease, high cholesterol, high blood pressure, and obesity, can also help your memory. Get enough protective nutrients from food, make the kind of lifestyle changes designed to funnel more oxygen and blood to your brain (like getting more exercise), add the kind of supplements we know benefit brain cells, and you could be answering *Jeopardy* questions well into your 80s. Also: Keep challenging yourself mentally, and you'll keep growing new connections between neurons, which keeps your brain's ability to learn and recall information strong.

It's worth noting that aging brain cells aren't the only reason for memory loss. One study from the University of California-Berkeley found that older people who thought they were losing their memory were instead having problems tuning out distractions that interfered with their ability to learn and remember things. The bottom line: If you don't pay attention to it in the first place, you won't remember it later.

Do This Now

If you've been forgetting everything except where you put your head, try these steps.

1. Go to bed 30 minutes earlier tonight and every succeeding night until you're getting as much sleep as you need. Follow the tips in the Insomnia entry (page 235) to ensure you get a good night's rest.

2. Before you engage in a task or activity in which you need to remember new information, close your eyes, empty your mind, and practice deep breathing for at least two minutes.

3. When you receive new information you need to remember, tune out everything else and stay actively focused on the information.

4. Begin taking 60 to 80 milligrams ginkgo two or three times a day. If you're taking a test of any sort, take a dose of 120 to 180 milligrams one or two hours beforehand.

5. Drink a cup or two of caffeinated coffee a day.

Why It Works

A large body of evidence supports the role of sleep in consolidating and cementing our memories. It also serves to enhance memories, restoring lost memories and producing additional learning. It's why a good night's sleep is so important if you're going to do well on a test the following day.

The deep breathing helps clear your mind and lower your stress hormones, both of which, studies find, can help your brain better absorb new information. Focusing all your attention on the information coming in helps it "stick."

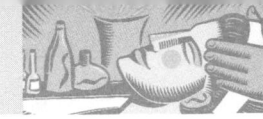

Ginkgo is a potent antioxidant and one of the most important herbs in our arsenal when it comes to memory and learning. One study on 31 postmenopausal women who took either 120 milligrams a day of ginkgo or a placebo found that those taking the supplement improved more on certain memory and attention tasks than those taking the placebo. If ginkgo alone doesn't do it for you, try adding 75 milligrams of the Chinese herb dang shen (*Codonopsis pilosula*), which one study found improved memory more than ginkgo alone.

Finally, studies find that coffee (more likely, the caffeine it contains) improves alertness and some forms of memory. Population studies even show lower levels of Alzheimer's disease in people who drink coffee.

Other Medicines
Herbs and Supplements

Bacopa. There's some evidence that this Ayurvedic herb can improve memory, probably through its strong antioxidant effects. In one study that gave healthy volunteers 300 milligrams of the herb or a placebo, the people who got the herb significantly improved the ability to process visual information, learn new material, and consolidate their memory (that is, transfer short-term memories to long-term storage). Follow package directions for dosage.

St John's wort. Memory problems can be related to mild underlying depression. In those instances, buy a St. John's wort supplement standardized to 0.3% hypericin or 2% to 5% hyperforin and take 300 milligrams three times a day. The herb can interact with prescription medications, so talk with your doctor before taking it.

Guarana and ginseng. Ginseng is a considered a "tonic" herb that benefits general health, while guarana, which contains caffeine, is a stimulant. One study compared an extract of guarana, 200 milligrams Panax ginseng, or both together in 28 healthy participants, and found that all three treatments improved the participants' ability to perform certain cognitive-related tasks throughout the day. Guarana had the greatest benefit on attention tasks, while ginseng and the combination of both herbs improved the memory task most.

Acetyl-L-carnitine. This amino acid is often included in "brainpower" and "memory boosting" supplements sold in drugstores. It plays numerous roles in helping to maintain the health of neurons, and may also improve production of the neurotransmitter acetylcholine, important in memory. Most studies on its use have been conducted in Alzheimer's patients, with some evidence that high daily doses can help slow the decline. Start with a modest dose of 200 milligrams two or three times a day.

Phosphatidylserine (PS). This is a naturally occurring fat we get as part of our normal diet. It's particularly important in enabling neuronal membranes to transmit electrical signals. In several studies in middle- to late-aged people with mild memory problems, the supplement consistently and significantly improved participants' ability to recall lists of words after two to four months of use. Take 200 to 300 milligrams a day in two or three divided doses.

Vinpocetine. This herb, derived from the Madagascar periwinkle, was developed in Hungary about 20 years ago. It's mainly used to treat people with a loss of blood flow to the brain, a key contributor to memory and learning problems. Although there aren't many human studies to go by, three studies show that taking vinpocetine can improve attention, concentration, and memory more than a placebo. Take 2.5 to 5 milligrams three times a day, increasing to 10 milligrams three times a day if you don't improve with the lower dose after four to six weeks.

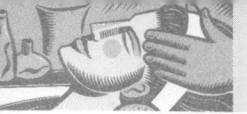

Other Approaches

Exercise. We know there's a connection between cardiovascular conditions like heart disease and brain conditions like Alzheimer's disease, likely related to the effects of oxidation, inflammation, and reduced blood flow to the brain. And we know that exercise improves cardiovascular conditions. Now comes evidence that exercise—whether it's get-your-heart-pumping aerobic activities or less intense, mind-body exercise like yoga and t'ai chi—can also improve cognitive ability.

In one study, researchers compared the memory function of 140 older adults who regularly practiced mind-body or cardiovascular exercises with those who didn't get any regular exercise. Those who did both exercises outperformed all other groups, while those who did either one still had better memory and learning ability than those who didn't exercise at all.

Prevention

Use your brain every day. Daily crossword puzzles, reading *The New York Times*, tackling challenging jigsaw puzzles, and playing chess or bridge can all help maintain sharp mental processes.

Watch your alcohol consumption. Too much can decrease your mental functioning (even without a hangover).

Watch your portion sizes. You know how you feel after the Thanksgiving meal, when your brain is about as stimulated as the congealed mashed potatoes? Well, to a lesser extent, that effect occurs any time you eat too much.

Eat whole grains and other low-glycemic index foods. Blood sugar swings can affect memory. In one Australian study, people who ate a breakfast designed to have minimal impact on blood sugar (centered on All-Bran cereal) scored higher on tests for mental alertness than those who ate a breakfast centered on cornflakes (which raises blood sugar). Avoid sugary foods that lack fiber. And see page 51 for more on low-glycemic diets, which help keep blood sugar levels steady.

Follow a brain-healthy diet. This is the same advice we gave in the Alzheimer's chapter. It means no more than 30 percent fat, with little or no trans and saturated fats, plenty of foods rich in vitamins E and C and beta-carotene (like dark green leafy and brightly colored vegetables), lots of fish, flaxseed oil, walnuts, and other sources rich in polyunsaturated fatty acids, and regular consumption of foods high in antioxidant flavonoids, such as tea, berries, pomegranates or pomegranate juice, and dark chocolate.

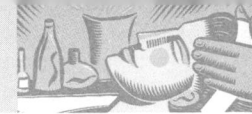

Migraine

There are headaches, and then there are migraines. Given the difference between the two, it almost doesn't seem right to classify a migraine as a headache. Prior to a migraine, you might be extra sensitive to light, smell, or sound. You might even experience flashing lights or partial loss of vision. During the attack, there's severe, throbbing pain, often on one side of the head, sometimes accompanied by nausea or vomiting. The misery can last for hours or even days, and can significantly interfere with your quality of life if you get migraines often.

Fortunately, there are effective prescription drugs that can stop a migraine in its tracks, and if you sense a migraine coming on, you'll want to take one instead of trying to "ride out" the migraine. For people who get frequent migraines, there are also drugs that can help prevent them—but they may come with a hefty price tag and potential side effects that can be serious. So if you're prone to migraines, pay special attention to the "Prevention" section of this entry. There are plenty of natural approaches to try before you decide to turn to these drugs.

Migraines don't just appear; they're instigated by triggers, including certain foods or drinks, the menstrual cycle, stress, muscle tension in the neck and head, exposure to bright lights, inadequate sleep, strong odors, even changes in the weather.

Do This Now

At the first inkling of a migraine, follow these steps to abort the attack or minimize its intensity.

1. Take one dose of a prescription medication such as Imitrex (sumatriptan), Zomig (zolmitriptan), or Maxalt (rizatriptan), also known as triptans.

2. If you don't have prescription medicine, take a dose of over-the-counter painkiller, such as naproxen (Aleve) or a product combining acetaminophen, aspirin, and caffeine, such as Excedrin. Take one Aleve or two Excedrin.

3. Dilute peppermint and lavender essential oils (about 3 to 5 drops in 15 to 20 drops of olive, avocado, or sesame oil) and rub on your temples, around your hairline, and across the back of your neck. You can even find these essential oils in rub-on sticks.

4. To relieve nausea as well as pain, take two 500-milligram capsules of ginger with a small amount of water, or suck on a dried ginger candy. For severe nausea, take the prescription antiemetic Tigan (trimethobenzamide) or Compazine (prochlorperazine) in either oral or suppository form.

5. If you feel that you can't keep anything down, put a few drops of peppermint essential oil on a tissue and sniff.

6. Use this acupressure technique: Rub the fleshy area between your thumb and first finger of your hand very firmly and rhythmically while sitting quietly with your eyes closed and breathing deeply for 5 to 10 minutes. As you breathe out, ease up on the pressure on your hand and imagine all pain in your head draining out as your breath relaxes.

7. Lie down in a dark room with an ice pack on the back of your neck and on your forehead. Picture yourself lying on a beach in the sun

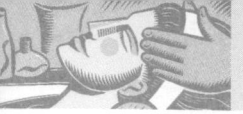

and feel the warmth centered on your hands and head. Continue feeling the warmth soak into your hands and head for 15 minutes.

Why It Works

Triptans, or selective serotonin-receptor agonists, have revolutionized migraine treatment. Taken at the first sign of a migraine, they can stop it in its tracks; even if you swallow them after the headache is in full force, they can cut the migraine's severity and duration.

They work by blocking the release of inflammatory substances from nerve endings and constricting swollen blood vessels in the brain. You can also get Zomig and Imitrex as a nasal spray (helpful if you are nauseated—you don't have to worry about keeping the drug down) and Imitrex as an injection. (Do not give yourself a shot of Imitrex during an aura, however.)

The lavender essential oil is relaxing, while the ginger and peppermint are well-known remedies for nausea. There's even some evidence ginger can help with the migraine itself, probably by blocking inflammatory substances called prostaglandins.

You can also make a cold compress with the lavender and peppermint oil. For every 6 ounces water, add 7 drops lavender oil and 3 of peppermint, then add ice cubes. Stir and dip a washcloth in the mixture. Use as a cold compress to the back of neck and forehead (be careful not to get it in your eyes—the peppermint can burn).

The acupressure technique acts on a specific acupuncture point to release stuck "chi," or energy, relieving pain. In one study of acupuncture on people with chronic tension and migraine headaches, those who received acupuncture had an average of 22 fewer days of headache a year, used 15 percent less medication, made 25 percent fewer visits to their doctor, and took 15 percent fewer sick days off. Meanwhile, a review of 16 studies on acupuncture for migraine and tension headaches found true acupuncture to be "significantly superior" to a placebo acupuncture.

Finally, if you're enduring a full-blown attack and have already taken medication, you need to give it time to work. A quiet, dark room helps, as does focusing your mind on something other than the pain.

Other Medicines
Prescription Drugs

Triptans are the preferred medication for migraine these days, but if they don't work, your doctor may prescribe other drugs, including:

Ergotamine derivatives. These drugs include Ergostat (ergotamine), Cafergot (caffeine plus ergotamine), and DHE (dihydroergotamine). They were the first-line treatment for migraine before the triptans arrived on the scene. They work by constricting blood vessels and interacting with serotonin receptors in the brain, like the triptans, but they have more side effects, including nausea and vomiting and muscle cramps. DHE is considered the most effective.

Midrin (isometheptene). Midrin also works by constricting blood vessels. Although generics are available, the branded version seems to be more effective.

Lidocaine 4% liquid. This numbing agent is taken as a spray squirted in the nostrils every two hours.

Prescription-strength nonsteroidal anti-inflammatories. Anaprox and Naprosyn are often the first choice.

Muscle relaxants. Although these drugs are not a first-line treatment for migraine, they're sometimes prescribed for severe migraines and may help abort a full migraine. At the very least, they'll help you relax and sleep—often the best cure for a migraine.

Reglan (metoclopramide). This antinausea drug can also help abort a migraine.

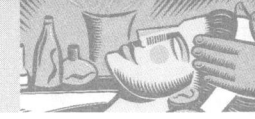

Other Approaches

Neck stretches. Tension in this area can trigger a migraine. At the first sign of a migraine, sit up straight in an armless chair. Grab the edge of the chair with your right hand and lean your neck over to the left, trying to place your left ear onto your left shoulder to stretch your neck muscles. Hold for 10 seconds, then repeat on the other side. Moving your hand back on the chair seat stretches muscles in the back of the neck; moving it forward stretches muscles in the front. To prevent migraines, do these stretches at least once a day.

Acupuncture. If you can get yourself to an acupuncturist before the full force of a headache hits, you might find relief. One study comparing acupuncture with Imitrex or a placebo injection found Imitrex and acupuncture were most effective in preventing an attack, but that the drug was more effective than the acupuncture at relieving the pain once the headache hit full force. Also, an analysis of 22 studies of acupuncture for the treatment of all recurrent headaches, including migraine, found it was more effective than a control or placebo.

Prevention

Identify and avoid your dietary triggers. Food and drink trigger migraines in up to 20 percent of patients. Specific foods include wine, dark beer, aged cheese, cashews, onions, chocolate, and processed meats, as well as food additives like sulfites, MSG, and tartrazine. Keep a headache diary and write down everything you ate before an attack, then look for patterns.

Wean yourself off caffeine, or limit caffeinated drinks to no more than three a day. Sudden decreases in caffeine consumption can trigger a migraine.

Maintain a regular sleeping and eating schedule. Too little or too much sleep, or going too long between meals, can trigger a migraine.

Take 1,000 milligrams magnesium aspartate before bed. Migraines happen because blood vessels in the head spasm and then get flabby, and the pain results from nerves firing in the head in reaction. Magnesium helps maintain the tone of blood vessels so this doesn't happen, and increases the amount of stimulation required to make nerves fire. If they don't fire, you won't feel any pain. Studies find many migraine patients are low in this mineral, and that daily supplementation can reduce the frequency and severity of attacks.

Take 200 milligrams riboflavin (vitamin B_2) twice a day. Although there aren't as many studies on its use as on magnesium, the studies that have been conducted show promising results. One compared daily use of riboflavin to a beta-blocker (a prescription drug sometimes prescribed for migraine prevention) for three months and found the number of headaches dropped about the same in each group. Another compared it to a placebo or aspirin and found 80 percent of those receiving the vitamin had half as many monthly headaches (or fewer) than those taking placebo.

Take 125 milligrams freeze-dried feverfew leaf once or twice a day. Several studies find daily doses of this can reduce the frequency and severity of migraines. It's thought to work by inhibiting chemicals that promote inflammation or making the blood vessels less reactive, so they don't dilate as readily when they shouldn't.

✺ What About...

Migralief?

Anecdotal reports suggest that this over-the-counter product, which contains riboflavin, magnesium, and feverfew, works well in preventing migraines, although there are no good clinical studies to prove it.

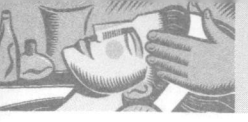

Take 75 milligrams of a butterbur extract twice a day. This is sold under the brand name Petadolex. Few studies have been conducted on its use for migraines, but one study in 33 patients who received either 50 milligrams of butterbur twice a day or placebo found that people who took the herb saw their migraine incidence drop from an average of 3.4 migraines a month to 1.8 migraines a month after three months (about a 45 percent drop), compared to a drop of approximately 15 percent in the placebo group.

For migraines triggered by your menstrual cycle, take 45 to 80 milligrams of soy phytoestrogens daily for at least three cycles. The theory here is that falling estrogen levels in the latter part of the menstrual cycle contribute to migraines, and moderating that drop with plant-based estrogens from soy could help. One study found the number of migraines dropped significantly in 10 women who took the supplement for three months, although there was no comparison to a placebo.

Take 3 to 6 grams of fish oil a day. There's some evidence these anti-inflammatory oils can reduce the incidence of migraines by reducing inflammation. And they're good for your heart, so there's no harm in trying them.

Visit a chiropractor. If your migraines are primarily triggered by stress or muscle tension in the neck and head, consider chiropractic. A study of 127 people with migraine found 22 percent had almost no migraines after two months of chiropractic. Another 50 percent said their headaches were much less severe.

Practice a relaxation therapy at least 15 minutes a day. Stress is a well-known migraine trigger, so it's not surprising that mind-body therapies can significantly reduce the frequency and severity of the headaches. One of the most effective therapies is biofeedback. By learning to consciously raise the temperature in you fingertips, for instance, you draw blood to your extremities and away from your head, which constricts the blood vessels there and helps abort an attack. Biofeedback is usually done in conjunction with guided imagery, in which you concentrate on peaceful mental images. One study compared 20 migraine patients who received biofeedback/relaxation therapy with a control group told to relax on their own. The biofeedback group significantly reduced the pain, depression, and anxiety associated with migraines compared to the control group. You'll need to see a professional to learn biofeedback, but then you can use the technique on your own.

See a psychologist for cognitive-behavioral therapy. This short-term form of therapy (weeks or months, not years) helps you change negative thought patterns that may be causing you stress—which, in turn, may be contributing to your migraines. It also teaches you how to alter your typical reactions to stressful or negative situations and reduce the effect the pain has on your life. Studies find this therapy works best in conjunction with medication—a true integrative approach.

Take preventive medication. If you're having frequent migraines that interfere with your quality of life, talk to your doctor about taking a medication on a daily basis to prevent them. Commonly used medications include beta-blockers like Inderal (propranolol), calcium channel blockers (like verapamil), ACE inhibitors, tricyclic antidepressants (Elavil), and antiseizure medications like Neurontin (gabapentin).

Try Botox for severe migraines. Several studies find this toxin, approved to treat wrinkles, can also prevent migraines. However, it's very expensive and your insurance probably won't pay for it.

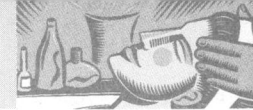

Muscle Soreness

You know the problem—you pushed yourself at the gym, turned over the garden on the first warm day in early spring, had a cleaning frenzy before the relatives arrived—and the next day you're so sore and stiff you can barely drag yourself out of bed. While researchers aren't quite sure what causes delayed-onset muscle soreness, they suspect it's the result of microscopic tears in your muscles, coupled with the inflammation that follows an injury.

You can't do much about the muscle tears except wait for the body to heal, but you can combat the inflammation in several ways. And please, take your soreness as a signal not to further overdo it. Gentle exercise is good right now, but overdoing it again could make you more vulnerable to muscle strains and other injuries.

Do This Now

After a bout of strenuous activity, or if you're already sore, do the following to reduce the pain and inflammation.

1. Give yourself an ice massage. Freeze a couple of inches of water in a Styrofoam cup and peel off the top of the cup, exposing the edge of the ice but leaving the bottom of the ice covered. Hold on to the bottom part of the cup and rub the exposed ice over the sore muscle. Always rub in the direction the muscle runs so you stretch as well as massage the muscle. Massage for 20 minutes at a time, several times a day, if the soreness is less than 48 hours old.

2. Take ibuprofen (400 to 600 milligrams) or Aleve (225 milligrams) throughout the day, following the package instructions, for up to two days after exertion.

3. Add 10 drops lavender, calendula, rosemary, eucalyptus, ginger, or St. John's wort essential oil to 1 ounce massage oil and gently rub into the sore muscle.

4. After the massage, rub a sports cream like Ben Gay or a natural product like Tiger Balm or White Flower oil (available at health food stores) into the sore area.

5. If it's been more than 48 hours since your strenuous activity, apply a heating pad for 20 minutes at a time several times a day.

Why It Works

The ice combats muscle inflammation and also numbs nerve endings, relieving pain. (But ice is of little use starting 48 hours after the injury, which is why we recommend switching to heat then.) The pain relievers also reduce inflammation.

Several studies find that post-exertion massage can greatly reduce muscle soreness. In one study in which 14 people exercised their arm hard enough to cause pain, half received a 30-minute massage and half rested. The massage group had less muscle pain, lower blood levels of creatine kinase (an indirect marker of muscle damage), higher blood levels of neutrophils (suggesting these inflammatory chemicals weren't at the injury site contributing to inflammation), and higher levels of cortisol during the night (the stress hormone cortisol is a natural anti-inflammatory; levels usually drop during the night and increase in the morning). The oils enhance the

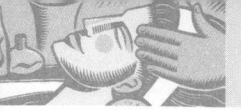

effects of the massage by increasing blood flow to the sore area, removing toxins and relieving pain. We want you to follow up the massage with a sports cream or natural salve, which also ease the ache and are thicker than the oils you used for the massage, so they stay on longer.

Other Medicines
Herbs and Supplements

Bromelain. Studies find this enzyme, derived from pineapple stems, reduces swelling and bruising. Take 500 milligrams two or three times a day.

Prescription Drugs

Ketoprofen lotion. This anti-inflammatory is typically prescribed in oral form for rheumatoid arthritis. Mixing it into a lotion or cream and applying it directly to the sore muscle minimizes the amount that gets into your bloodstream, reducing toxic strain on your liver. The cream has to be mixed by a compounding pharmacy (a pharmacy that creates drug mixtures) and ordered by your doctor. The strength of the cream should be 10 percent.

Other Approaches

Exercise. Call it the hair of the dog that bit you. Studies find that gentle exercise or stretching can relieve muscle soreness—as long as you don't overdo it. Try to focus on the parts of your body that aren't as sore. So, for instance, if your arms are sore from the weightlifting session, take a walk.

Warm bath. Ideally, spend 20 minutes in a whirlpool or Jacuzzi. If your best option is a home bathtub, add 1/2 to 1 cup Epsom or Dead Sea salts, along with 15 drops lavender, calendula, rosemary, eucalyptus, ginger, or St. John's wort essential oils.

WARNING

A Downside of Birth Control Pills

Although women generally experience less inflammation than men after exercise, there's some evidence that women who are taking oral contraceptives, which increase estrogen levels, may find their muscle recovery after exercise delayed.

Arnica 30X. This homeopathic remedy is well studied for its ability to reduce pain and inflammation. Follow the package directions, taking every 15 to 30 minutes for the first two hours after exertion, then once an hour for the next eight hours, then three to four times during the following 24 hours.

Prevention

Load up on antioxidants. Several studies find that taking antioxidants, especially vitamin C, for two weeks before beginning a new exercise program or subjecting your muscles to unusual strain can minimize muscle soreness and help maintain muscle function. Take a combined product containing 1,000 milligrams of vitamin C, less than 400 IU of vitamin E, and at least 5,000 IU of beta-carotene.

Start slowly. You wouldn't run a marathon without training first, so why would you spread a truckload of mulch after sitting on the couch all winter?

Warm up before you begin. Some light stretching and walking enhances blood flow to your muscles and stretches them, reducing the risk of injury.

Mix up your workouts. If you're doing weight or resistance training, don't work the same muscle groups every day.

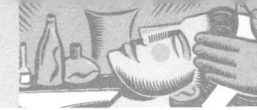

Nicotine Addiction

We don't need to give you another reason to quit smoking—there are plenty of them throughout this book. But the fact is, if quitting were easy, few people would be smoking today. Despite what the big tobacco executives once swore, nicotine is an addictive substance. Smoking is also psychologically addictive. That's why you need all the tools at your disposal to help you quit the habit.

Luckily, we've become very good at learning the best ways to help people stub out their cigarettes for good. We urge you to take advantage of that knowledge.

Do This Now

Once you've made up your mind to quit smoking, follow this advice to start off on the right track.

1. Make a list of reasons why you want to quit.

2. Now set a quit date and let your support system (family, friends, doctor) know about it.

3. Get a prescription for a low dose of bupropion and begin taking it two weeks before your quit date.

4. List the "cues" that lead to your smoking, such as having a drink or cup of coffee, finishing a meal, talking on the phone, etc. Now list other things you can do besides smoke in those instances. For example, when talking on the phone, keep your hands busy by folding laundry or wiping counters. Instead of sitting with a cigarette after a meal, go for a walk. And if you're used to a cigarette and a cup of coffee, switch to tea.

5. As your quit date approaches, slowly cut back your smoking by waiting an extra five minutes when the first craving hits. The next day, extend that time to 10 minutes, then 20 minutes, then 45 minutes, then an hour. By the time your quit date arrives, you should have cut back significantly on the number of cigarettes you're smoking.

6. On your quit date, throw out all your cigarettes and all ashtrays and lighters.

7. Begin using a nicotine-replacement product such as a nicotine patch, gum, or nasal spray.

Why It Works

The list of reasons to quit is obviously motivating. Whenever a cigarette craving hits, pull out the list and reread it. Your other list will help you avoid the smoking "traps" that dot the course of your day.

Studies find that people who set quit dates and don't smoke on that date are 10 times more likely to still be smoke-free six months later than those who smoke on their quit date. By informing everyone in your life of the date, you enlist their support and also put pressure on yourself to follow through. A good idea is to choose a date that has some personal meaning, like your child's birthday (you want to be around for many more birthdays), or your own (a present to yourself). Ideally, pick a time when you know your stress level will be manageable.

Bupropion, often prescribed at higher doses for depression, can significantly increase the odds that you'll still be smoke-free after six months to a year. Overall, studies find it can nearly double

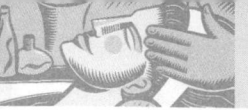

✍ What About...

Weight Gain?

We won't lie to you—when you quit smoking, you can gain weight unless you take steps to prevent it. The weight gain comes for two reasons. First, smoking increases your metabolism slightly. It returns to normal when you stop. Second, many people subconsciously substitute food for cigarettes when they try to quit. So it's important that you find low-calorie choices to snack on when an oral craving hits. Carrot and celery sticks (because they have a cigarette shape and take a while to chew) and grapes (because they keep your hands occupied) are good bets. If you really need to keep your mouth busy, try sugar-free lollipops or candies.

rates of smoking cessation compared to placebo, and, an added bonus, it may help prevent the weight gain that often follows quitting. The drug acts on dopamine receptors in the brain, which are involved in addiction.

Adding the patch or gum boosts your chances of success further, helping wean you off nicotine. Studies find greater success rates in people who use these products than in those who try to quit cold turkey. Follow the directions carefully, and *don't smoke* while using these products. If you have heart disease or high blood pressure, make sure to talk to your doctor before using them. Even though nicotine replacement products are sold over the counter, check with your insurance company about reimbursement. Many policies cover all or part of the cost.

Cutting down on your smoking before your quit date should make it easier to quit. Other ways

to help yourself smoke less include switching to a brand you don't like, buying one pack at a time and keeping it in an inconvenient place, and not smoking at all in your car and house so they become smoke-free *before* your quit date.

Other Medicines
Herbs and Supplements

Milk thistle. This herb helps detoxify and strengthen the liver, important when you're quitting smoking and your body is trying to rid itself of nicotine and other smoking-related toxins. Take 175 milligrams of standardized extract two or three times a day for two weeks.

St. John's wort. This herb is traditionally used to treat anxiety and depression. It can be very helpful when you're coping with withdrawal symptoms from nicotine addiction. Buy a product standardized to 0.3% hypericin or 2% to 5% hyperforin and take 300 milligrams three times daily. St. John's wort can interact with prescription medications such as birth control pills and heart medications, so talk with your doctor before taking it.

Other Approaches

Regular exercise. Regular exercise as part of any smoking cessation program serves two functions: decreasing stress and helping prevent the weight gain that often accompanies quitting. One option: Every time you feel like lighting up, take a walk, spend 10 minutes on the stationary bicycle, or go pull weeds in the garden.

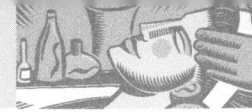

Restless Legs Syndrome

You may know it as the urge to move or jerk your legs when you're sitting or lying still, especially at night. Restless legs syndrome (RLS) occurs when brain cells send false signals of pain, discomfort, tingling, and itchiness to nerve endings in the legs (and vice versa). Moving turns off these signals, but the creepy-crawly sensations return as soon as you're still again.

The syndrome is thought to result from an overproduction of the brain chemical dopamine during the day, which leads to an underproduction at night.

Do This Now

If your itchy, jerking legs keep you awake:

1. Get out of bed and walk for 10 minutes.

2. Sit on the edge of the bed and draw circles with your toes.

3. Knead your calves, thighs, and feet with a mixture of 15 drops lavender oil in 1/4 cup massage oil.

4. Before you try to sleep again, pack bags of towel-wrapped frozen vegetables or ice packs around your legs.

Why It Works

Walking stimulates the nerves in your legs, turning off the creepy-crawly signals to your brain. The toe circles do the same and also stretch the legs and feet. The massage relaxes the muscles. Finally, the cold compresses numb nerve endings while you sleep. The towels should absorb most of the moisture as the ice thaws.

Other Medicines
Herbs and Supplements

Valerian and passionflower. When taken together, these herbs relax muscles and improve sleep. Take 600 milligrams standardized valerian and 300 milligrams passionflower before bed.

Folic acid. In one small study, researchers found that women with RLS were deficient in this B vitamin, required for proper brain and nerve function. Supplementing helped. Take 400 to 800 micrograms a day, along with a 50-milligram B complex supplement.

Magnesium and calcium. These minerals decrease spasms and quiet abnormal nerve messages. Take 150 to 300 milligrams magnesium and 300 to 600 milligrams calcium a half-hour before bed. Give this several weeks to work.

Prescription Drugs

Dopamine agonists. These drugs, including Mirapex (pramipexole), Permax (pergolide), and Requip (ropinirole), return dopamine levels to normal.

Other Approaches

Exercise. Moderate exercise—such as walking or yoga—can improve symptoms, whereas excessive exercise makes them worse.

Prevention

Limit caffeine. It increases dopamine levels.

Quit smoking. Nicotine is another daytime dopamine raiser.

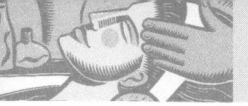

Sore Throat

If you have a sore throat, it's quite likely you have a viral infection. (See Colds on page 82.) Since only time can cure the virus, our self-help approaches focus on easing the pain.

Do This Now

For fast relief of throat pain, rest your voice and do the following.

1. Mix 1 tablespoon salt in 1 cup warm water until dissolved, then gargle.

2. Suck on an herbal throat lozenge that contains slippery elm. One brand is Thayer.

3. Take 100 milligrams Tylenol, 750 milligrams aspirin, 400 milligrams ibuprofen, or 225 milligrams Aleve.

Why It Works

Gargling with salt water remains one of the simplest, most effective remedies for a sore throat. The warmth increases blood flow to the throat, which helps fight infection, and the salt washes away dead cells. Boost your gargle with a squeeze of lemon, which shrinks swollen throat tissue.

Slippery elm coats mucous membranes like those in the throat. The painkillers relieve pain and, except for the Tylenol, reduce swelling.

Other Medicines
Herbs and Supplements

Warm chamomile tea. Chamomile fights inflammation and even acts as a mild sedative. Make a double-strength tea by steeping 2 tea bags in 1 cup boiling water. Gargle with and sip the tea. Add honey for more relief.

Herbal throat sprays. These sprays, such as Singer's Saving Grace, contain a variety of throat-soothing ingredients. Formulas may include soothing and anti-inflammatory herbs such as chamomile and licorice, throat-coating herbs like slippery elm and marshmallow, glycerin (a natural vegetable-based lubricant), or honey (an antiseptic that also coats the throat and draws and retains moisture—a good thing if you have a dry, scratchy throat). Spray into the mouth two or three times every one to four hours.

Throat Coat. This clinically tested herbal tea contains slippery elm, marshmallow, and other throat-soothing herbs.

Over-the-Counter Drugs

Lozenges containing benzocaine. These temporarily numb the pain.

Other Approaches

Humidifier. Adding moisture to the air reduces throat dryness, which helps relieve pain.

Lemon and honey. Sip hot water mixed with 1 teaspoon lemon juice and a bit of honey. The acidity of the lemon juice encourages production of saliva, bathing the throat. The honey pulls moisture from swollen throat tissue.

Heating pad. Apply a heating pad to the throat or wrap the throat in warm flannel (put it in the dryer for five minutes or microwave for 30 seconds) or a towel dipped in hot water and wrung out. The heat increases blood flow, relieving pain.

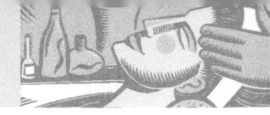

Sprains and Strains

Technically, you have a sprain if you've stretched or torn a ligament (a band of fibrous tissue that connects two or more bones at a joint) and a strain if you injured a muscle or tendon (tissue that connects muscle to bone). Either way, a sudden twist, fall, or blow to the body has created pain, swelling, bruising, and stiffness. Roughly 73 percent of people with sprains suffer recurrent sprains, making preventive steps a must.

Do This Now

Do this now to reduce pain and inflammation.

1. Apply an ice pack for 20 minutes at a time four to eight times a day.

2. Rub arnica ointment and an ointment containing comfrey onto the injured area.

3. Wrap an Ace bandage around the injured area tight enough to be snug but not so tight that you cut off blood circulation.

4. If the strain is around a joint, elevate the joint so it's above the level of your heart. For example, rest your leg on a few pillows piled onto a footstool.

5. Take oral arnica 30C every 15 to 30 minutes after an injury (follow package directions) for four hours, then four times a day for the first 48 hours.

6. Take ibuprofen (400 to 600 milligrams) or Aleve (225 milligrams) every four hours up to two days.

Why It Works

The ice, compression wrap, elevation, and pain relievers reduce swelling, inflammation, and pain. The compression wrap also helps protect your joint from another injury.

The arnica remedies and comfrey cream reduce bruising and pain and may speed healing. Arnica curbs inflammation, as does comfrey, which also stimulates the reproduction of cells to promote the growth of healthy new tissue. (Don't use comfrey on broken skin.)

Other Medicines
Herbs and Supplements

Bromelain. This enzyme, derived from pineapple, reduces swelling, pain, and tenderness. Take 500 milligrams at the time of injury and then twice a day for three more days. Make sure the supplement contains at least 2,000 MCU (milk clotting units) or 1,200 GDU (gelatin dissolving units), and wait at least an hour after a meal before taking it.

Glucosamine. This natural anti-inflammatory is well known for easing arthritis pain, but it can also speed healing of sprains and strains. Take 1,500 milligrams four times a day for the first few days after your injury. Check with your doctor first if you have diabetes; it may interfere with blood sugar control.

Prevention

Wear a brace while you exercise for at least six months to help prevent another sprain.

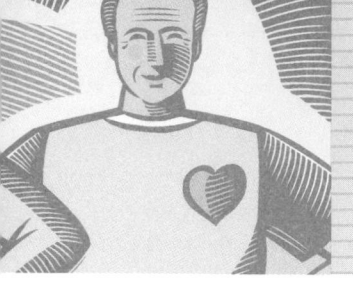

Alzheimer's Disease

Many people view aging like a game of Russian roulette—if you're unlucky enough to land on the chamber with the bullet, you'll get Alzheimer's, and if you do, you're out of luck because there are no treatments.

If you think this way, fortunately, you're wrong on several fronts.

Today we have a number of medications that can slow the progression of the disease, and a vaccine under development. We're also making great strides in understanding the possible causes of Alzheimer's. We now know lifestyle plays a role, which means there are concrete steps you can take to reduce your risk.

One key discovery: The same conditions that increase your risk of heart disease, including high cholesterol, high blood pressure, high levels of the amino acid homocysteine, and being overweight, also increase your risk of Alzheimer's.

Why? We're not quite sure. But it may have to do with the importance of healthy blood flow to the brain. If that blood flow is compromised because of clogged or narrowed blood vessels, less oxygen gets to the brain and fewer waste products leave it. Detritus builds up, possibly leading to the abnormal clumps (called amyloid plaques) and tangled bundles of fibers (called neurofibrillary tangles) found in the brains of Alzheimer's patients.

Cholesterol may also play a role. In animals, high cholesterol leads to extra plaque in the brain, as well as extra plaque in the arteries. And

sure enough, people who regularly take statin drugs to lower their cholesterol are less likely to develop Alzheimer's than people who don't.

So if you're worried about developing Alzheimer's, or even if you've recently been diagnosed, taking steps to reduce your risk factors for heart disease (described on page 268) can also reduce your risk of Alzheimer's and, quite possibly, slow the progression of the disease if you have it.

Alzheimer's is a disease ideally suited for integrative medicine. In one study of 35 people with mild dementia and depression, an approach using antidepressants, drugs for Alzheimer's, and nutritional supplements, along with some changes in diet and mild physical exercise, not only significantly slowed mental decline for two years, but even improved memory and other cognitive functions.

Our Best Advice

The earlier you're diagnosed with Alzheimer's, the earlier you can start treatment. This, in turn, not only slows progression of the disease, but also buys you time to benefit from new treatments that may be just around the corner.

1. Start taking a cholinesterase inhibitor such as Aricept (donepezil) along with the NMDA inhibitor Namenda (memantine) as prescribed by your doctor.

2. Begin taking 80 milligrams ginkgo two or three times a day.

3. Take 400 IU vitamin E and 1,000 milligrams vitamin C daily.

4. Take a daily B vitamin supplement containing at least 800 micrograms folic acid, 400 micrograms vitamin B_{12}, and 250 milligrams niacin.

Why It Works

As of late 2005, there were two classes of drugs for Alzheimer's: cholinesterase inhibitors, including Aricept (donepezil), Exelon (rivastigmine) and Reminyl (galantamine), and NMDA (N-methyl-D-aspartate) inhibitors, in which one drug, Namenda (memantine), has been approved.

Cholinesterase inhibitors work by increasing the amount of the neurotransmitter acetylcholine in the brain, which helps brain cells communicate. These drugs work best when prescribed early in the disease (which is why early diagnosis is so important). Studies find they can slow the progression of the disease, freeing up caregivers and reducing their stress.

Namenda is thought to work by regulating the activity of glutamate. This brain chemical affects learning and memory, helping the brain process, store, and retrieve information. Studies find Namenda can also slow mental decline when used either alone or in combination with Aricept, and it seems to work even in people in the moderate to severe stages of the disease.

Ginkgo seems to work just as well as cholinesterase inhibitors in slowing mental decline. Studies find the herb could delay the loss of abilities needed to cope with everyday life by 10 months after 26 weeks of treatment and by 21 months after a year of treatment. The herb probably works by protecting brain cells from oxidative damage, strengthening blood vessels, and, possibly, preventing the formation of amyloid plaques, one of the hallmarks of the disease.

Remember oxidative stress, Super Threat #2 from Part 2 of this book? Today the evidence is clear that oxidative stress damages brain cells, contributing to Alzheimer's. In fact, many people with Alzheimer's and other forms of dementia have low levels of antioxidants in their blood. That's why we recommend the antioxidant vitamins E and C.

One major study published in the *New England Journal of Medicine* gave 341 people with moderately severe Alzheimer's disease either Cognex (tacrine)—an older drug rarely used these days—vitamin E, the drug plus the vitamin, or a placebo for two years. Treatment with either the drug or the vitamin slowed progression of the disease significantly more than treatment with the placebo. Other studies find that taking vitamins E and C together significantly reduces the risk of Alzheimer's in healthy people.

Why the B vitamins? Because they help control levels of the amino acid homocysteine, a heart disease risk factor and also an Alzheimer's threat. Elevated homocysteine levels double the risk of developing Alzheimer's disease. B vitamins break down homocysteine so there's less of it in your body. If you don't get enough B vitamins, you may have too much homocysteine. Studies find that lowering homocysteine levels with vitamin B_{12}, folic acid, and vitamin B_6 can not only reduce the risk of Alzheimer's but also improve the mental status in people who have Alzheimer's and high levels of homocysteine.

Other Medicines
Herbs and Supplements

Phosphatidylserine (PS). This is a naturally occurring fat we get as part of our normal diet. It's particularly important in enabling the membranes of brain cells to transmit electrical signals within the cell and to other brain cells. Although most positive studies have been conducted on people with mild memory problems—not Alzheimer's—we still think it's a good option for Alzheimer's patients, along with traditional medical treatment. Take 100 to 300 milligrams a day.

Vinpocetine. This supplement, derived from the Madagascar periwinkle, was developed in Hungary about 20 years ago. It's mainly used to treat people with a loss of blood flow to the brain, a key contributor to memory and learning problems. Although there aren't many human studies on its use, three studies show that taking vinpocetine can improve attention, concentration, and memory in people with memory problems more than a placebo. Take 5 milligrams three times a day, increasing to 10 milligrams three times a day if necessary.

Acetyl-L-carnitine. This amino acid is often included in "brainpower" and "memory boosting" supplements sold in drugstores. It plays many roles in helping to maintain the health of brain cells, and may also improve production of the neurotransmitter acetylcholine. In studies on Alzheimer's patients, there is some evidence that high daily amounts like those we recommend here can help slow the inevitable decline. Take 1,500 to 3,000 milligrams in two or three divided doses throughout the day. *Note:* this *not* the same thing as L-carnitine. Also, avoid products with "D" carnitine.

Melatonin. Evening doses of melatonin can improve two common symptoms of Alzheimer's: sleep problems and "sundown syndrome," in which the person becomes agitated as darkness arrives. A review of four studies in which people with Alzheimer's were given 3 milligrams melatonin a day for 21 days as the sun set found that most people who took the supplement showed less "sundowning" behavior and slept better. Start with 1 milligram a day at sunset, gradually increasing the dose (up to 3 milligrams) until you see a benefit.

Other Approaches

Cognitive activities. Keep exercising your brain as long as possible. We know more intellectually active people are less likely to develop Alzheimer's in the first place, so we think that maintaining that activity as long as possible may help delay the disease's progression. In Europe, there are "memory clinics" that use this approach on people with various forms of dementia, and a program in Florida brings together people in the early stages of dementia for a college-level course covering nutrition, mental fitness, stress reduction, communication, and information about the course of the disease. The course provides people more control over their disease, helps them learn to make lifestyle changes that could slow the disease's progression, and improves their mood, self-esteem, and independence.

Massage and therapeutic touch. Many people with Alzheimer's go through stages in which they become very agitated, wander, and exhibit disruptive behavior. Several studies suggest that massage therapy and therapeutic touch (in which practitioners hold their hands close to a person without making physical contact in an effort to correct imbalances in the person's "energy field") can soothe this agitation and reduce the disruptive behavior. One study found that they also reduced levels of the stress hormone cortisol.

Aromatherapy. Aromatherapy won't slow the progression of the disease, but it can help calm agitated behavior. In one study involving 15 severely demented and agitated people in a nursing home, researchers filled the air of the Alzheimer's unit with the scent of either lavender oil or a placebo for two hours a day. After the aromatherapy, 9 of the 15 patients were significantly

less agitated. Another study using lemon balm oil applied to the face and arms twice a day showed similar results. Try a room diffuser plugged into the wall, or mix 10 to 20 drops of either oil in a 6-ounce bottle of filtered water with a tablespoon of plain vodka or grain alcohol. Shake, then spray the room and/or the bedclothes prior to sleep.

Prevention

Get 30 minutes of physical activity a day. Doing so could reduce your risk of Alzheimer's by 50 percent—even more if you increase the amount of activity.

Take a baby aspirin every day. We've recommended this elsewhere to protect you against cardiovascular disease; studies also suggest that regular use of nonsteroidal anti-inflammatories like aspirin or ibuprofen can cut your risk of Alzheimer's by about one-third. A baby aspirin, or 81 milligrams, a day is all you need.

Exercise your mind. Certain activities that stretch your mind, like chess or crossword puzzles, actually help rewire your brain, increasing the number of synapses, or connections, between brain cells. One study found such activities could lower your risk of developing Alzheimer's disease or any other form of dementia by as much as 75 percent.

Maintain a healthy weight. One long-term study of 1,500 adults found those who were obese in middle age were twice as likely to develop dementia in later life.

Get your cholesterol under control. See the entry on high cholesterol (page 284) for specific tips and advice.

Follow a brain-healthy diet. That means no more than 30 percent fat, with little or no trans and saturated fats, plenty of foods rich in vitamins E and C and beta-carotene (like dark green leafy and brightly colored vegetables), lots of fish, flaxseed oil, walnuts, and other sources rich in polyunsaturated fatty acids, and regular consumption of foods high in antioxidant flavonoids, such as tea, berries, pomegranates or pomegranate juice, and dark chocolate.

Take this vitamin trio. Take a B vitamin complex to maintain normal homocysteine levels. Also take 400 IU vitamin E and 1,000 milligrams vitamin C a day. One study of 4,740 Utah residents ages 65 and older found taking both vitamins daily for three years reduced the prevalence of Alzheimer's 78 percent.

Take 1 to 2 grams fish oil daily. When researchers followed 815 people ages 65 to 94 for several years, they found that those who ate fish once a week or more were 60 percent less likely to develop Alzheimer's than those who never or rarely ate fish. Fish oil capsules ensure you get the omega-3 fatty acids found in fish.

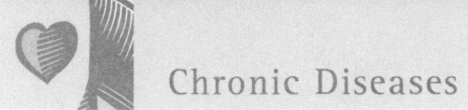

Attention Deficit Hyperactivity Disorder

There's been more controversy swirling around this disorder than pretty much any other condition in this book—about who has it, what causes it, and how to treat it. We do know that it coincides with physical chances in the brain (MRI studies find that brains of children with ADHD are smaller than brains of children without the condition) as well as imbalances in dopamine and norepinephrine, brain chemicals that are critical to our ability to pay attention, maintain focus, and control impulses.

People with ADHD generally have higher levels of a protein that drains the brain of dopamine. When dopamine levels are low, so are levels of norepinephrine.

ADHD affects your ability to do everything from listening to a teacher's lecture to safely driving a car. Get into the work world—where you're expected to continually jump between tasks, manage your time, and keep several balls in the air simultaneously—and you can imagine the potential difficulties.

The disorder affects an estimated 7.5 percent of school-age children, according to a study published in the journal *Pediatric and Adolescent Medicine* in 2002. And, contrary to what we used to believe, one doesn't just outgrow it. Researchers estimate that about 4.5 percent of adults have ADHD, a number that's increasing as awareness of the condition in adults grows.

While drugs like Ritalin (methylphenidate) and other stimulants have been used effectively for more than 50 years, we believe an integrated approach that includes therapy and behavioral training for children and adults, and medication if needed, works best.

Our Best Advice

Here are the first steps we recommend after an ADHD diagnosis.

1. Talk to your doctor about whether taking a low-dose stimulant like Ritalin or the newer nonstimulant drug Strattera (atomoxetine) is appropriate.

2. If your child has ADHD, check with your local school system or mental health provider for parent training classes and sign up. Also try to find a teacher who has received special training in classroom behavior modification methods for children with ADHD.

3. If you're an adult and you aren't taking stimulant medication, try drinking two or three cups of coffee a day, unless it gives you trouble sleeping.

4. For two weeks, cut out all processed foods, especially those high in preservatives, dyes, and other additives, and eat only fresh, organic foods.

5. Take 1 to 2 grams fish oil a day, along with 2 grams evening primrose, borage, or black currant oil.

Why It Works

The evidence on medication as part of a comprehensive approach to treating ADHD is among the strongest in all of pediatric psychiatric medicine, with more than 160 randomized clinical trials showing that short-term use of stimulants improves symptoms in 65 to 75 percent of

children compared to only 5 to 30 percent of those receiving a placebo. Although it might seem counterintuitive to give a stimulant to a child who is hyperactive, these drugs actually reduce hyperactivity by balancing levels of dopamine and serotonin, associated with a sense of well-being.

The major risk with stimulants: Long-term use in children can affect their growth. Unlike Ritalin, Strattera is not a stimulant. Rather, it works on dopamine receptors in the brain, enabling the chemical to stick around longer. Other advantages: It only needs to be taken once a day because its effects last for 24 hours. Although there is no long-term research yet on its use (it was approved in 2002), it works just as well as stimulants in children and adults.

Adding behavioral therapy to drug treatment could allow some children to reduce the amount of medication they take, according to the largest study of long-term use of stimulants, involving 600 children. The therapy includes training parents to provide more structured forms of discipline and to change their expectations of their children, professional counseling by therapists trained in treating ADHD, and rewarding kids for positive behaviors. There's also very good evidence that training teachers in classroom management of children with ADHD can improve children's performance. Keep this in mind

though: In the study, medications plus behavioral therapy worked better than intensive behavioral therapy alone.

Caffeine is a natural stimulant that can provide some benefits in people with ADHD. Of course, it's not as effective as stimulant medication.

Although well-designed studies show no benefit from special "ADHD diets," there is some evidence that the condition, or, at least, the behavior, may be related to certain food allergies. That's why we recommend limiting processed foods, which often have dyes and other additives. that could trigger a response. Try eliminating all such foods for two weeks. If you notice a significant improvement in your child, he or she may have an additive-related allergy.

We recommend the oils because they are rich in fatty acids. There's some evidence that some children with ADHD, particularly those who are hyperactive, have significantly lower levels of key fatty acids found in fish oil and certain foods like flaxseed. In one study in which 50 children with ADHD who had low levels of these fatty acids took a fatty acid supplement (including vitamin E) for four months, some of their ADHD symptoms improved.

We're not sure exactly which combination of fatty acids is most important, but other studies find supplementing with just one fatty acid had no benefits. That's why we recommend a combination of fish oil and one of the other oils, rich in a fatty acid called gamma linolenic acid (GLA).

✌ What About...

Sugar?

The myth that sugar creates hyperactive children just won't go away, despite numerous studies showing no connection between sugar and behavior. While limiting your child's sugar intake is a good idea from a nutritional and dental standpoint, there's no evidence that it does anything for ADHD symptoms.

Other Medicines
Herbs and Supplements

Zinc. There is some evidence that children with ADHD might have low levels of zinc. The mineral is involved in the production of melatonin, the so-called sleep hormone. Melatonin also plays an important role in regulating levels of the brain chemical dopamine. So, the thinking goes, low zinc levels could ultimately lead to low dopamine levels. In one six-week study, children who received 55 milligrams a day of zinc sulfate along with their stimulant medication exhibited fewer ADHD-related behaviors compared to those who just took the drug. Take 20 to 50 milligrams a day, but don't go any higher without consulting your physician.

Iron. Iron deficiencies, although relatively uncommon in children, can lead to behavioral problems. Ask your doctor to check your child's iron levels and, if they're low, recommend a supplement. Don't supplement on your own.

Prescription Drugs

In addition to Ritalin and Strattera, already described above, children and adults with ADHD may benefit from other medications, including:

Tricyclic antidepressants. One of the most studied medications for ADHD outside of stimulants, these drugs (primarily Elavil and Norpramin) are often prescribed in low doses. Like Strattera, they keep dopamine around in the brain longer. Studies find they can be as effective as the stimulants, even more so in people for whom stimulants have no benefit. However, they aren't used as much in children anymore, because they can lead to some heart problems. Other side effects include dry mouth, constipation, sedation, and weight gain.

Wellbutrin (bupropion). This is another antidepressant that affects dopamine receptors in the brain. In one study of 109 children with ADHD, kids taking this drug improved more than those taking a placebo. Another trial comparing the drug to Ritalin found both drugs improved ADHD symptoms similarly. Bupropion, however, can induce tics and skin rashes in some children.

Antihypertensives. These drugs, including clonidine and guanfacine, are primarily used to treat high blood pressure, but studies find they're

---

Diagnosing ADHD

In Children

Diagnosing ADHD in a child requires cooperation among the child's parents, teacher and doctor, and should be done by a qualified therapist or pediatric developmental specialist. There are three main types of ADHD:

Predominantly inattentive, in which a child doesn't pay attention to details or makes careless mistakes, has problems sustaining attention, doesn't appear to listen, struggles to follow instructions, and has difficulty with organization, among other symptoms.

Hyperactive-impulsive, in which the child fidgets and squirms and has trouble staying in his seat, is hyperactive, talks a lot, blurts out answers, has problems waiting or taking turns.

A combination of the two.

In Adults

In adults, common ADHD symptoms include:

- Memory problems
- Problems persisting on tasks
- Problems regulating emotions and motivation
- High variation in task or work performance
- Chronic lateness and poor perception of time
- Becoming easily bored
- Low self-esteem and high anxiety
- Depression and mood swings
- Problems with keeping a job
- Relationship problems
- Substance abuse
- Risk-taking behaviors
- Poor time management

---

also effective in some kids with ADHD. And in one study of 62 children and teenagers with ADHD, the drug helped them sleep better.

Other Approaches

Neurofeedback. The evidence is growing for the use of this type of biofeedback, also called EEG biofeedback, to "reprogram" the brains of children with ADHD so they can focus better. In one study of 100 kids between ages 6 and 19 with ADHD—all taking the same medication—half also had weekly EEG biofeedback sessions. During these sessions, they learned to deliberately change their brain activity by playing special video games, using their brain waves to control the game.

While a year's worth of counseling and medication relieved some symptoms of ADHD among the children, researchers found that only the kids who also received the biofeedback training managed to hold on to those gains after going off the medication. In fact, all the biofeedback kids cut their medication by at least half, and 40 percent were able to stop taking it altogether. A regular biofeedback practitioner may not have the extra training and specialized equipment to treat ADHD; ask ahead of time. Large academic medical centers are most likely to offer this therapy.

Computer training. A computer program called RoboMemo trains children to improve their working memory. This is the form of memory that enables you to focus on future goals, solve problems, and control your attention. One study found that daily training with the program can improve children's performance on certain cognitive tasks while reducing symptoms of inattention and hyperactivity. Currently, RoboMemo is available only in Scandinavian countries, but the program's manufacturer, CogMed Cognitive Medical Systems, plans to sell an English version.

Relaxation therapy. Several very small studies suggest that relaxation therapies like deep breathing, hypnosis, meditation, and progressive muscle relaxation can reduce hyperactivity in children. It makes sense.

Prevention

Turn off the TV. In research from the University of Washington in Seattle, every hour of TV toddlers watched increased their risk of later attention problems 10 percent. Researchers suspect early and intense TV watching molds children's brains in such a way as to later affect the kids' ability to pay attention. TV, with its rapid scene changes, quickly passing images, and stimulating sounds and colors, may condition the brain to expect that high level of stimulation.

Congestive Heart Failure

"Heart failure" sounds about as bad as any medical condition can get, but it's not always so dire. In fact, people with a mild case lead relatively normal lives with few limitations. On the other hand, there are those on the other end of the spectrum who can barely get out of bed.

In CHF the heart isn't very efficient at pumping blood. Instead of coursing through your body with speed and aplomb, blood and other fluids back up into your lungs and other tissues, causing "congestion" and preventing the rest of your body from getting the oxygen-rich blood it needs.

CHF can be managed, and our goal is to help you resume as normal a life as possible. Make no mistake—you will likely need pharmaceutical treatments. But there's more you can do, and we'll share those ideas here. Remember that any degree of heart failure needs to be taken seriously, so it's important that you talk with your doctor about any of the treatments here before trying them.

Our Best Advice

Follow these recommendations to keep your disease from getting worse and maintain your quality of life.

1. Get checked for conditions that can occur at the same time as CHF and complicate your care. These include depression and sleep apnea. Follow your doctor's recommendations to address them. Of course you should also address coronary artery disease, which most cases of CHF stem from.

2. Weigh yourself every day and call your doctor if you gain or lose more than two pounds in a day.

3. Take between 400 and 900 milligrams hawthorn extract a day. If you take the higher amount, split it into two doses during the day. Use an extract standardized to 2.2% flavonoids or to 18.75% oligomeric procyanidins. Try HeartCare from Nature's Way.

4. Take 100 milligrams coenzyme Q_{10} twice a day with food, or take the capsule form, made with oil.

Why It Works

About a third of heart failure patients show signs of depression, with one in seven suffering from major depression. That creates a double whammy. Not only is depression debilitating by itself, but studies find it further weakens the heart by damaging blood vessels and affecting the nervous system and heart rhythms.

The connection could be related to the fact that people who are depressed are less likely to take their medicine, or from a suspected association between depression and blood clots, possibly due to inflammation or decreased movement (when you're depressed, you tend to be less physically active). Whatever the connection, heart failure patients with major depression are twice as

TIME TO WORRY

If you have congestive heart failure, get to the emergency room at the first sign of chest pains or shortness of breath, preferably by ambulance. If you feel any extra or irregular heartbeats, sit quietly for a few moments and breathe deeply to see if the symptoms dissipate. If not, call your doctor immediately.

WARNING

Don't take licorice in any form. Licorice can increase fluid and salt retention, exactly what you want to avoid. Most U.S. "licorice" candy is really anise-flavored and therefore safe. But the European version is usually real licorice, so stay away. Also avoid St. John's wort if you're taking the heart medication digoxin. The herb interferes with digoxin absorption.

likely to die within a year of diagnosis than those who aren't depressed.

Apnea, the sleep disorder that causes frequent breathing interruptions, is both a risk factor for heart failure and a common complication for those already suffering from CHF. Studies find an increased risk of death from both conditions.

We want you to weigh yourself daily because an overnight weight gain of two pounds or more means you're retaining fluid, a danger sign with congestive heart failure, while a sudden weight loss could signify you're on too high a dose of your diuretic. Fluid accumulation leads to swelling of various parts of your body, including your legs and abdomen. More seriously, fluid can accumulate in your lungs, causing breathing difficulties. Generally, your doctor will increase your diuretic dose.

Hawthorn is a widely studied and frequently used herbal heart treatment, with an abundance of evidence indicating its benefits for heart failure patients. One study of 40 heart failure patients with the less serious Class 1 and Class 2 stages of the disease found the extract significantly improved participants' ability to engage in physical activities. Just as important, it seems to be safe and well tolerated, making it a good complement to more intense pharmacological medications. The herb probably works via antioxidant flavonoids that seem to improve blood flow, strengthen blood vessels, and help your body use oxygen.

Coenzyme Q_{10}, or CoQ_{10}, helps your heart cells use energy, important in a heart that isn't pumping enough blood. Studies find that heart failure patients often have low levels of CoQ_{10}, and that supplementing can improve the heart's pumping action.

Other Medicines
Herbs and Supplements

Vitamin B complex. Diuretic drugs used to treat heart failure sometimes deplete your body of thiamine, an important B vitamin. Low thiamine levels can make heart failure worse, and some evidence suggests supplementing can improve heart function even in advanced heart failure patients. If you're taking diuretics, take 50 milligrams of a B-complex vitamin daily. If your thiamine levels are low, consider taking a thiamine-only supplement, up to 200 milligrams daily.

Magnesium. Magnesium helps regulate heartbeats, so an imbalance can increase the risk of dangerous arrhythmias, or irregular heartbeat. Commonly prescribed medications for heart failure such as diuretics and digoxin can contribute to low magnesium levels. That's probably why several studies find supplementing with magnesium can reduce or even eliminate arrhythmias in heart failure patients. Take 20 to 100 milligrams magnesium daily.

❧ Helpful Hint

An Alternative to Hawthorn

If you find you have trouble with hawthorn's occasional side effects—nausea, sweating, or gastrointestinal discomfort—try the hawthorn-based homeopathic preparation Cralonin, which at least one study found helped heart failure patients manage physical activity better.

L-carnitine. This is another nutrient that boosts heart-cell energy, thereby improving your heart's pumping ability. Your heart imports L-carnitine from the liver and kidneys, but that supply might not be enough. Take 1 gram twice a day.

L-arginine. Supplementing with this amino acid helps maintain kidney function, a key concern with heart failure patients. More dramatic, however, is its ability to improve poor blood flow, a cause of constant fatigue. In one study, 21 heart failure patients did much better in exercise tests after taking 9 grams L-arginine for seven days. Start with 2 grams three times a day. If you see no improvement after two to four weeks, gradually increase up to 5 grams, three times a day. Make sure your doctor knows if you're taking potassium-sparing diuretics or are prone to herpes outbreaks before starting on this supplement.

Prescription Drugs

If you have congestive heart failure, your doctor will probably prescribe one or more of these:

Diuretics. These drugs, including Thalitone (chlorthalidone), Lasix (furosemide), and Lozol (indapamide), maintain safe fluid levels and reduce high blood pressure.

Digoxin. Digoxin boosts heart contractions and helps prevent arrhythmias.

ACE inhibitors. These drugs reduce the amount of enzymes that tighten blood vessels, enabling blood to flow better and the heart to pump more efficiently. They also help control fluid buildup, maintain a healthy sodium balance, and increase potassium levels.

WARNING

Watch what you wash your pills down with. Studies find grapefruit juice can interfere with the action of numerous heart failure medications.

Beta-blockers. These drugs reduce your heart rate and the force of the heart's contraction, thus reducing the heart's demand for oxygen.

Nitrates. This is an older treatment usually used for chest pain, but it can also help your heart pump blood by dilating blood vessels and minimizing the extra resistance that sometimes occurs during the heartbeat cycle, which slows the blood's exit from your heart.

Other Approaches

Salt restriction. You'll need to limit yourself to as little as 1 1/2 teaspoons salt, or less than 3,450 milligrams sodium, a day if your condition is severe. Remember, this amount includes the salt in processed foods as well as the salt you yourself add to food.

Pomegranate juice. This antioxidant-rich juice is thought to act much like an ACE inhibitor to limit fluid retention. Try a product like POM Wonderful or add water to 2 ounces of pomegranate concentrate and drink daily.

Deep breathing or meditation. Studies find that practicing deep breathing can help in heart failure by improving oxygen flow through the bloodstream. The relaxation effects also reduce the heart-damaging effects of stress hormones. Meditation, with its emphasis on relaxation and breathing, can impart similar benefits.

Exercise. One study that put 35 men and women with advanced heart failure on a 10-week exercise program found their physical endurance significantly improved. In another study, volunteers who exercised for 20 minutes a day gained a stronger heart-pumping capacity after six months. Check with your doctor first. You may need to exercise in a medically supervised setting, such as a cardiac rehabilitation program.

T'ai chi. This gentle martial art combines the benefits of exercise with stress reduction and breathing exercises. In one study of 30 heart

failure patients, those who took a 12-week t'ai chi course reported a higher quality of life than those who didn't.

Acupuncture. When you have heart failure, your nervous system reacts, treating it as a stress and releasing stress hormones that cause the heart to beat faster, but not better. Acupuncture calms that stress response.

Prevention

The biggest contributor to heart failure is coronary artery disease, or CAD, (more on this on page 268), so your top prevention priority is to avoid risk factors for CAD, such as high blood pressure, smoking, obesity, and high cholesterol. Here are some heart-disease prevention strategies that specifically apply to heart failure:

Control your diabetes. Congestive heart failure and diabetes often coexist in older adults because uncontrolled diabetes damages heart function. More on diabetes on page 276.

What About...

Creatine?

Because creatine supplementation increases muscle endurance, there's some evidence it can help heart failure patients overcome fatigue during physical activity. However, it can negatively affect kidney function (already compromised with heart failure), so we don't recommend it.

Eat more fish. Researchers followed 4,738 heart-healthy older adults for more than a decade and found that those who ate broiled or baked (not fried) fish once or twice a week were 20 percent less likely to develop heart failure. The connection is probably due to high amounts of heart-healthy omega-3 fatty acids in fish, as well as to the fact that if you're eating fish, you're not eating red meat, with its artery-clogging saturated fat. Aim to eat fatty fish (such as salmon or tuna) at least twice a week. Buy wild, not farmed, fish if you can afford it.

Coronary Artery Disease

You can measure a country's economic progress in several ways: Its gross domestic product. The number of cars per capita. The education level of its citizens. Or, its rate of coronary artery disease. CAD is truly a disease of the Western lifestyle, brought on by high-fat diets, wide waistlines, cigarette smoking, and grinding stress. The inflammation that contributes to CAD (remember inflammation, Super Threat #1, from Part 2?) is exacerbated by all that modern life offers, including fatty meats, processed foods, and desk jobs that discourage exercise.

Cancer may be scarier, but the fact is, more people die from CAD than from any other disease.

The mechanism is fairly simple. Plaque—a collection of dead cells, cholesterol, and other gunk—builds up on the walls of coronary arteries. This process is helped along by inflammation, which makes LDL ("bad") cholesterol denser and stickier and more likely to glom onto those walls. As the plaque grows, it narrows the artery and impedes the flow of blood to the heart. A piece of ruptured plaque or a clot that forms on top of the plaque could block the flow altogether (and also trigger more inflammation as the body sends immune cells to the rescue). The result: a heart attack. CAD can also lead to congestive heart failure (page 264).

If lifestyle is a main contributing factor for CAD, it's also a main treatment approach. So be prepared to change your diet, manage your stress, and get more exercise.

Our Best Advice

To control CAD and help prevent a first or second heart attack, as well as reduce the incidence of angina, or chest pain, do the following.

1. Take 81 milligrams buffered aspirin daily with food.

2. Take 1 to 2 grams fish oil daily.

3. Make olive oil, vegetables and fruit, whole grains, and fish the mainstays of your diet.

4. Spend at least 30 minutes a day in some sort of physical activity. Walking, bicycling, swimming, working out with weights, gardening—all have been found to reduce your risk of CAD, heart attack, and stroke.

5. Choose one stress management technique (such as yoga, meditation, qi gong, or t'ai chi) and practice it every day.

Why It Works

When plaque ruptures, numerous cells rush to the site to repair the damage. Among them are platelets, particles that help blood clot. But the last thing you want in a coronary artery is a blood clot. Aspirin helps prevent clots. It also quells the inflammation that contributes to artery blockage. Because daily aspirin use carries some risks, talk to your doctor before starting.

The heart benefits of fish oil, rich in omega-3 fatty acids, are many, including reducing the risk of irregular heart beats that could lead to sudden death, reducing the risk of blood clots, and, most important, reducing inflammation.

Southern Europeans have protected themselves from CAD for centuries by emphasizing plant-derived oils (especially olive oil) and fish oils over animal fats like butter, whole grains over refined grains, and plant-based food over red meat and dairy. Today we call this approach to eating the Mediterranean diet. One analysis of no

fewer than 147 studies dealing with diet and heart disease found "compelling" evidence that this eating strategy helps fight CAD.

Olive oil alone contributes to CAD protection; recent evidence finds it has significant anti-inflammatory powers, much like aspirin. It's also rich in antioxidants called phenols, shown to retard the buildup of LDL cholesterol on coronary arteries. Choose extra virgin olive oil; it's higher in antioxidants and tastes better.

Regular moderate exercise decreases the risk of death from CAD by improving circulation, enabling your body to use oxygen more efficiently, and helping you lose excess weight. In one of many studies showing the benefits of exercise, CAD patients who exercised had healthier arteries, had lower cholesterol and triglyceride levels, and could exercise longer than patients who didn't.

Believe it not, chronic stress contributes to CAD (to learn why, read about Super Threat #5 in Part 2). Amazingly, getting those stress hormones under control not only reduces the risk of CAD but can actually help open up clogged arteries.

Other Medicines
Herbs and Supplements

Hawthorn. This herb is one of the most widely prescribed heart remedies in Europe. It improves blood flow by relaxing blood vessels. It also strengthens the heart's pumping powers, helping prevent a serious complication of CAD, heart failure, which brings with it shortness of breath. Take 60 milligrams three times a day of the Crataegutt extract found in products such as HeartCare by Nature's Way.

B vitamins. Supplementing with vitamins B_6, B_{12} and especially folic acid reduces levels of homocysteine, a protein associated with heart disease. (In fact, in one study, people with the most homocysteine in their blood had double the heart attack risk of people who had the least.)

Take a B complex vitamin supplement that contains at least 400 micrograms folic acid, 50 milligrams vitamin B_6, and 500 micrograms B_{12} daily. If you've had angioplasty, in which the surgeon inserted a stent to prop open the artery, talk to your doctor before taking these supplements; some studies suggest that high doses like those we recommend could raise the risk of restenosis, in which the artery becomes clogged again.

Coenzyme Q_{10} (CoQ_{10}). Levels of this natural substance, found in many foods and in every cell of the body (especially the heart), are frequently low in heart disease patients. It helps maintain healthy heart muscle tissue and also acts as an antioxidant. Most research emphasizes its benefits for those with heart failure, but several small studies indicate it can help angina sufferers better tolerate physical activity. Take 100 to 300 milligrams a day.

L-carnitine. This amino acid, highly concentrated in the cells of the heart, helps those cells generate energy and use oxygen more efficiently. Studies find taking 500 milligrams three times a day helps angina patients exercise longer and more safely. We recommend 1 gram twice a day.

Arginine. Another amino acid, arginine can also help CAD patients. Studies find that taking 6 to 8 grams a day can help them better tolerate exercise with less risk of chest pain. It seems to work by increasing nitric oxide production, which improves blood flow by dilating blood vessels.

✌ Helpful Hint

Drink Your Grapes

You don't need to drink red wine to get the benefits of its most important antioxidant, resveratrol. It's also abundant in dark grape juice, table grapes, and blueberries.

Prescription Drugs

Nitrates. Fast-acting nitrates, such as nitroglycerin, are pills or sprays used to abort an angina attack. Nitrate medications also come in slow-acting preparations like patches and ointments, which provide longer-term angina prevention.

Beta-blockers. These are the drugs of choice for older CAD patients with angina. They help prevent chest pain and heart attacks by lowering blood pressure and reducing the heart's demand for oxygen. Commonly prescribed beta-blockers include Sectral (acebutolol), Tenormin (atenolol), and Zebeta (bisoprolol).

ACE inhibitors. Drugs such as Altace (ramipril), Vasotec (enalapril), and Lotensin (benazepril) open up arteries by interfering with production of the vessel-constricting chemical angiotensin. This reduces the risk of a heart attack, especially for people whose CAD is accompanied by heart failure or diabetes.

Calcium channel blockers. These drugs lower blood pressure and slow the heart rate, but they're generally less effective against angina than ACE inhibitors and beta-blockers. Some calcium channel blockers, such as Norvasc (amlodipine) and Cardene (nicardipine), however, do appear to help angina patients.

Other Approaches

Surgery. Two major but common surgical procedures eliminate artery blockages that cause CAD. They are:

• **Angioplasty.** This minimally invasive procedure is now performed far more often than bypass surgery in the United States. A narrow tube is threaded from the groin into the coronary artery and a tiny balloon is inflated in the artery. The balloon clears the blockage by pressing the plaque against the vessel wall. Then a metal tube called a stent is implanted in the vessel to keep the artery open. Today, stents come coated with special drugs to prevent the plaque from reforming.

• **Bypass surgery.** This procedure transplants sections of artery from elsewhere in the body to create detours, or bypasses, around blocked arteries. It's much more invasive than angioplasty because it involves opening up the chest, so it carries higher risks and requires a much longer recovery time. Still, most people are out of the hospital in three to five days. Why would anyone go with bypass surgery instead of angioplasty? One reason: A recent study found that bypass delivered longer-lasting results than angioplasty, which opens up relatively small sections of artery. With angioplasty, repeat procedures may be necessary.

Enhanced external counterpulsation (EECP). Common in China and making inroads here, EECP is a noninvasive alternative to angioplasty and bypass surgery. Pressurized cuffs are placed around the leg and inflated and deflated. This alters blood flow to the heart, improving heartbeat efficiency. Studies find it reduces angina episodes in 73 percent of CAD patients. A typical EECP course consists of 35 one-hour daily treatments.

✑ What About...

Chelation Therapy?

Chelation therapy uses injections of an organic chemical called ethylenediaminetetraacetic acid (EDTA) that dissolves artery-clogging plaques by depriving them of calcium. Sounds good, but despite anecdotal reports of success, clinical trials testing chelation therapy have found no cardiovascular-related benefits. A large trial was under way in 2005 through the National Institutes of Health; we'll know more when it's completed.

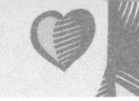

Flaxseed. Flaxseed is the richest food source of omega-3 fatty acids and lignans, an antioxidant. Together they retard plaque buildup, the hallmark of CAD. Take 1 tablespoon of flaxseed oil daily, or include 3 tablespoons of the freshly ground seeds in meals throughout the day (try it sprinkled over salads or yogurt, or mixed into sauces).

Prevention

Maintain a healthy weight. Obesity, especially belly fat, increases your chances of coronary artery disease, probably by increasing the risk of other contributors to CAD, including high cholesterol, high blood pressure, and diabetes. As you read in Part 2, belly fat also contributes to inflammation, a major risk factor for CAD.

Stop smoking. Smoking greatly increases your risk for CAD and at least doubles your risk of a heart attack. The tobacco smoke constricts blood vessels and weakens blood's ability to carry oxygen to the heart. It also raises cholesterol levels and encourages blood clotting. See the Nicotine Addiction entry (page 251) for advice on quitting.

Control your blood pressure and cholesterol. These are serious risk factors for CAD. See pages 280 and 284 for advice.

Prevent or control diabetes. Diabetes increases inflammation, which contributes to CAD, and damages the lining of blood vessels, making plaque buildup more likely.

A healthy diet and regular exercise are your frontline defenses, but also consider Glucophage (metformin), especially if blood sugar levels are already high. Studies suggest this medication not only helps prevent diabetes in people with insulin resistance or metabolic syndrome but may also protect against heart disease directly, probably by decreasing blood fats known as triglycerides.

Consume alcohol in moderation. Whether alcohol is good or bad for you depends on how

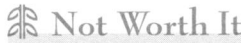 **Not Worth It**

Vitamin E Supplements

Eating foods rich in vitamin E (such as seeds, nuts, olive oil and green leafy vegetables) appears to reduce the risk of CAD. However, there's very little solid evidence to suggest the same benefit from supplements. A huge study of nearly 40,000 women found little difference in heart disease incidence between those who supplemented with 600 IU of vitamin E every other day for 10 years and those who took none.

much you drink. Studies find that light daily consumption (one drink for women, two for men) can protect against CAD. We don't quite know how, but one possibility is that it increases production of nitric oxide, thus improving blood flow. It also seems to prevent blood clots. If you like it, quaff red wine, whose antioxidants are believed to work together with the alcohol itself to provide strong heart protection. Just don't drink too much alcohol or the risks will quickly outweigh the benefits.

Drink your antioxidants. Antioxidants make cholesterol less harmful to arteries. Green tea and black tea, dark grape juice, and pomegranate juice are all rich in antioxidants. A study of more than 3,000 Saudi Arabians found those who drank the most black tea every day were least likely to develop heart disease. Other studies find similar results with green tea.

Take a daily multivitamin. Among the likely benefits of taking a daily multi are a lower homocysteine level and less oxidation of "bad" cholesterol (remember, oxidation makes cholesterol more likely to stick to artery walls). Aside from the all-important B vitamins, make sure it includes magnesium, potassium, and zinc. A growing body of research finds that people with low levels of those minerals are more likely to develop heart disease.

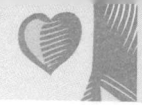

Depression

Many people refer to themselves as "depressed" when they simply mean they feel sad. But depression goes way beyond ordinary sadness. It disrupts your entire life, affecting your appetite, sleep, work, and relationships for weeks, even months.

Today we know that depression is not "all in your head," but the result of certain chemical changes in the brain. According to one theory, prolonged or acute stress triggers depression in susceptible people by damaging or destroying brain cells, creating static in the brain's communication network.

That static prevents messages from getting to and from brain cells via chemical messengers called neurotransmitters. When these messengers, including dopamine, serotonin, and norepinephrine, don't make their way from one brain cell to another, communication breaks down, eroding mood and triggering a variety of symptoms. The aim of most prescription drugs and many herbal remedies is to lift depression by strengthening this communication network, raising levels of particular neurotransmitters to improve the ability of your brain cells to process signals.

The non-drug therapies we discuss in this entry may help with mild to moderate depression; more severe depression will require prescription medication, but, as always, lifestyle and other alternative approaches can work synergistically with medication to improve your condition.

Do This Now

When you're feeling low and depressed, start here to begin working your way back to a positive, stable mood.

1. Talk to your doctor about your depression. Today depression is very treatable with medication, therapy, or both.

2. Take 300 milligrams St. John's wort (standardized to 0.3% hypericin or 2% to 5% hyperforin) three times daily.

3. Even if you don't feel like moving, force yourself to get at least 30 minutes of exercise every day, preferably outside in the sunlight.

4. Take 1 to 2 grams fish oil supplements or 2 tablespoons flaxseed or flax oil daily.

Why It Works

Depression is one of the most treatable diseases doctors see, with some doctors and researchers estimating recovery rates as high as 98 percent, given the right treatment. Yet a major study published in the *Journal of the American Medical Association* found that less than half of all people suffering from depression nationwide receive adequate treatment. "Adequate" means at least eight half-hour sessions of counseling with a mental health professional, or treatment with antidepressant drugs for at least 30 days combined with four visits to any type of physician. Don't try to work your way out of your depression on your own—that's dangerous.

Hyperforin, a main ingredient in St. John's wort, lifts mood in the same way as many prescription antidepressants, by coaxing brain cells to take up more mood-elevating brain chemicals like serotonin, which brain cells produce and reabsorb like a sponge. Many studies show this herb works as effectively as low-dose prescription antidepressants, without the side effects of dry

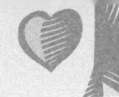

GETTING TESTED

There are no real tests for depression, just symptoms to watch for. See your doctor as soon as possible if you have been experiencing any of the following for two weeks or more.

- Persistent sad, anxious, or "empty" mood
- Feelings of hopelessness, pessimism
- Feelings of guilt, worthlessness, helplessness
- Loss of interest or pleasure in hobbies and activities that were once enjoyed, including sex
- Decreased energy, fatigue, being "slowed down"
- Difficulty concentrating, remembering, making decisions
- Insomnia, early-morning awakening, or oversleeping
- Appetite and/or weight loss or overeating and weight gain
- Thoughts of death or suicide; suicide attempts
- Restlessness, irritability
- Persistent physical symptoms that do not respond to treatment, such as headaches, digestive disorders, and chronic pain

mouth and diminished sex drive. St. John's wort can interact with prescription medications such as birth control pills and heart medications, so talk with your doctor before taking it. You can take it along with antidepressant drugs.

Although depression can leave you nearly catatonic on the couch, force yourself to put on some walking shoes and get outdoors; the effort will be worth it. Numerous studies show that a combination of aerobic exercise (such as walking) and strength training (such as weightlifting) works best at boosting mood. In one study of 24 depressed breast cancer survivors, 10 weeks of aerobic exercise (four days a week, 30 to 40 minutes per session) significantly reduced depression and anxiety compared to a control group that

didn't do any exercise. In addition to aerobic exercise and weight training, studies show that t'ai chi and yoga can also help improve mood. Walking outside brings an extra benefit: exposure to sunlight, which studies show can boost mood.

Finally, studies link low levels of omega-3 fatty acids with depression. In fact, some researchers attribute higher rates of depression in our society in part to modern-day farming and livestock-raising practices that have nearly eliminated this fat from the food supply, leaving most of us deficient. Supplements of oils highs in omega-3s may help. In one study of 28 people with a major depressive disorder, those who supplemented with omega-3 fatty acids were significantly less depressed after eight weeks than those who took a placebo.

Other Medicines
Herbs and Supplements

Ginkgo biloba. This herb increases blood flow to the brain, which can boost energy and improve concentration. Research hasn't yet linked this herb directly with mood, but one study found it improved attention and memory (common problems when you're depressed) in one week. In another study, the herb improved some of the sexual side effects some prescription antidepressants can cause. Take 40 to 80 milligrams of an extract standardized to 24% flavonoids and 6% terpene lactones two to three times a day.

B vitamins. The B vitamins folate and B_{12} help the brain convert amino acids into mood-boosting brain chemicals such as serotonin. People older than age 60, whose bodies may poorly absorb these vitamins, and vegetarians, who may not get enough B vitamins through their diets, may benefit most from supplements. Take 800 micrograms folate and 400 micrograms vitamin B_{12} daily as part of a B vitamin complex.

Zinc. Low zinc levels may trigger a drop in immunity that affects your mood. In one study of

14 depressed people, those who took a zinc supplement in addition to a prescription antidepressant were significantly less depressed after six weeks than those taking only the antidepressant. Take 25 milligrams daily.

S-adenosyl-L-methionine (SAMe). Like prescription antidepressants, SAMe boosts levels of brain chemicals involved with mood. It works about as effectively as prescription medications, and tends to kick in faster (within one to two weeks) than prescription drugs, which may take three or more weeks to begin working. Take 200 milligrams twice a day for one week. If you don't feel better after one week, increase the dosage another 200 milligrams for a week. Continue to increase the dosage by 200 milligrams until you feel better, up to 1,200 daily milligrams.

5-hydroxytryptophan (5-HTP). This molecule increases levels of the mood-boosting brain chemical serotonin. Studies find it significantly improves mood compared to placebo. Take 50 milligrams three times daily.

Prescription Drugs

Antidepressants. There are more than 20 of these drugs on the market. They generally start to work within three to six weeks, first lifting physiological symptoms such as insomnia, poor appetite, and fatigue, then boosting mood. If one doesn't help within three weeks, talk to your doctor about switching to another. You may even find you need to combine two or more. Also, if your antidepressant triggers side effects such as dry mouth, headache, or low sex drive, talk to your doctor. You might be able to switch to an antidepressant that poses fewer side effects.

Other Approaches

Psychotherapy. Studies show that psychotherapy can be just as effective as prescription medications in treating mild to moderate depression. Of the many types of psychotherapy, the two with the most research behind them are cognitive-behavioral therapy and interpersonal therapy.

Cognitive-behavioral therapy teaches you how to change thinking and behavior patterns that contribute to depression. For example, you learn how to reframe thoughts from negative to positive. Interpersonal therapy teaches you how to better handle your relationships with others, particularly those that may be contributing to your depression.

Journal writing. Writing down your thoughts, feelings, and daily events can help you better cope with stressful situations. In one study, 20 people who were depressed wrote about their emotions and reactions daily for four months. Psychiatric nurses who evaluated the journals determined that the daily writing episodes helped participants better cope with stressful life events.

Electroacupuncture. This modern-day twist on acupuncture, in which the acupuncture needles are attached to a device that generates electrical pulses, boosts mood by increasing levels of certain neurotransmitters in the brain. In one study completed on 106 depressed people, 15 minutes of electroacupuncture performed three times a week for one month significantly reduced fatigue and improved sleep and mood compared to a control group that received a sham form of acupuncture.

Massage therapy. In one study of 32 people with depression, those who underwent three one-hour massage sessions spaced two to three days apart found their moods much improved compared to a control group that didn't get a massage.

Bright light therapy. This therapy works best for people with seasonal affective disorder, a type of depression triggered by lack of sunlight during the winter months. You either sit outside up to two hours a morning or use a light box that delivers 10,000 lux of full-spectrum white light for one and a half to two hours.

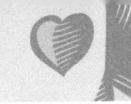

Biofeedback. A biofeedback called neurofeedback teaches you to alter your brain wave patterns in a way that leads to a better mood.

Posture. Believe it or not, improving your posture can improve your mood. When you stand up straight, you tend to think more positively, according to one study of 24 people.

Music. Listening to music you enjoy can reduce stress, slow your heart rate, and help you focus on your feelings. In one study, people with a major depressive disorder who listened to soft music for two weeks were significantly less depressed after the study than those who did not listen to music.

Prevention

Unfortunately, once you suffer one bout of depression, you have a 70 percent chance of becoming depressed again at some point during your lifetime. You can decrease those odds with the following strategies.

Stay on your antidepressants. Once you start taking an antidepressant, continue to do so for at least six months after you feel better to reduce your risk of relapse, and don't stop taking it without your doctor's okay.

Learn to relax. Stress can lead to and worsen depression, so do yoga, meditation, or other relaxation techniques on a regular basis.

Follow a mood-friendly diet that includes plenty of foods rich in omega-3 fatty acids (specifically, flaxseeds, flaxseed oil, cold-water fish). Keep simple sugars, alcohol, and caffeine to a minimum.

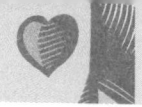

Diabetes, Type 2

Think of type 2 diabetes as an extreme form of insulin resistance (described in detail on page 48). In type 2 diabetes, your pancreas usually still makes some insulin—the hormone that helps blood sugar enter cells—but your body isn't very good at using it. That leaves more blood sugar, or glucose, floating around in the bloodstream. Some people with type 2 diabetes can control their blood sugar level with diet and exercise alone; others (usually those who've had the disease for years) also need oral medication or, eventually, insulin shots.

Our goal is to provide you with the top integrative therapies to enable you to remain medication free or, with your doctor's approval, reduce the amount you're taking. If you're able to move from insulin to an oral medication, we'll consider that a success. Do not go off your medication without first discussing it with your physician.

You also need to consider other health conditions that often coexist with diabetes. For instance, many people with type 2 diabetes are overweight, so see Obesity on page 291. You're also more likely to develop high cholesterol and coronary artery disease, so also see those entries on pages 284 and 268. And, because diabetes is first and foremost an inflammatory disease, read up on inflammation on page 38.

Our Best Advice

Our best advice concentrates on nonmedical treatments that can increase the effectiveness of diabetes drugs or insulin, or help you use less.

1. Add at least one high-fiber food (like a vegetable, whole fruit, beans, or whole grain rice, cereal, or pasta) to every meal.

2. At least once a day, substitute a low-glycemic food for a higher glycemic choice, like whole grain bread for white bread, a bran muffin for a bagel, whole wheat pasta for regular white pasta, etc.

3. After checking with your doctor, start exercising at least 20 minutes a day.

4. Start meditating 15 minutes a day or take yoga class three times a week.

5. Take a multiple vitamin/mineral every day.

Why It Works

Fiber slows the speed at which your stomach empties after a meal, which also slows the rise in blood sugar that happens after you eat. It's best to get your fiber from food (fruits, vegetables, whole grains, legumes). An excellent source is oat bran. One study found that simply eating a slice of oat bran bread with meals improved post-meal blood sugar and cholesterol levels in people with diabetes. Aim for about 2 ounces of oat bran a day for best results.

If you just can't stomach enough fiber-rich food, take 5 to 10 grams of a fiber supplement such as psyllium or guar gum before meals. *Caution:* Fiber supplements can make it difficult for your body to absorb drugs and other supplements, so take your pills at least an hour before, or several hours after, taking a fiber supplement.

The glycemic index ranks foods according to how quickly the carbohydrates they contain increase blood sugar levels—the lower the score, the slower the rise in blood sugar. High-fiber foods are usually relatively low on the glycemic index. Stick with a diet high in vegetables and

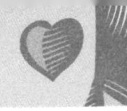

fruit, whole grains, and other high-fiber foods like beans, oats, and bran, and you'll do well. An article that evaluated 16 clinical trials on the effects of a low-glycemic diet on blood sugar found that such diets significantly reduced levels of fructosamine, a marker indicating blood glucose levels over two or three weeks, as well as total and LDL ("bad") cholesterol.

Exercise makes your body more sensitive to insulin; in other words, it essentially helps to reverse your diabetes (it helps stave off the disease as well). In addition to lowering your blood sugar, it also lowers your risk of heart disease, which is high if you have diabetes. We're not talking about marathons here—20 to 30 minutes a day of physical activity, ideally a mix of aerobic exercise and strength training—is all it takes.

Exercise also helps by decreasing the production of stress hormones, which raise blood sugar. Meditation and yoga lower stress hormones too. Studies from Duke University find such relaxation techniques can significantly reduce blood sugar levels in people with diabetes.

Finally, the multivitamin/mineral is important to counteract oxidative stress, a main culprit behind many diabetes-related complications, including heart disease and nerve damage. (Read more about oxidative stress starting on page 44.)

Particularly important vitamins/minerals include vitamin E (400 IU a day), vitamin C (500 to 1,000 milligrams a day), magnesium (300 to 600 milligrams a day), and zinc (30 milligrams a day). If you can't find these amounts in one supplement, take separate supplements.

Two studies found that taking a daily combination of these four micronutrients for three months significantly decreased blood sugar levels while increasing levels of "good" HDL cholesterol and reducing blood pressure. An added benefit of a daily multivitamin is that it seems to reduce your risk of infections, which is higher if you have diabetes.

Other Medicines
Herbs and Supplements

Prickly pear cactus. In Latin American cultures, people eat the ripe fruit of this cactus fried or in shakes to lower blood sugar levels. More and more grocery stores stock such exotic fruits these days, but if you can't find it, buy it as a juice or powder. Several small studies find prickly pear cactus can lower blood sugar levels, possibly because it contains components that work similarly to insulin. If you eat it as a food, aim for ½ cup of cooked cactus a day. Otherwise, follow label directions.

Fenugreek. This spice is commonly used in Indian cuisine and as part of Ayurvedic medicine. It actually belongs to the legume family (as do peanuts), and its high fiber content (it's 50 percent fiber) is a major reason for its blood sugar lowering benefits. Plus, studies find it increases the release of insulin from the pancreas. In one well-designed study, 25 people newly diagnosed with diabetes received either a fenugreek seed extract or followed a special diet and exercise program. After two months, blood sugar levels in both groups dropped about the same. An added bonus? Fenugreek can also reduce cholesterol levels. Mix 50 grams of powdered fenugreek with water to make a gruel, or take 1/2 to 1 tablespoon of a defatted fenugreek seed powder or two fenugreek pills before meals. Don't worry if your urine smells like maple syrup while you're taking it; that's normal.

Cinnamon. Researchers from Pakistan, the birthplace of cinnamon, found that people with type 2 diabetes who took between 1 and 6 grams (about 1/4 to 1 1/2 teaspoons) of cinnamon for 40 days had blood glucose levels 18 to 29 percent lower than those who didn't take any cinnamon (the more cinnamon, the lower the blood sugar levels). Try mixing the spice into coffee or tea, sprinkling it over cereal, yogurt, or cottage cheese, and adding to baked goods and even sauces.

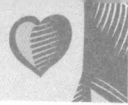

Bitter melon. This South American fruit/vegetable (it's referred to as both) has been used as a diabetes treatment in folk medicine for centuries—and for good reason. Animal and human studies find it can reduce blood sugar levels, most likely through a chemical in the plant that acts like insulin. Buy bitter melon capsules and follow the package directions.

Gymnema sylvestre. This plant has been used to treat diabetes in Ayurvedic medicine for thousands of years. Chewing the leaf or even holding the extract in your mouth for a minute suppresses your ability to taste sweetness for more than an hour, reducing the amount of food (and calories) you take in during your next meal. You can find several products on the market that take advantage of this action, including gums called Sweet Relief and SugarFighter. Gymnema also boosts the release of insulin from the pancreas, and may enable you to take less diabetes medicine. Take 400 milligrams of a gymnema extract twice a day.

Bilberry. Not only does a tea made with this herb reduce blood sugar levels in animal studies, but the fruit of the plant, rich in antioxidants called anthocyanidins, also seems to help prevent damage to very tiny blood vessels. This damage is common in people with diabetes, resulting in a nerve-related complication called neuropathy, as well as the eye problem called retinopathy. Take 80 to 160 milligrams of an extract standardized to 25% anthocyanidins in divided doses.

Prescription Drugs

In addition to injectable insulin, several oral drugs are available for the treatment of type 2 diabetes. These include:

Sulfonylureas. Sulfonylureas are the oldest class of oral diabetes drugs. The newer drugs within this class, such as Amaryl (glimepiride), are less likely to induce hypoglycemia, or dangerously low blood sugar. They work by stimulating your pancreas to make more insulin, so only use them if the insulin-producing beta cells in your pancreas still work.

Biguanides. The most commonly prescribed biguanide is Glucophage (metformin). It seems to work by reducing the amount of glucose the liver releases and helps insulin push glucose into muscle cells. Don't use it if you have kidney failure or congestive heart failure.

Thiazolidinediones. Avandia (rosiglitazone) and Actos (pioglitazone), help your muscles take in more glucose, thus reducing the amount of glucose your liver releases, although not as much as metformin. There's some evidence it may also help maintain the pancreas's ability to produce insulin, which often weakens over time. Downsides are that they take up to a month to begin working (four months for maximum effect), and can cause weight gain. Stay away if you have congestive heart failure.

Alpha-glucosidase inhibitors. Used rarely these days, Precose (acarbose) and Glyset (miglitol) slow the absorption of carbohydrates. They have to be taken throughout the day as soon as you start eating. They also cause gas and bloating, side effects that may disappear once you've been using them awhile.

Meglitinides. Prandin (repaglinide) and Starlix (nateglinide) help the pancreas make more insulin, but only when blood sugar is high—a

❦ Helpful Hint

Sweeten With Stevia

The leaves of stevia, a Mexican herb, make an excellent sweetener whether or not you have diabetes (you can buy the herb in extract form as a dietary supplement). If you have diabetes, there's some evidence that stevia can also increase the release of insulin from the pancreas, helping lower blood sugar levels.

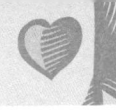

plus over the sulfonylureas because they reduce the risk of hypoglycemia. They're taken before meals so they work right when you need them.

Incretins. This is the newest class of diabetes drug. The first drug, Byetta (exenatide) was approved in April 2005, and others are coming. Given by self-injection with a prefilled pen, it enhances the effect of hormones secreted by the intestines that signal the pancreas to make more insulin. It also prevents the liver from releasing stored glucose, and slows the rate at which food enters the intestine, further blunting any post-meal glucose spikes. There's also some evidence these drugs can help maintain the health of insulin-producing cells in the pancreas. Byetta even suppresses the appetite and may therefore help with weight loss. It's often prescribed along with oral diabetes medications (although it may also be prescribed alone), and is taken before breakfast and dinner.

Other Approaches

The right ratio of macronutrients. In addition to choosing from low-glycemic foods, follow the standard diet recommended for people with diabetes: 40 to 50 percent of your calories from complex carbohydrates (whole grains, fruits, vegetables, beans and legumes, i.e., low-glycemic), 20 to 30 percent from protein (limit meat and substitute soy and seafood whenever possible to reduce saturated fat); and 20 to 30 percent from fats, particularly "good" (monounsaturated) fats like olive and canola oil.

Onions and garlic. Make these a regular part of your diet. Animal and a few human studies find the fragrant vegetables can lower blood sugar as well as cholesterol and blood pressure.

Green or oolong tea. A small study of 20 people with type 2 diabetes found that those who drank 1 1/2 quarts of oolong tea a day for 30 days significantly reduced their blood sugar levels and their levels of fructosamine (a marker that provides information about your glucose levels over the past two to four weeks) compared to when they drank only water. In lab animals, there's evidence in animals that green tea helps cells soak up more glucose.

Prevention

Follow a high-fiber, low-glycemic diet. Make it high in dietary magnesium sources, like leafy green vegetables and whole grains, which studies find can reduce the risk of diabetes. At the same time, decrease the amount of meat in your diet, particularly processed meats like bacon and cold cuts. Studies find the higher your consumption of these foods, the higher your risk of developing type 2 diabetes.

Maintain a normal body weight. Being overweight or obese is probably the greatest risk factor for type 2 diabetes. See Obesity (page 291) for our best recommendations on maintaining a normal weight.

Take a yoga class. One study of 98 people with a variety of illnesses, including diabetes, found that nine days of yoga classes reduced blood glucose, total and LDL ("bad") cholesterol levels, and triglycerides, while increasing HDL ("good") cholesterol, likely due to yoga's ability to reduce the effects of stress on the body.

High Blood Pressure

High blood pressure is one of those conditions that sound relatively harmless—but it's anything but. It not only increases your risk of stroke and heart attack, which you probably know, but also dementia, kidney disease, bone loss, vision problems, and impotence.

Blood flows through arteries with remarkable force. If you have high blood pressure, that force is even higher than normal because the vessel walls have been narrowed by plaque or the arteries have become stiff and less accommodating (or both). Either way, the heart must work harder to pump that blood, possibly leading to heart failure.

The high-pressure flow of blood can scar the artery walls over time. This is bad news because scarred walls give artery-clogging plaque a much better foothold than smooth ones do. If your blood vessels aren't very elastic and don't contract and expand easily, the pressure of the blood can knock loose a piece of that plaque, or a blood clot, which could travel to your brain and cause a stroke, or block a coronary artery and cause a heart attack.

If you're between 40 and 70 years old, every increase of 20 mm/Hg of systolic blood pressure (the top number) or 10 mm/Hg in diastolic blood pressure (the bottom number) *doubles* your risk of cardiovascular disease. On the other hand, bring your blood pressure down to normal and you reduce your risk of stroke 35 to 40 percent, your risk of heart attack 20 to 25 percent, and your risk of heart failure more than 50 percent.

Aim for a reading below 120/80 mm/Hg. Today, anything between 120/80 and 139/89 is considered prehypertensive, meaning you're at risk for high blood pressure; 140/90 and above means high blood pressure.

We believe strongly that the best approach to treating high blood pressure is one that combines drugs, if warranted, with self-help strategies—including relaxation techniques and changes to your diet. As with many of the chronic diseases we discuss, the lifestyle changes that work to treat the condition also work to prevent it.

Our Best Advice

1. Follow the Dietary Approaches to Stop Hypertension (DASH) diet. That means keeping saturated fats (from animal and dairy products) as low as possible, switching to non- or low-fat dairy, choosing whole grains over refined flour products like white bread, and eating 8 to 10 servings of fruits and vegetables daily.

2. If you smoke, stop.

3. Avoid alcohol. The heart benefits of moderate drinking do not apply if you have high blood pressure.

4. Get out for a 30-minute walk, bike ride, or swim every day.

5. Meditate for 15 minutes once or twice a day.

Why It Works

The DASH diet was originally developed by the National Institutes of Health (NIH) and tested on 459 adults with a wide range of blood-pressure readings. Both systolic and diastolic readings dropped dramatically after only two weeks on the diet. Expect to see your own pressure drop 8 to 14 points in the same time period.

Key to the DASH diet is replacing cholesterol-raising saturated fat (found in fatty meats, poultry skin, and full-fat dairy products) with good fats like olive oil. A large survey from Spain found the more olive oil people consumed, the lower their risk of hypertension. Another study from Italy found using olive oil every day enabled people with high blood pressure to take less medication. Certain substances in olive oil probably enhance nitric oxide levels, helping blood vessels dilate and improving blood flow.

The generous servings of fruits and vegetables also play a big role in your blood pressure control. The extra fiber helps reduce blood cholesterol (so there's less to stick to artery walls) and the high levels of plant antioxidants prevent LDL cholesterol from oxidizing, making it less likely to stick to vessel walls. In one study of 56 people who followed a higher-salt version of the DASH diet for a year, the half who also increased their fruit and vegetables intake were the only ones whose blood pressure didn't rise.

Reducing refined white-flour foods and saturated fat also helps you shed extra pounds, which always helps lower blood pressure. However, you can gain the benefits even if you don't lose weight; studies find the DASH diet's benefits are independent of weight loss.

You must quit smoking. Nicotine narrows arteries, increasing the pressure blood exerts on them. A revealing look at this effect comes via a study of 40 healthy volunteers, half chronic smokers, half of whom had never smoked. Once they lit up, their heart rate and blood pressure shot up, regardless of smoking history.

With alcohol, there's always a trade-off between moderate drinking's heart protective effect and its blood pressure elevating effect. But if you already have high blood pressure, the choice is clear: Cutting back on the booze significantly lowers blood pressure.

Meanwhile, regular moderate exercise by itself can decrease systolic blood pressure (the top number) by 3.5 points or more, and diastolic blood pressure (the bottom number) by 2 points or more. This is true regardless of your starting weight. Practice steady, rhythmic activities—like walking, jogging, swimming, or cycling—for at least a half hour most days of the week. And, as always, talk to your doctor first before beginning any exercise program.

Finally, the connection between stress and blood pressure is clear. That's why we recommend transcendental meditation (TM), a form of meditation in which you sit quietly and repeat a single word or sound. It can significantly lower blood pressure by decreasing the release of stress hormones and relaxing blood vessels. See page 60 in Part 2 for instructions.

TIME TO WORRY

While even mild hypertension (140/90 mm/Hg to 159/99 mm/Hg) needs to be taken seriously, blood pressure readings of 160/100 mm/Hg indicate "Stage 2" hypertension and put you in immediate danger of stroke and heart attack. About two thirds of strokes and half of all heart attacks happen to people with Stage 2 hypertension. Get yourself to a hospital immediately so doctors can bring your pressure down.

Other Medicines
Herbs and Supplements

Soy. We're not quite sure just how soy lowers blood pressure, but it could have something to do with a powerful antioxidant in soy called genistein. Regardless, soy works. In one study of more than 300 people, those who supplemented with 40 grams of isolated soy protein daily for 12 weeks saw their blood pressure drop an average of 7.88 mm/Hg systolic and 5.27 mm/Hg diastolic. There are many ways to get isolated soy

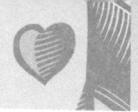

protein. Buy the powder and add it to shakes or even baked goods—the study participants got theirs in cookies! You can also get good results over time from drinking four 8-ounce glasses of soy milk daily.

Folic acid. Folic acid, a B vitamin, seems to ease the stiffness in the large blood vessel that carries blood out of your heart. In one study of 41 people with high blood pressure, those who took 5 milligrams of folic acid a day for three weeks found their systolic pressure dropped an average of 4.7 points. Take 5 milligrams a day.

Fish oil. The good fats known as omega-3 fatty acids, which are abundant in fish such as salmon and mackerel, are important components of the DASH diet. But you can also get the benefits from fish oil capsules. Studies find at least 2 grams a day (but preferably 4 to 6 grams) can reduce blood pressure, probably by making blood vessels more flexible. Fish oil supplements also lower triglyceride levels, an extra heart benefit.

Hibiscus flower. When 39 people with high blood pressure drank a cup of hibiscus tea every morning for a month, their average blood pressure dipped from about 139/91 mm/Hg to 124/80 mm/Hg. That was essentially the same improvement 36 other people in the same study achieved with daily doses of the blood pressure drug Capoten (captopril). The effects are likely due to the herb's diuretic properties and ability to slightly relax blood vessels. Researchers made the tea with 10 grams of dried flower steeped in hot water, but you can buy hibiscus tea bags in health food stores and online, or take supplements of hibiscus extract. Drink a cup a day or follow package directions for the supplement.

Potassium. Potassium reduces blood pressure by helping your kidneys flush sodium out of your body. Sodium increases the amount of fluid in your body, thus increasing the amount of blood and the pressure through vessels. Many experts consider getting adequate potassium levels even more critical to managing blood pressure than reducing sodium. If your blood pressure is already high, you may be potassium depleted, especially if you're taking diuretics that deplete the mineral. In addition to supplementing with 1.5 to 3 grams of potassium a day, add more high-potassium foods like bananas, cantaloupes, tomatoes, dried beans, and nuts to your diet.

Prescription Drugs

Diuretics. These drugs, which help your body get rid of excess fluid and salt, are considered the first-line therapy for high blood pressure, safely lowering pressure, reducing your risk of heart attack and stroke, and protecting against blood clots. Although they're the oldest and least expensive blood pressure medication, a landmark 2002 study found they worked better than newer alternatives such as ACE inhibitors, beta-blockers, and calcium channel blockers, and cost much less. Don't be surprised if you wind up taking more than one diuretic.

The most commonly prescribed diuretics for high blood pressure are the thiazides, such as

What About...

Aspirin?

Although low-dose aspirin is often recommended to reduce the risk of heart attack and stroke in high-risk people, some studies suggest it may actually raise blood pressure, especially in people taking drugs like ACE inhibitors. Low-dose aspirin (81 milligrams) may be fine—an Italian study of 142 people with high blood pressure found no difference in blood pressure between those who took a low-dose aspirin every day and those who didn't—but avoid taking higher doses of aspirin or any other nonsteroidal anti-inflammatory drug, such as ibuprofen, on a regular basis.

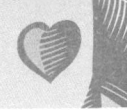

WARNING

Stay away from herbal licorice supplements or candy flavored with real licorice. They raise blood pressure (which is why licorice is sometimes used to treat low blood pressure).

Diuril (chlorothiazide), Hygroton (chlorthalidone), and Lozol (indapamide). But doctors sometimes prescribe potassium-sparing diuretics, such as Midamor (amiloride) and Aldactone (spironolactone) to avoid depleting that important mineral.

Other Approaches

Salt control. Cutting way back on salt is beneficial for many people with high blood pressure. Not only does sodium (found in salt) increase fluid retention, but it's also thought to stimulate secretion of hormones that damage blood vessels. But not everybody benefits from salt reduction. It depends on whether you're "salt-sensitive." If you are, you can usually reduce your blood pressure an average of 6 systolic and 2 diastolic points by limiting your sodium intake to no more than 3 grams, or about 1 1/2 teaspoons of salt. (Remember that the salt in packaged foods counts too.) Give it a month to see a benefit. If your blood pressure doesn't change, you're probably not salt-sensitive.

Chocolate. Here's a remedy you'll like—eat a small dark chocolate bar every day. Dark chocolate is rich in flavonols, antioxidants that reduce blood pressure by improving blood vessel function. When 20 volunteers ate a 3.5-ounce bar of dark chocolate every day for a week, their systolic blood pressure dropped an average of 12 points and their diastolic pressure dropped an average of 8.5 points. When those same participants switched to white chocolate (which contains no flavonols), their blood pressure didn't change. Make sure you use real, bitter dark chocolate, with a high percentage of cocoa, and not sweetened commercial candies. Also, compensate for the extra calories by cutting calories from elsewhere in your diet.

Stress reduction. The link between stress and elevated blood pressure is clear, and job-related stress is a major culprit. But by taking advantage of a workplace stress reduction program, you can lower your blood pressure significantly—by 10.6 points systolic and 6.3 diastolic, according to one study. The program might include counseling on how to refocus your emotion in a positive way, as well as techniques for responding positively to stressful situations. Check with your human resources department for programs in your area. If you don't have an employer, ask your doctor, local hospital, senior center, or YMCA about stress-reduction training.

Qi gong. This ancient Chinese mind-body exercise also seems to help lower blood pressure, perhaps by reducing stress and the release of stress hormones. A small study of 36 middle-aged people with high blood pressure found significantly lower blood pressure after eight weeks of two 30-minute qi gong routines a day. Traditional Chinese Medicine practitioners and licensed acupuncturists usually offer qi gong training.

Prevention

Get your weight under control. Being overweight doubles your risk of developing high blood pressure. So maintaining a healthy body weight, or shedding excess pounds if you need to, helps you avoid hypertension. It doesn't take much loss—just 10 percent of your total body weight (20 pounds if you weigh 200 pounds) can make a huge difference.

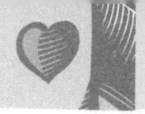

High Cholesterol

Here's the truth: A high cholesterol level does not automatically doom you to a heart attack or stroke. In fact, half the people who have heart attacks don't have high cholesterol (although they may have other risk factors, such as inflammation). That said, high cholesterol *does* increase your risk of heart disease and stroke, not to mention Alzheimer's disease and, for men, erectile dysfunction. So it pays to bring it down.

"Cholesterol" isn't as simple as high and low. There are "good" (HDL) and "bad" (LDL) types of cholesterol. (Good cholesterol sweeps bad cholesterol out of the body, so high levels of this kind are actually beneficial.) And that's not all: We now know that "bad" cholesterol comes in different forms, some of which are more dangerous than others. For instance, small, dense LDL particles are the stickiest and the most likely to glom onto artery walls. If you have a lot of inflammation and oxidative stress (Super Threats #1 and #2), you're more likely to have this type.

Target levels of "bad" cholesterol keep getting lower and lower, especially for people at high risk for heart disease. In fact, current target levels are so low, it may not be possible for many people to achieve them through a healthy diet alone, especially if high cholesterol is in your genes. That's one reason more and more people are taking cholesterol-lowering statin drugs.

But most statins don't increase "good" cholesterol—and this is one area where integrative approaches such as exercise and niacin can be helpful. Statins also don't do much for high levels of dangerous blood fats called triglycerides, which is where fish oil can help. Fish oil also decreases inflammation, now considered a major risk factor for heart disease along with high cholesterol.

The bottom line: Lowering high cholesterol should be viewed as part of a larger journey toward healthier arteries.

You may want to try to manage your cholesterol first with diet and supplements before turning to a statin. Even if you're taking a statin, some of these strategies could help you take lower doses of the drug (with your doctor's approval). Use these ideas as part of a complete cholesterol-lowering strategy with the help of a doctor trained in natural medicine.

Note that we don't have a separate "Prevention" section in this entry; following the dietary, exercise, and stress reduction recommendations here is the best way to prevent high cholesterol.

Our Best Advice

If your cholesterol is high but you don't need medication yet, follow our best advice to lower it and reduce your risk of heart disease.

1. Eat a bowl of oatmeal several mornings a week, and stock up on oat grain bread.

2. Spread the bread with 2 tablespoons Benecol (or another sterol spread) instead of butter or margarine. If you don't use the spread, take a supplement with 1 to 2 grams of sterols a day.

3. Sprinkle a teaspoon of crushed flaxseed over cereal, yogurt, salads, eggs, etc., at least once a day, and use flaxseed oil in salad dressings.

4. Stock up on low- or no-fat versions of milk, sour cream, yogurt, salad dressing, cheese, cream cheese, and mayonnaise if you use it.

5. Eat fish, tofu, or bean-based meals several times a week.

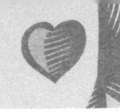

6. Take a 30-minute brisk walk every day.

7. In addition to a multivitamin, take the following supplements: 5 to 10 milligrams policosanol twice a day, a garlic supplement standardized to 500 milligrams allicin twice a day, and 50 to 100 milligrams niacin once a day, particularly if your HDL levels are low.

8. Set the alarm on your watch or computer to beep every hour. When it does, close your eyes and practice deep breathing for three minutes.

Why It Works

We want you to eat oats and flaxseed because they're terrific sources of soluble fiber, which studies find can significantly reduce LDL levels. (Flaxseed is also rich in valuable omega-3 fatty acids, which you've read about elsewhere.) Soluble fiber works by forming a gel in your stomach and small intestine that absorbs some of the cholesterol and fat from the food you eat, so less of it reaches your bloodstream. Plus, a chemical reaction related to eating fiber reduces the amount of cholesterol your liver makes.

Spreads like Benecol contain sterol, a plant-based compound similar to cholesterol. It's so similar, in fact, that it competes with real cholesterol for space on receptors that let cholesterol be absorbed by the body—and it usually wins, resulting in lower blood cholesterol levels. Studies find two to three grams a day (less than 2 tablespoons) of one of these spreads can reduce total and LDL cholesterol levels 9 to 20 percent.

Cutting way down on saturated fat is key if you want to lower your cholesterol. This is the type of fat abundant in cheese and other full-fat dairy foods (like ice cream), some red meat, and chicken skin. For every 1 percent increase in saturated fat in your diet, your LDL increases by 2 percent.

Fill your plate instead with veggies, and use fish, beans, and tofu as lean protein sources.

Why? They each have cholesterol-lowering properties, which meat doesn't have. Fish lowers total cholesterol and also helps prevent dangerous blood clots. Beans are chock-full of cholesterol-lowering soluble fiber. And studies find 25 grams of soy protein a day can reduce cholesterol levels about 5 percent.

One thing a healthy diet can't do is raise your levels of "good" HDL cholesterol—but exercise can. It can also lower your triglycerides and your stress hormones, which you'll read more about in a minute. It even increases the size of cholesterol particles, making them less dangerous.

As for the supplements we recommend: Policosanol, a mixture of alcohols purified from sugarcane, works like a natural statin. Studies find that 5 to 10 milligrams a day lowered cholesterol levels as well as several statin drugs did. Plus, the supplement has a good track record; users followed for more than three years had no negative side effects.

Niacin is a B vitamin that can reduce LDL cholesterol 15 to 20 percent, as well as reducing

✐ What About...

Red Yeast Rice?

This yeast is a natural statin. It's so similar to statin drugs, in fact, that the FDA decided it was a drug and shouldn't be sold as a supplement. It ordered the red yeast extract Cholestin off the market in 2002. Cholestin is still being sold under the same name, but it now contains a different active ingredient. You can, however, still find red yeast extract in some health food stores and online.

Red yeast rice is much cheaper than statins and may have fewer side effects. But remember that there's not nearly as much research into this supplement as there is into statins, which are among the most well-researched drugs in the world. Don't take it if you're already taking a statin.

triglyceride levels. Plus, it's one of the few supplements or drugs that increases HDL levels. We're starting you off on a relatively low dose, which can be increased. But don't take more than 150 milligrams without your doctor's supervision, and avoid sustained-release niacin because it can cause liver problems in high doses.

Garlic's cholesterol-lowering effects have been mixed in studies, but that seems to be due to differences in the type of supplements used. We recommend Kwai or Kyolic brands. An added bonus? Garlic can lower blood pressure, too. Either eat two to five fresh cloves a day (try them roasted with some olive oil and spread on whole grain bread), or take an extract standardized to contain 1.3% allicin.

Why the deep breathing? You may be surprised to learn that chronic stress can raise cholesterol. One reason is that stress hormones signal fat cells to release stored fatty acids, which are converted to cholesterol. They also prompt the liver to release triglycerides, which also end up as cholesterol. So reducing stress is key.

Other Medicines
Herbs and Supplements

Artichoke leaf extract. A German study found dried artichoke leaf extract reduced total cholesterol an average of 18.5 percent and LDL 22.9 percent. The herb is thought to work by limiting the amount of cholesterol the liver makes while encouraging the conversion of cholesterol into bile acids. Take 1,800 milligrams a day in two or three divided doses.

Guggul. This herb works by sending more cholesterol to the liver for absorption, thus reducing blood cholesterol levels. In one study of 205 people, the majority of those taking 500 milligrams guggul a day for 12 weeks saw their cholesterol and triglyceride levels plummet an average of 24 percent, and HDL levels increased in

> ### ✐ What About...
>
> #### Eggs?
> Eggs are not the devils they've been made out to be. You no longer have to avoid them. In fact, eggs pack a nutritional powerhouse in a relatively small number of calories. For the best benefits, though, choose free-range eggs. When *Mother Jones* magazine tested eggs from free-range chickens versus those from commercially raised chickens, it found the free-range eggs had up to twice as much vitamin E, six times as much beta-carotene, and four times as many omega-3 fatty acids. Plus, they averaged just half the cholesterol the USDA lists for eggs from commercially raised hens.

60 percent of them. Other studies find combining guggul supplements with a healthy diet high in fruits and vegetables can reduce cholesterol levels as much as some commonly used medications. Give guggul time to work; it can take up to four weeks before you see improvement.

Prescription Drugs

Statins. The drugs, including Lipitor (atorvastatin), Lescol (fluvastatin), Mevacor (lovastatin), Pravachol (pravastatin), and Zocor (simvastatin), along with an extended-release form of lovastatin called Altocor, work by partially blocking an enzyme that controls how quickly your body produces cholesterol. They also increase your body's ability to strain LDL cholesterol from your bloodstream and bring it to your liver, which breaks it down for excretion from the body.

Fibrates. These drugs enable your liver to absorb more fatty acids, thus reducing triglyceride production. They're also used to increase HDL levels, but they are probably the least effective drug at reducing LDL levels. Don't take with statins; they can cause muscle damage.

Cholesterol absorption inhibitors. The first drug approved in this drug class, Zetia (ezetimibe), lowers cholesterol by preventing the intestine from absorbing it. It is usually paired with a statin. Studies find the two together can reduce cholesterol levels 25 percent more than statins alone.

Actos (pioglitazone). This drug is approved for treating type 2 diabetes and insulin resistance, but it can also reduce dense LDL cholesterol—a more dangerous form of LDL cholesterol—particularly in people with metabolic syndrome.

Bile acid sequestrants. This is the oldest class of drugs for reducing cholesterol. They work by removing bile acids in the intestines so they can't be reabsorbed and carried back to the liver, where they are turned into cholesterol. Drugs include cholestyramine, sold under the brand names Questran, Prevalite, and LoCholest, and Colestid (colestipol). Studies find they lower LDL about 15 to 30 percent with relatively low doses while slightly increasing HDL levels. They may be prescribed with a statin. Bile acid sequestrants aren't used very often these days because of side effects, including bloating, heartburn, and an increase in triglyceride levels.

Other Approaches

Weight loss. Losing as little as 10 pounds can reduce cholesterol levels 5 to 8 percent.

The Portfolio diet. Think of this as the ultimate cholesterol-lowering diet. Invented by

> ❧ Helpful Hint
>
> ### Take CoQ$_{10}$ With Your Statin
>
> If you're taking statins (or red yeast rice), add 100 milligrams a day of coenzyme Q$_{10}$, more if you already have some form of coronary artery disease. Statins seem to reduce your body's ability to produce this enzyme, which is required to help cells use energy.

Canadian researchers, it combines all the food elements of various cholesterol-lowering diets into one dietary "portfolio." It's low in saturated fat and high in plant sterols and soluble fiber (from foods like oats, barley, and legumes), and it includes soy and nuts. By the way, it's vegetarian. It also requires three doses a day of psyllium. In a study, the Portfolio diet was almost as effective as a diet very low in saturated fat *combined with* a statin drug. You can learn more about it at portfolioeatingplan.com.

Pomegranate juice. Studies find that drinking 40 grams a day of concentrated pomegranate juice can significantly reduce total and LDL cholesterol levels. Pomegranate juice is also powerfully antioxidant—more so even than red wine—so it makes cholesterol less dangerous to arteries (see Super Threat #2 in Part 2).

Tea. Like drinking pomegranate juice, drinking a couple of cups of black or green tea can help you in more than one way: by modestly lowering cholesterol, and by acting as an antioxidant to make cholesterol less dangerous to arteries.

HIV and AIDS

Not long ago, HIV and AIDS were death sentences, plain and simple. But in the past 10 years, thanks to pharmaceutical drugs, we've managed to turn both into treatable chronic diseases.

HIV (human immunodeficiency virus) infection is caused by a type of virus called a retrovirus. It sets its sights on the immune system, crippling immune cells called CD4 T cells, whose job it is to signal other immune cells to destroy invaders. The virus essentially takes over these cells, forcing them to make copies of the virus. It may also force cells to produce a chemical that turns off healthy T cells, effectively shutting down much of the immune system.

Once this happens, your body is helpless against the thousands of infectious agents you encounter millions of times a day. So you may develop numerous infections, neurological conditions, and cancers, one of which will eventually kill you if you don't rein in the virus. Full-blown AIDS (acquired immunodeficiency syndrome) develops when you have an "AIDS-defining" illness or when blood tests show your number of CD4 T cells has dropped below a certain level.

As with most serious diseases, conventional medicine is your first line of defense. Expect to take a cocktail of prescription drugs—so many you'll really need to get organized. But supporting the immune system is also key, which is where lifestyle changes and some supplements come into play.

Our Best Advice

Once you learn you're infected with HIV, follow these steps—along with the other advice throughout this entry—to keep the amount of virus in your system as low as possible.

GETTING TESTED

If you have had unprotected sex with someone who might be infected with HIV, or think you might be infected with HIV, get tested. It's quick and painless. Most clinics wipe a swab around your mouth, then insert it into a vial containing a chemical solution. The results are available within 20 minutes.

1. Make sure your health professionals and sexual partners know about your condition.

2. Find an infectious disease specialist who specializes in HIV patients.

3. Follow your medication instructions to the letter. Do not skip doses, take doses late, or take doses out of order.

4. Begin taking a multivitamin that contains at least 20 milligrams vitamin B_1, 20 milligrams vitamin B_2, 25 milligrams vitamin B_6, 100 milligrams niacin, 50 micrograms vitamin B_{12}, 500 milligrams vitamin C, and 400 to 800 micrograms folic acid.

5. Also take 800 IU vitamin E, 200 micrograms selenium, and 30 milligrams beta-carotene plus 5,000 IU preformed vitamin A daily.

6. Follow the dietary advice starting on page 66 in Part 2 to help bolster your immune system.

Why It Works

HIV infection requires a doctor up-to-date on the latest treatments, which is why we recommend finding a specialist (usually an infectious disease specialist). Of course, HIV is transmissible through sex, so you need to inform any sexual partners.

When your doctor decides to start treating you with antiretroviral drugs is more a question of art than of science. There's a risk that starting too early could make the virus develop a resistance to the drugs. But starting too late could let the virus gain a stronghold the drugs can't break. Generally, it depends on your current immune status (including your CD4 counts), the rate at which your infection is progressing, and your ability to take the medicine as directed.

The goal of medical treatment is to suppress the virus, keeping it from replicating and slowing or even halting the progression of the disease. Even small decreases in the amount of virus in your system, called your viral load, can make a big difference in your CD4 counts and your overall health. However, if you don't follow your drug regimen exactly, the virus can become resistant to the drugs, limiting future treatment options. Other medicines (not described here) are aimed at preventing secondary infections or cancers that occur as the result of your weakened immune system.

We want you to take the multivitamin and other antioxidants for several reasons. First, about one third of people with HIV are deficient in these micronutrients. Second, your suppressed immune system opens you up to significant damage from inflammation as your body tries to fight off infections; this, in turn, increases free-radical production (see Super Threat #2, oxidative stress, in Part 2). Numerous studies find that free radicals increase the virus's activity and its ability to take over T-4 cells.

Antioxidants neutralize free radicals, and high doses can reduce viral load. In one study, HIV-positive volunteers who took 800 IU vitamin E daily saw their viral load drop and their CD4 levels improve slightly. Another study found HIV-positive people who took 200 micrograms selenium a day were much less likely to be hospitalized for infections than those receiving a placebo. In a third study, of more than a thousand

> ## Antiretroviral Drugs
>
> Today HIV is treated with a cocktail of drugs that act against various enzymes or proteins that help keep the virus alive and replicating. You're given a "cocktail" so the virus can't escape by becoming resistant to just one drug. The drugs include:
>
> - AZT, Retrovir, Combivir, and Trizivir (zidovudine)
> - 3TC, Epivir, Combivir, Trizivir (lamivudine)
> - d4T, Zerit (stavudine)
> - ddI, Videx, Videx EC (didanosine)
> - ABC, Ziagen, Trizivir (abacavir)
> - ddC, Hivid (dideoxycytidine)
> - Viread (tenofovir)
> - Emtriva (emtricitabine)
> - Sustiva (efavirenz)
> - Viramune (nevirapine)

pregnant women infected with HIV, those who received a daily multivitamin were 39 percent less likely to progress to the final stage of AIDS or die of complications from the disease than those who received a placebo.

Finally, weight loss is a major problem for people with HIV and AIDS, and weight loss further depresses the immune system. The dietary advice we gave for Super Threat #4, immune stress, helps bolster the immune system.

Other Medicines
Herbs and Supplements

N-acetyl-cysteine (NAC). This amino acid contributes to the production of glutathione, a powerful antioxidant, as well as acting as an antioxidant itself. Many people with HIV have low glutathione levels, possibly due to nutritional

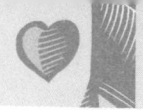

issues, although a protein produced by the HIV virus may also contribute to its loss. In one seminal study on NAC conducted by Stanford researchers, 27 HIV-positive men took about 4,400 milligrams of the supplement a day for two to eight months. After two years, those receiving NAC were much more likely to still be alive than those who never took it (this was in the days before antiretroviral drugs). Even men who didn't take NAC were still more likely to survive if they had higher glutathione levels to start with. Take 4,400 milligrams a day.

Korean red ginseng. One study in HIV-positive people treated only with this herb (which we don't recommend doing) found their CD4 counts remained steady or even increased while taking the herb. Another study found that taking Korean red ginseng along with the HIV drug zidovudine reduced rates of viral resistance to the drug compared to people taking only zidovudine.

L-glutamine. When you have HIV, your body uses large amounts of this amino acid, possibly in making immune cells. This, in turn, leaches glutamine from muscle cells, leading to the muscle wasting and weight loss often seen in people with HIV. One study found that supplementing with 40 grams of L-glutamine plus antioxidants over three months resulted in a weight gain of nearly five pounds in people who took the supplements versus those who took a placebo.

Coenzyme Q$_{10}$. Levels of this antioxidant substance, found in all the body's cells, are often low in people with HIV. There's some evidence that supplementing with 200 milligrams a day can improve immune system markers and reduce the risk of secondary infection.

Arginine. This amino acid enhances immune system activity. One small study in HIV-infected people found it boosted activity of natural killer cells, immune cells that, among their other functions, destroy cells infected with viruses. Take 8 grams daily.

Other Approaches

Stress management. Living with a chronic disease, especially HIV/AIDS, is not easy. Mind-body therapies such as cognitive-behavioral therapy, meditation, and relaxation training can help you deal with the stress, provide some relief from symptoms, and improve your mood. Better still, according to several studies, they may also improve your immune function. One study of 25 men with HIV found those who spent 10 weeks learning stress management techniques had significantly higher immune markers (including CD4 counts) after 6 to 12 months than a control group.

Most medical centers and community health programs offer stress management training. Consider adding a massage to those approaches; one study found that HIV-positive people who received a weekly whole-body massage coupled with stress management used less medical care and felt their health was better overall than those who received only a massage or no intervention.

Acupuncture. About one-third of people with HIV or AIDS develop peripheral neuropathy, or nerve pain in the legs. You can read more about various treatments for nerve pain on page 330, but a few studies also find significant benefits to acupuncture for HIV-related neuropathies. There's also good evidence that it can improve your sleep, often a problem for people with HIV. And, as you know, lack of sleep further suppresses your immune system.

Prevention

Use condoms for all sexual activity. And before having sex, find out your partner's HIV status and sexual history (it's possible to be infected but not yet have a positive test result).

Don't share intravenous drug needles with anyone. Of course, we don't recommend using recreational drugs to begin with.

Obesity

Only someone who has spent the last few years on a desert island could not know that we're in the midst of an obesity epidemic. Today more than 6 out of 10 American adults are overweight or obese. The culprit? Too many calories coming in from food and beverages, and not enough calories being used up through exercise.

Although it would be easy to blame obesity on lack of willpower, it's not quite that simple. Part of your weight is hard-wired into your genes; put certain people into the right environment and the pounds pile on. And today's environment seems designed to encourage weight gain, from suburban neighborhoods that require a five-mile car ride for a gallon of milk to labor-saving devices that now go as far as robotic vacuums. Meanwhile, cheap, high-fat, high-sugar food is everywhere we turn.

Think a few extra pounds won't hurt anything but your self-esteem? Actually, nothing except smoking is worse for your health than being overweight. It contributes not only to heart disease and diabetes but also to sleep disorders, cancer, and other conditions. Remember inflammation, Super Threat #1? Fat cells secrete inflammatory chemicals, which contribute to just about every health woe you can imagine.

Obesity also speeds up the aging process. At the same time, aging itself increases the risk of obesity. That's because as you age, you lose muscle mass, which slows your metabolism.

Don't worry about becoming super-model skinny. You don't actually have to be considered thin to improve your health. Losing just 5 to 10 percent of your weight can make a big difference. In this entry, we show you how to do that. One thing we don't want you to do is crash diet. Yo-yo dieting, in the long run, is worse than not dieting at all.

Our Best Advice

Losing weight is not an overnight proposition but a daily effort. Here are our top recommendations to help you fight and win the battle.

1. Whenever you eat, start with half your normal portion size. For instance, if you normally have a whole bagel for breakfast, start with half a bagel. Wait 20 minutes after finishing before deciding if you're still hungry. Chances are, you won't be.

2. If you're eating on a plate, fill half your plate with fruits and vegetables, leaving one quarter for whole grains and the other quarter for protein.

3. Eat a piece of fruit before you start lunch and a salad with low-fat or fat-free dressing before you start dinner.

4. Make sure you get some protein and a little bit of fat with every meal.

5. Get at least 25 grams of fiber daily.

6. Eat breakfast every morning, preferably a high-fiber cereal or a high-fiber liquid shake.

7. Substitute water, skim milk, and low-calorie sodas and juice for regular soft drinks, juices, and whole milk.

8. Make a list of 10 things to do when hunger hits and it's not mealtime. Keep the list on the fridge in plain sight.

9. Take a daily 45-minute walk.

10. Find a friend to be your weight-loss buddy or join a weight-loss group like Weight Watchers.

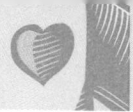

Why It Works

Decreasing your portion sizes is the single best move you can make if you're trying to lose weight, particularly in this age of super-sizing. Studies find that we eat what's in front of us, regardless of how hungry we are. So start small and don't reach for seconds until at least 20 minutes have passed—about the time it takes for a feeling of fullness to reach your brain.

This is particularly important in restaurants, where the adage seems to be "more is better." We suggest asking the waiter to put half your meal in a box before you even touch it. Better still, limit your meals out. We all tend to eat far more calories and fat in a restaurant than we do at home.

Fruits and vegetables are naturally very low in calories, so by eating more of them, there's less room on your plate (and in your stomach) for higher-calorie starches and meat. That said, protein is important. It makes you feel full longer than carbohydrates (including fruits, vegetables, and starches) do.

Stepping Up Your Efforts

Walking is an excellent way to burn calories, and pedometers are an excellent way to motivate yourself to walk more. These little gadgets, which clip onto your belt or waistband (some pricier models even work when you put them in your pocket) count every step you take, motivating you to take more of them. Knowing it's there tracking your every move gives you the extra push you need to take the stairs instead of the elevator and take that extra loop around the park. On average, most people take only 2,000 to 3,000 steps a day. Studies find adding 2,000 steps a day helps maintain your current weight, while 8,000 to 10,000 steps a day (about 5 miles) helps the pounds drop off.

Fiber is a key element of any weight-loss diet. Like fat and protein, fiber fills you up—but it's not digestible, so it contains no calories. It also slows down the conversion of food into blood sugar so you avoid blood sugar spikes that have been shown to contribute to weight gain.

A good way to get a healthy dose of fiber is to eat breakfast. Look for a cereal that contains at least 5 grams of fiber per serving. Breakfast does more than provide fiber, though. Studies show that eating breakfast helps you eat less food later in the day—and fewer total calories. And it kicks your body's metabolism into gear again after a night of fasting.

Eating breakfast is a habit that most successful dieters have in common. It helps rev your metabolism. Watch your portion size, though; a serving of cereal should be about one cup.

Our drinks add to our love handles. Consider this: The average American consumes 245 calories a day from soft drinks. If this describes you, you could lose 25 pounds a year just by switching from Coke to water or skim milk. Even switching from 2 percent to 1 percent milk cuts out about 20 percent of the calories.

Too often we eat not because we're hungry but because we're bored, anxious, mad, or tired. Instead of reaching for food, we want you to try taking a walk, calling a friend, cleaning out a closet, or paying a couple of bills first. We think you'll find that the urge to eat will pass.

As for the exercise part of the equation: People who exercise as well as cutting calories have an easier time losing weight and keeping it off than people who diet exclusively. Burning an extra 250 calories a day, about the amount used in a brisk 45-minute walk, lops off about 26 pounds a year, as long as you don't replace those calories with food.

Finally, it's hard to lose weight on your own. When researchers at Columbia University in New York assigned 413 overweight and obese men and women to either a self-help program in which

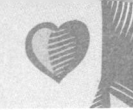

they met twice with a nutritionist and then followed a program on their own, or Weight Watchers, after two years those going to Weight Watchers lost more than those going it alone. It doesn't have to be a formal program like Weight Watchers; an online friend or diet support group can also help.

Other Medicines
Herbs and Supplements

Green and oolong tea. These teas have some of the best evidence behind them when it comes to supplements for weight loss. They increase your metabolism so you burn calories faster instead of storing them as fat. The effect is likely due to a combination of flavonoids (antioxidants) called catechins and caffeine. One study using a green tea extract standardized to 25 percent catechins found it increased participants' daytime metabolism 5 percent.

Calcium, magnesium, vitamin D. Losing weight can trigger bone loss, so make sure you're supplementing with 500 to 600 milligrams of calcium twice a day. Choose a calcium supplement that also contains magnesium and vitamin D.

Prescription Drugs

Meridia (sibutramine). This is the most commonly prescribed weight-loss medication. Originally developed as an antidepressant, it appears to work by interfering with chemical signals in the brain that regulate hunger. It works, but it's not a magic pill; you still have to diet and exercise. Side effects include increased heart rate and blood pressure, as well as dry mouth, insomnia, and nausea.

Xenical (orlistat). This drug works by preventing your body from absorbing fat. One two-year study found people taking Orlistat lost an average of 6 percent of their body weight after

What About...

Weight-Loss Supplements?

When the Food and Drug Administration banned the sale of products containing ephedrine in 2004, many supplement manufacturers turned to other herbs that also contain stimulants. One is bitter orange, reputed to speed metabolism. However, only one study comparing the herb to a placebo has been published, and a careful review of that study found no evidence that it was effective for weight loss. Also, the herb could lead to high blood pressure and increase your risk of a heart attack. Another commonly marketed weight-loss herb is country mallow, an Indian herb that contains about 1 percent ephedrine. There are no published studies on its effectiveness for weight loss.

a year, compared with an average 2 percent loss in the placebo group. The side effects can be a turnoff, however, including oily stool, diarrhea, gas, and bloating.

Glucophage (metformin). This drug is typically prescribed for people with type 2 diabetes, insulin resistance, or polycystic ovary syndrome (PCOS), but some studies find it can also help people with these conditions lose weight.

Other Approaches

Low-fat dairy foods. These foods, such as low-fat milk and yogurt, are rich in both protein and calcium, and there's a good body of research suggesting that a diet high in calcium can boost weight-loss efforts.

Surgery. One of the fastest-growing surgeries in the country is bariatric surgery, in which the stomach is either stapled or banded (gastroplasty), which reduces the amount of food that enters the stomach, or partially bypassed (gastric bypass) so calories aren't absorbed. These

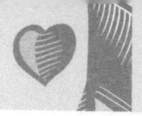

procedures carry risks, however, including infection, malnutrition, and a 1 percent risk of death from the surgery itself. Bariatric surgery is recommended only as a last resort for people who are morbidly obese, i.e., with body mass indexes in the high 30s or higher.

Acupuncture. The few studies conducted on acupuncture for weight loss generally find it can be a beneficial addition to a weight-loss program. One study combined laser acupuncture (which uses laser beams instead of needles) with a low-calorie diet and found that people who used the two approaches together lost more weight than the people who just cut calories. A couple of studies on auricular acupuncture, which uses acupressure points on the ear, found those receiving the treatment lost more weight and had less appetite than those receiving a sham version. Researchers theorize that acupuncture may suppress appetite by stimulating a section of the vagal nerve (one of the many nerves that carries messages to and from the brain) and increasing levels of serotonin (a neurotransmitter that plays a role in appetite).

Food diary. It takes work, but keeping a food diary is an almost surefire way to lose weight. Write down everything you eat and drink (even the cream you poured into your coffee), when you ate it, and how you felt at the time. Studies find using a food diary can help you eat 15 percent less. In fact, people who keep a food diary almost always begin to lose weight, even if they don't consciously change their eating habits. The diary makes you think twice before grabbing a high-calorie treat. It also makes you more aware of what you're really eating and reveals patterns you may not be aware of—you may snack more than you imagined, for instance, or eat when you're tired.

Osteoporosis

Osteoporosis can seem like a vague, far-off threat until the day you push open a heavy door and fracture your wrist, or discover that your favorite pants no longer fit because you've lost two inches thanks to compression fractures in your spine.

That day is just the end result of a process that began back in your youth. You see, bone operates like a bank. In your teens and twenties you're putting "money" into the bank as bone-building cells called osteoblasts build bone faster than cells called osteoclasts break it down. As you age, however, the balance shifts, especially in women (when estrogen levels drop after menopause, bone breakdown speeds up). Osteoporosis doesn't just strike women, though; men get it too.

If over the years you've managed to build up an extra-strong supply of bone via weight-bearing exercise (which helps calcium work) and good nutrition (calcium and vitamin D are key), you have more bone "in the bank" and can afford to lose some without any dire consequences. But if your bone has been weakened already because of medications like steroids, a sedentary lifestyle, a lack of calcium in your diet, or your genes, you need to do everything you can to slow or reverse bone loss.

Our Best Advice

Here's our best advice if you've been diagnosed with osteoporosis. Much of this advice also applies if you're at very high risk of the disease, even if you haven't been officially diagnosed (see "Getting Tested" on page 297 and "What's Your Risk?" on page 298).

1. Begin taking a prescription medication to improve bone mineral density.

2. Take 1,500 milligrams of calcium a day in three or four divided doses, along with 10 milligrams of manganese, 15 to 45 milligrams of zinc, 3 milligrams of boron, and 1 to 2 milligrams of copper.

3. Take at least 400 IU vitamin D a day, up to 800 IU. (For convenience, look for a calcium pill that also contains vitamin D.)

Why It Works

As recently as 10 years ago, there was little doctors could do to treat osteoporosis. Now there are several medications that, coupled with lifestyle changes, can slow or even reverse bone decline. Talk to your doctor about which one is right for you. (See "Bone-Building Drugs" on page 296.)

Calcium is critical: In the five years after menopause, women who don't get enough of this mineral lose about 2 percent of bone a year. Supplementing with 1,000 to 1,500 milligrams a day can cut this loss in half. We recommend taking calcium in divided doses because studies find the mineral is best absorbed when you take no more than 500 milligrams at a time. There are different forms of calcium. If you take calcium carbonate or calcium phosphate supplements, take them with food for best absorption; others can be taken without food. If you are taking acid-blocking drugs for heartburn or peptic ulcer, stick with calcium citrate because it's most easily absorbed.

Manganese is also important; studies find women with osteoporosis have lower levels of

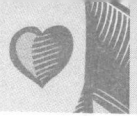
this mineral, required for bone formation. Add it to calcium and it improves bone mineral density more than calcium alone. Don't take more than 11 milligrams a day of manganese, however, because it could build up in your system and cause neurological damage.

Zinc also improves bone-building activity and seems to work best in combination with manganese, copper, and calcium. Copper slows bone turnover by inhibiting osteoclasts (bone-gobbling cells). Boron seems to improve the way your body absorbs calcium.

While calcium can reduce bone loss, it only increases bone density when taken with vitamin D (which is really a hormone) or the prescription osteoporosis drugs mentioned in "Bone-Building Drugs" (see box). In one large study of 87,000 nurses, researchers found that women who got the most vitamin D in their diets or through supplements were least likely to experience fractures. As you age, your body becomes less effective at creating vitamin D from sunshine. People 70 and over should aim for 700 IU a day.

Other Medicines
Herbs and Supplements

Magnesium and potassium. Although the evidence is still accumulating, a growing number of researchers think magnesium and potassium are important minerals in preventing and treating osteoporosis. The two seem to work together to regulate blood calcium levels (so your body doesn't snatch calcium from bone). Take 1/3 to 1/2 the amount of calcium you're taking as your magnesium dose. So if you're taking 1,500 milligrams calcium, aim for 750 milligrams magnesium. And take about 10 milligrams potassium.

Soy isoflavones. These plant-based estrogen-like compounds are thought to help protect bone the way a woman's natural estrogen does. Even though there's no clear evidence yet that proves

---

Bone-Building Drugs

These are powerful drugs with potential side effects. Talk to your doctor about which one is the best for you.

Bisphosphonates. Fosamax (alendronate) and Actonel (risedronate) reduce bone loss, increase bone density, and decrease the risk of spine, wrist, and hip fractures. Take on an empty stomach with 6 to 8 ounces of water first thing in the morning, then don't eat or take other pills for at least 30 minutes. Stomach pain and heartburn are common side effects of these drugs.

Selective estrogen receptor modulators (SERMs). Evista (raloxifene) increases bone mass and reduces the risk of spinal fractures. An added benefit: Studies suggest the drug may reduce the risk of some breast cancers by 65 percent.

Miacalcin (calcitonin). Recommended for women more than five years beyond menopause. Studies find this drug slows bone loss, increases spinal bone density, and may relieve pain associated with bone fractures. You take it daily as a nasal spray.

Parathyroid hormone. Forteo (teriparatide) is the only osteoporosis drug shown to stimulate bone formation as well as increase bone mineral density. The downside? It has to be injected daily, usually into the thigh or lower abdomen (you do this yourself at home with an injector pen), and studies find it slightly increases the risk of bone cancer in animals.

---

supplementing with soy isoflavones or with soy protein reduces the risk of fractures, we still recommend you eat or supplement with 20 to 60 grams of soy protein containing 80 to 90 milligrams of soy isoflavones daily.

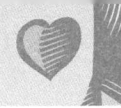

Ipriflavone. In a two-year Italian study involving 453 women ages 50 to 65 with decreased bone density, those who took 600 milligrams of ipriflavone plus calcium daily maintained their bone density; those who took calcium alone experienced significant bone loss. Ipriflavone can also help with the back pain associated with osteoporosis. *Warning:* Some studies find that it can reduce the numbers of certain immune system cells. If you're taking this supplement on a regular basis, make sure your doctor knows and tests your white blood cells levels every six months. Take 200 milligrams three times a day.

Other Approaches

Strength training. The shearing force put on bone by strength training (such as lifting dumbbells) helps increase bone density better than any other type of exercise. One study of 36 postmenopausal women that compared 30 minutes of strength training a day twice a week to walking four times a week found strength training increased bone density 1 percent in the spine and hip—a significant amount—along with a 14 percent improvement in balance. Walkers had only a slight increase in spine density and no improvement in hip density. (Walking may not increase bone density, but it's still important for *maintaining* bone density, and it's good aerobic exercise for your heart. Our point here is simply that strength training is even more important for bone health, so you shouldn't ignore it.)

Fall assessment. A fall poses the greatest risk to your overall health, mobility, and independence when you have osteoporosis because you could break a bone and need to be hospitalized. Get a "fall assessment," performed by a physician or rehabilitation specialist. He or she will evaluate everything from the medications you take to your lifestyle in terms of their potential contribution to falls, and make suggestions on how to reduce your risk (for instance, by keeping your home well lit, wearing sturdy shoes, and using devices to assist in mobility).

Prevention

In addition to taking calcium and vitamin D daily, follow this advice to prevent osteoporosis.

Drink your milk. Other good dietary sources of calcium are low-fat dairy products, canned salmon, sardines with the bones, and dark-green leafy vegetables.

Switch to tea. Tea contains several compounds that may benefit bone, including fluoride, isoflavones, polyphenols, and tannins. One study found men and women who drank green or oolong tea for at least six years had higher bone density throughout their body, while other studies find lower risks of hip fracture and increased bone density in people who drink black tea.

GETTING TESTED

Bone density tests are the only way to detect low bone mass and monitor the effectiveness of osteoporosis treatments. The most commonly used test is dual energy X-ray absorptiometry, or DEXA. It's painless and takes only about 15 minutes. It measures bone at the most common fracture sites—the spine, hip, and wrist.

If you have a high risk of osteoporosis (see "What's Your Risk?" page 298) you should begin screening at age 60. Otherwise, annual screening starting at age 65 should do.

Bone density results are read as "T-scores," which measure how far your bone density deviates above or below the average bone density value for a young, healthy, white woman. A T-score at or below -2.5 results in a diagnosis of osteoporosis; a T score between -1 and -2.5 results in a diagnosis of osteopenia, or low bone density.

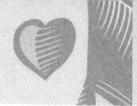

Sign up for Pilates classes. Although any kind of weight-bearing exercise—walking, weightlifting, calisthenics, running—can reduce your risk of osteoporosis by helping to maintain bone mass, Pilates also improves balance, which can reduce fractures resulting from falls. T'ai chi and yoga also improve balance.

Get enough protein. Despite long-held beliefs that too much protein leaches calcium from bone, protein is critical for strong bone. In fact, it makes up half of bone tissue. Studies find that getting enough protein through your diet protects against osteoporosis. Protein supplements given to elderly people with hip fracture reduce bone loss and shorten hospital stays. About 0.5 milligram of protein per pound of body weight should do, although some experts recommend up to twice that amount. Three ounces of roasted chicken breast contains 26.37 grams protein; a cup of milk contains 34.42 grams.

Stop smoking, and limit your alcohol consumption. Tobacco and alcohol both interfere with bone health.

What's Your Risk?

Many factors increase your risk of osteoporosis. Among the most important:

- A family history of osteoporosis
- A thin body frame or a body mass index (BMI) less than 20
- Being white, Asian, or female
- Having certain medical conditions, like anorexia, Cushing's syndrome, Turner's syndrome, or any condition that affects your body's ability to absorb or use nutrients
- Taking medications including steroids, gonadotropin-releasing hormone agonists or antagonists, cyclosporins, chemotherapy, and anticonvulsants.

Minimize your use of aluminum-containing antacids. They can interfere with the effects of calcium and other bone-building minerals.

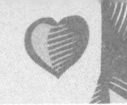

Parkinson's Disease

Perhaps no disease more clearly represents the terrible toll oxidation can take than Parkinson's disease. It's a neurodegenerative disease, meaning it damages brain cells, impairs function, and gets worse over time. Parkinson's tends to strike earlier than Alzheimer's (average age at diagnosis is 57) and affects nearly every system in the body. The disease is marked by increasing muscle tremors, followed by slowness of movement, stiffness, and problems walking. About one-third of people with Parkinson's go on to develop dementia.

The hallmark of the disease is the destruction of dopamine-producing neurons (brain cells) in a small part of the brain called the substantia nigra, or SN, which controls movement. Thus, the main goal of medical treatment is getting the brain to produce more dopamine, replacing dopamine, or finding ways to keep existing dopamine around longer.

Because the disease wasn't even described until early in the 19th century, and because its prevalence has grown in Western countries along with our own growth in industrialization, many researchers suspect that toxins in the environment contribute to its development via oxidation (see Super Threat #2, oxidative stress, in Part 2). However, there's obviously something else going on, or everyone would have it. And it seems there is: People with Parkinson's seem to have higher levels of rogue electrons that escape control when brain cells make energy. These electrons become free radicals, which damage those dopamine-producing brain cells.

Plus, studies find that the SN areas in the brains of people with Parkinson's are abnormally low in glutathione, a powerful antioxidant needed to reduce oxidative stress in that part of the brain. In fact, glutathione is so vital to sustaining cellular life that once levels drop severely, the cell nearly always dies.

Although there's no cure for Parkinson's, there are medications that can help. And you can also take extra measures to slow oxidation and help retard the disease's progression.

Our Best Advice

No matter where you are in your Parkinson's diagnosis, follow this advice to slow further progression.

1. Begin taking 100 milligrams coenzyme Q_{10} three times a day, gradually increasing to 1,200 milligrams a day.

2. Also take 400 IU vitamin E and 1 to 2 grams vitamin C daily (in two to four divided doses of 500 milligrams).

3. Follow a low-fat, low-calorie diet high in fruits, vegetables, and beans.

4. Drink several cups of green tea a day.

5. Get at least 20 minutes a day of physical activity three days a week. A good option is walking back and forth in the shallow end of the pool. If you find you can't exercise on your own, get your doctor to write you a prescription for physical therapy. Add a session of t'ai chi once a week.

Why It Works

Cells contain tiny "furnaces" called mitochondria, which produce energy for the cell. A by-product

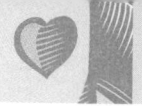
of this energy production is spare electrons. If these electrons escape the cell, they become free radicals, which cause oxidative damage in the brain. Coenzyme Q_{10}, an antioxidant found in every cell of the body, traps the spare electrons in the mitochondria, where they are used to produce the next round of energy. Obviously, its role is important. But studies find significantly low levels of coenzyme Q_{10} in the mitochondria of brain and blood cells in Parkinson's patients, which is why we recommend supplements. Animal studies find it protects dopamine-producing brain cells.

In one of the few published trials in humans, of 80 people with Parkinson's who weren't taking any medication yet, those who took coenzyme Q_{10} for 16 months (or until their condition got so bad they needed medication) became less disabled in this time period than those who got a placebo. The results were so encouraging that the government is now funding large clinical trials to evaluate the supplement as a potential treatment for early-stage Parkinson's.

We also recommend vitamins E and C. In one study, very high doses of vitamin E (3,200 IU) and vitamin C (3 grams a day) delayed Parkinson's patients' need for medication by about 35 months. We don't routinely suggest such high doses of vitamin E—it can increase the risk of heart disease—so talk to your doctor about what dosage is safe for you (we know that 400 IU is safe). You can take high doses of vitamin C on your own, but don't take more than 500 milligrams at one time.

Your diet can help too. Fruits and vegetables provide antioxidants to minimize oxidative damage. We suggest 9 to 12 servings a day. Don't panic! A serving is as little as a small glass of fruit or vegetable juice, a medium-sized piece of fruit, or 1/2 cup cooked vegetables or cut-up fruit or veggies. Keep your fat and calories low to reduce your risk of heart disease, which some studies suggest is

> ### 🌿 Helpful Hint
>
> ## Cut Back on Burgers and Chicken
>
> If you're taking a drug containing L-dopa, limit the amount of protein in your diet. Studies find that low protein intake (0.5 grams per kilogram of weight per day) can improve control of symptoms throughout the day, while high intake (10 grams/kilogram/per day) exaggerates what's known as the on/off pattern, when the drug temporarily stops working. So, for instance, if you weigh 150 pounds (68 kilograms), you shouldn't get any more than 34 grams of protein daily, about the amount in half a large chicken breast.

more deadly if you also have Parkinson's. Plus, eating fewer calories reduces oxidation.

The beans come into play because they can increase levels of the chemical levodopa (which eventually turns into dopamine) in the brain and reduce movement problems like shaking and stiffness, particularly in people with early or mild stages of Parkinson's. Aim for about 8 ounces (1 cup) of beans a day.

Green tea gives you heaping doses of polyphenols, antioxidant chemicals that help sop up free iron molecules. Some research suggests these iron molecules may contribute to the oxidative damage that causes Parkinson's. Plus, the tea contains theanine, which laboratory studies find can increase dopamine levels. Aim for three or four cups a day.

Regular exercise not only helps slow the loss of movement, but also improves mobility and mood. We recommend walking and suggest you walk to a recording of a metronome (or a very rhythmic song) to maintain a regular gait.

T'ai chi helps improve balance and prevent falls. In one study, a one-hour class once a week for 12 weeks slashed the risk of falls in half, a benefit that lasted at least a year after the class ended.

Other Medicines
Herbs and Supplements

Marijuana. Although the medical use of marijuana is controversial and still illegal in most states, there's good anecdotal evidence that smoking marijuana can reduce the shakiness and stiffness of Parkinson's. The prescription form of the active ingredient in the herb doesn't seem to have any benefit.

Mucuna pruriens. Compounds in the seeds of this Ayurvedic herb act pretty much like those in the standard Parkinson's drug. We particularly recommend this supplement for people in the early stages of the disease to delay the time until you need prescription medication.

In one small study of eight patients whose symptoms were not controlled well with medication, those who took 30 grams of this herb a day had higher levels of levodopa (L-dopa) than those who just took the medication, and the L-dopa lingered in the brain longer. The results led the researchers to suggest that this plant source of L-dopa might have some advantages over the prescription drug in long-term Parkinson's treatment. Don't, however, take it if you're already taking an L-dopa medication.

B complex vitamin. L-dopa raises levels of homocysteine, an amino acid linked to heart disease. To reduce your levels if you're taking the drug, take a B complex vitamin containing at least 800 micrograms folic acid, 400 micrograms B_{12}, and 50 milligrams B_6.

Omega-3 fatty acids. One study found that daily doses of evening primrose oil relieved tremors in people with Parkinson's, while another found wheat germ oil could improve symptoms. Both oils are rich in omega-3s. However, because they contribute to oxidation, be sure to also take the antioxidant vitamins C and E that we already recommended. Take 1 to 2 grams of either oil every day.

Prescription Drugs

Sinemet (carbidopa-levodopa). This is the main drug used in treating Parkinson's. It combines L-dopa and carbidopa, a drug that blocks action of an enzyme that breaks down dopamine. The carbidopa reduces some of the side effects that can result from L-dopa alone, including nausea and vomiting, and enables more of the L-dopa to get to the brain, so you can take a smaller dose. Sinemet's use is somewhat controversial, however, because there's some evidence it may actually contribute to damage of dopamine-producing neurons by increasing oxidation.

Eventually—after about two or three years on average—Sinemet stops working in some patients during certain times of the day. A longer-lasting form of the drug called Stalevo may get around this.

Dopamine agonists. These drugs include Parlodel (bromocriptine), Permax (pergolide), Mirapex (pramipexole) and Requip (ropinirole). They enhance the action of dopamine receptors on cells so they're more responsive to the dopamine that's available. The drugs can be taken alone or with Sinemet.

MAO inhibitors. These drugs do two things for people with Parkinson's. They keep dopamine in the brain longer by inhibiting an enzyme, monoamine oxidase, that plays a role in breaking it down. They also protect neurons from further oxidative damage, which can slow the progression of the disease. The most studied drug in this class is selegiline (Carbex and Eldepryl).

Anticholinergics. These drugs, which include trihexyphenidyl (Artane and Trihexane), benztropine, and procyclidine, reduce muscle tremors.

Symmetrel (amantadine). Also prescribed for viral infections, this drug increases dopamine levels in the brain and keeps dopamine available to brain cells longer. It's generally taken only short-term in early-stage Parkinson's, after which it usually stops working.

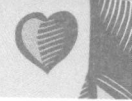

Other Approaches

Deep brain stimulation. This surgical procedure involves implanting a battery-operated device into the brain to electrically stimulate areas that control movement, blocking the abnormal nerve signals that lead to classic Parkinsonian symptoms. Studies find significant improvements in the quality of life of people with Parkinson's after the procedure, particularly in terms of movement. This procedure is very invasive, however, and is not recommended until late in the disease.

Surgery. Several surgical procedures have been developed to treat the movement disorders of Parkinson's, including procedures that destroy small parts of the brain, stem cell transplants to replace damaged neurons, and the surgical infusion of growth factors to stimulate production of certain chemicals in brain cells.

Alexander Technique. This therapy teaches you to change how you move in order to release tension and improve your balance. A 2002 study found that combining it with medical therapy could improve symptoms in people with Parkinson's more than medical therapy alone.

Acupuncture. Although clinical studies show no difference in benefits between acupuncture and placebo in relieving the muscle-related symptoms of Parkinson's, they do show it can help with sleep, often a problem for those with the disease. We recommend at least one trial of acupuncture to see if it helps relieve any symptoms or improve sleep.

Medical spa therapy. Ask your doctor for a prescription for this therapy, which combines water therapy with medical massage and other physical therapy. One small study in 31 people with Parkinson's found that three weeks of medical spa therapy significantly improved several Parkinson's-related symptoms, as well as psychological status.

Prevention

Get your caffeine. In one study, men who didn't regularly drink coffee were five times more likely to develop Parkinson's than those who did. Other studies find that high tea consumption reduces Parkinson's risk. The connection is related to caffeine, researchers say. Green tea doesn't contain as much caffeine as coffee, but it does contain some, and it also has brain-protecting antioxidants called polyphenols.

Eat your vegetables. A diet high in antioxidant-rich fruits and vegetables reduces the risk of Parkinson's, probably by protecting brain cells from oxidative damage.

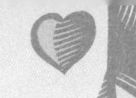

Peripheral Vascular Disease

Hardening of the arteries isn't only a problem for the heart; the same process can occur in the blood vessels of the legs. Called peripheral vascular disease (PVD), or peripheral arterial disease (PAD), it carries the same risk of heart attack and stroke as coronary artery disease (described on page 268). In fact, if you have this disease, you probably also have coronary artery disease.

Like coronary artery disease, PVD results from a buildup of cholesterol, dead cells, and other debris that gradually narrows blood vessels, limiting blood flow. While this causes angina, or chest pain, in people with coronary artery disease, it causes leg pain in those with PVD. That makes exercising, even walking, difficult.

The goal of conventional and complementary treatments is to avoid more serious problems (such as coronary artery disease if you don't already have it, heart failure, heart attack, and stroke), and to improve blood flow in your legs so you can go about your daily tasks with less pain and more stamina.

Controlling high blood pressure, one of the greatest risk factors for stroke, heart attack, and heart or kidney failure resulting from PVD, is key. See High Blood Pressure (page 280) for specific advice.

Our Best Advice

To help open up the arteries in your legs and prevent dangerous blood clots, we recommend the following four steps.

1. If you smoke, stop immediately.

2. Take 120 to 240 milligrams a day of ginkgo biloba divided into two or three doses.

Choose a ginkgo product that contains the EGb 761 extract, standardized to 24% flavone glycosides and 6% terpene lactones, such as Ginkgold.

3. Begin supplementing with 1,500 milligrams L-propionylcarnitine, a form of the amino acid carnitine, every day. Gradually increase the dose over the next four to six weeks to 4,000 milligrams a day.

4. Start an exercise program, such as walking, cycling, or swimming, most days of the week. Start with whatever you can do and gradually work your way up to at least 20 minutes a day.

Why It Works

Quitting smoking is especially vital for anybody with PVD because nicotine in the blood narrows arteries—the last thing you need when your arteries are already filling with gunk. Only diabetes and high blood pressure increases your risk of a heart attack or stroke more than smoking when you have PVD.

Ginkgo improves blood circulation by preventing particles in the blood called platelets from sticking together and forming blood clots. An analysis of nine studies on the herb concluded that its blood-thinning action definitely helped ease PVD leg pain.

L-carnitine that's been slightly modified into the L-propionylcarnitine form helps blood flow by relaxing vessel walls. Several studies confirm that it helps people with PVD participate in more physical activity without pain. One of the larger studies followed 485 people for a year. At the

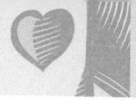
beginning of the study, they couldn't walk even 275 yards without pain. On average, those who supplemented were able to double their pain-free walking distance.

That's important, because regular exercise, which improves blood circulation in the legs, is key to controlling PVD. Starting an exercise program can be difficult if your legs hurt, however, so a structured program supervised by a cardiac rehabilitation expert is best. If that's not practical, exercise on your own until pain hits, rest until it goes away, then begin again.

Other Medicines
Herbs and Supplements

Fish oil. Supplementing with 3 to 5 grams of fish oil a day in either liquid or capsule form fights PVD in several ways. First, the fatty acids keep platelets from clumping together. They also reduce levels of triglycerides, blood fats that can increase the risk of blood clots.

Folic acid. Take 800 milligrams of this B vitamin daily. It relaxes blood vessels and reduces levels of homocysteine, an amino acid linked to heart disease. Studies also suggest that folic acid helps create new blood vessels, providing new blood routes around partial blockages.

Policosanol. A nutrient extracted from sugarcane, policosanol serves as a natural alternative to statins, the most commonly prescribed drug for high cholesterol. Studies find that supplementing with 10 milligrams policosanol twice a day reduces cholesterol levels, so there's less cholesterol to clog blood vessels in the legs. In one study, researchers gave 56 people with PVD either 10 milligrams policosanol a day for six months or a placebo, and found that those receiving the supplement were able to walk almost twice as far without limping as before they started the study.

TIME TO WORRY

If you experience sudden numbness, intense pain, inexplicable weakness, no pulse, a bluish color, and/or a cool feeling in your leg, call 911. You may be experiencing a rare but very serious kind of blood clot called an acute occlusion, which can lead to tissue death or gangrene, even amputation or death.

Over-the-Counter Drugs

Aspirin. Taken daily in low doses, aspirin has been found to be as effective in preventing stroke and heart attack in people with PVD as the prescription antiplatelet drugs described below. Take one or two baby aspirin a day, or 100 to 200 milligrams buffered aspirin. If you experience stomach irritation, or if you're among the approximately 40 percent of PVD patients who don't respond to low-dose aspirin, talk to your doctor about these prescription alternatives.

Prescription Drugs

Statins. These well-known cholesterol-lowering medications are especially helpful for people with PVD, who usually have high cholesterol. In fact, people with PVD who don't take statins are more likely to have a heart attack than those with coronary artery disease who do take them. What's more, research also indicates that statins, especially Zocor (simvastatin), provides benefits for people with PVD beyond cholesterol lowering. They seem to reduce inflammation in the arteries, and possibly enable the growth of new blood vessels.

Pletal (cilostazol). This medication heads a class of drugs called phosphodiesterase inhibitors, which relax blood vessels to improve blood flow, thus easing leg pain.

Antiplatelet drugs. Antiplatelet medications are key for controlling PVD because they make it harder for platelets to clump together, creating artery-blocking clots. Two commonly prescribed drugs in this class are Plavix (clopidogrel) or Ticlid (ticlopidine).

Other Approaches

A low-fat diet. As with any cardiovascular condition that includes partially blocked arteries, you need to reduce the amount of fat in your diet. That doesn't necessarily mean a severely low-fat diet. In fact, a year-long study of 45 people with PVD who followed either the very low-fat (less than 10 percent) Pritikin diet or the easier-to-follow American Heart Association low-fat diet (which focuses on limiting saturated fat rather than total fat) found similar improvement in pain-free walking for each.

Make fruits and vegetables the centerpiece of your diet, along with olive oil and fish, and reduce the amount of saturated fat from red meat, poultry skin, and regular dairy products.

Acupuncture. Cardiac rehabilitation experts have begun using electrical acupuncture, which stimulates acupuncture sites with small pulses of electricity, to ease pain and enhance blood flow in people with PVD. Although the scientific evidence is still thin, either traditional needle acupuncture or electrical stimulation of acupuncture points is worth a try.

Pneumatic compression. Similar to enhanced external counterpulsation therapy used for coronary artery disease (described on page 268), this treatment uses a special boot to cover your lower leg. The boot is inflated and deflated in conjunction with the resting phase of the heartbeat to exert pressure on the vessels, boosting blood flow. Better blood flow, in turn, increases the release of nitric oxide, which dilates blood vessels, improving circulation.

In a study published in 2005, 20 people with PVD who were having problems walking received 2 1/2 hours of pneumatic compression a day for three months. They improved far more than a similar group who only received aspirin and exercised. Plus, the pneumatic compression group maintained their improvement for at least a year after the therapy ended.

Prevention

Follow a heart-healthy diet and lifestyle. Your best strategy for avoiding PVD is to make the same lifestyle adjustments we've already suggested for people with the disease, such as diet and exercise. For instance, quitting smoking slashes your risk of developing PVD in half. In fact, studies find, 4 out of 10 people with PVD can blame their condition on smoking.

Rheumatoid Arthritis

Pain, inflammation, and swelling of the joints are the hallmarks of this disease, which can strike anyone at any age, including children. Unlike osteoarthritis (described on page 333), which primarily results from years of damage to the joints and cartilage (the cushioning material that separates joints from bones), rheumatoid arthritis (RA) is an autoimmune disease, in which the immune system basically goes haywire.

RA is typically triggered by a bacterial or viral infection that, in turn, trips some genetic switch. Once that switch is turned on, the immune system begins attacking the cartilage and other soft tissue that line the joints, as well as other connective tissue throughout the body—even the supportive tissue surrounding blood vessels and present throughout the lungs. Without appropriate treatment, the disease leads to terrible deformity, pain, and, eventually, premature death.

It sounds bad indeed, but thanks to tremendous advances in our understanding of the immune system and the inflammatory response in the past decade, we have an arsenal of new drugs to treat RA. These drugs, especially when combined with certain lifestyle changes and other integrative approaches, can make a real difference.

Do This Now

When your rheumatoid arthritis flares, bringing pain and swelling, rest your joints as much as possible, and follow this advice for short-term relief.

1. Take willow bark, the equivalent of 240 milligrams salicin daily, per package directions, in two or three divided doses. The pill form is sold under the name Asalixx, available online at www.bionoricausa.com or by calling 800-264-2325. (You can't find this product in most drugstores.)

2. Take a warm bath to which you have added 1 cup Epsom salts with 10 drops of one or more of the following essential oils: peppermint, juniper, lavender, or rosemary.

3. Begin taking 3 grams fish oil and 3 grams of either evening primrose oil, borage oil, or black currant oil a day.

Why It Works

The way to stop your pain is to stop the inflammation around the joint. NSAIDs (nonsteroidal anti-inflammatory drugs) like aspirin and ibuprofen do that, but they can harm your stomach. In fact, studies find that people with RA are nearly twice as likely as people with osteoarthritis to develop serious complications like peptic ulcers from NSAIDs. That's why we recommend willow bark, from which aspirin was first derived. It's easier on the stomach while still providing many of the same anti-inflammatory effects. One study found it was just as effective as a common prescription NSAID in people with RA.

If the willow bark doesn't contain your pain, your doctor may also prescribe one of many prescription NSAIDs available. Because they don't prevent destruction of the joint, however, expect them to be just one of several medications you take.

The warm bath with Epsom salts and essential oils is wonderful for relaxing the muscle around the joint and bringing more blood to the area. Plus, heat tends to change the perception of pain in the joint, so it hurts less. And the moisture helps the heat penetrate more deeply. The oils

have anti-inflammatory benefits and contribute to increased blood circulation.

We want you to take the fish oil and other oils because they are rich sources of GLA, which has strong anti-inflammatory effects. Numerous studies of GLA-rich oils find consistent benefits— primarily less joint tenderness and inflammation. Some studies find that people who take these supplements can reduce the dose of their NSAIDs or even stop taking them altogether.

For convenience, try taking the oils in liquid form rather than capsules, since you'd have to swallow a lot of capsules to get this dose. Also aim to get 2 teaspoons of olive oil in your diet a day. One study found that ingesting olive oil (which also has anti-inflammatory properties) along with fish oil supplements improved RA symptoms more than fish oil on its own.

Other Medicines
Herbs and Supplements

Valerian. When RA symptoms flare, you may have trouble sleeping. This herb, well documented for improving sleep, can help. Take 600 to 900 milligrams standardized to 0.04% valerinic acids at bedtime for at least four to six weeks.

Ginger. Ginger's ability to reduce inflammation is pretty amazing. (And you thought it was just a cooking herb!) You'll need to take quite a lot, though (enough that you need to buy the capsules of dried root instead of cooking with ginger). Take 4 grams of the dried root a day.

Antioxidants. To prevent the oxidative damage that can lead to inflammation (you read about oxidation in Part 2), take an antioxidant multivitamin supplement containing 500 milligrams vitamin C, 200 to 400 IU vitamin E, 200 micrograms selenium, and 2,500 to 5,000 IU beta-carotene.

Zinc. Some studies find low levels of this mineral in people with RA, and one study found that

supplementing improved symptoms. Take 25 to 50 milligrams a day along with 2 to 4 milligrams copper. Why add the copper? Not only can large doses of zinc deplete copper, which your body needs, but there's some evidence that copper may have some anti-inflammatory effects.

Calcium and vitamin D. People with RA have an increased risk of osteoarthritis, made even greater by the drugs they take. So be sure to take 1,500 milligrams calcium in divided doses, and 400 to 800 IU vitamin D daily (the older you are, the higher the dose you need).

Prescription Drugs

Glucocorticoids. Also called corticosteroids, these immune-suppressing steroid drugs, particularly prednisone, used to be the primary treatment for RA. And low daily oral doses, as well as injections directly into the affected joint, still form an important component of treatment. There's even some evidence that low-dose steroid use may slow the rate of joint damage. But the benefits of these drugs always have to be weighed against the negatives—which are significant. The drugs can increase the risk of osteoporosis and high blood pressure. They can also lead to weight gain, bloating, high blood sugar levels, and cataracts, as well as atherosclerosis, or hardening of the arteries.

Disease-modifying antirheumatic drugs (DMARDs). These drugs can actually prevent or reduce joint damage if you start them early enough. Some are slow-acting; others work faster but may have more powerful side effects. Drugs in this category include Plaquenil (hydroxychloroquine), Azulfidine EN-tabs (sulfasalazine), methotrexate, gold compounds, Cuprimine (penicillamine), and Arava (leflunomide), These are powerful drugs, all with their own pros and cons. For instance, hydroxychloroquine can damage your vision, while methotrexate, a

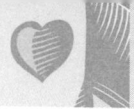

chemotherapy drug, can lead to liver or lung damage. Gold compounds can cause dangerous rashes and affect the liver and lungs, and penicillamine can cause nerve disorders. You'll need to discuss with your doctor which one is best for you, then monitor your symptoms closely.

Tumor necrosis factor (TNF) inhibitors. The newest class of drugs for RA, these work by blocking the release of inflammatory chemicals. Three drugs are approved in this category: Enbrel (etanercept), Remicade (infliximab), and Humira (adalimumab). All three are given by self-injection. They are often given in conjunction with methotrexate (see above). One study found that Humira combined with methotrexate was about five times more effective than methotrexate alone.

Compared to other DMARDs, the TNF inhibitors seem to have very few serious side effects beyond immune suppression, but they haven't been on the market long enough for doctors to determine what, if any, the long-term side effects might be.

Other Approaches

Low-allergenic diet. There's some evidence that food allergies may play a part in autoimmune illnesses like RA. In one study, people with RA who followed a diet that excluded common allergens like grains, nuts, milk, and eggs for 10 to 18 days found their symptoms significantly improved. Adding the foods back made their symptoms worse. Other studies find similar results, with corn, wheat, bacon/pork, oranges, milk, oats, rye, egg, beef, and coffee being the most common problem foods. Many of these foods contribute to the production of arachidonic acid, which provides fuel for inflammation. That's also why studies find vegetarian diets can improve RA symptoms.

Surgery. If your joint damage is severe and you're in a great deal of pain, you may need

✿ Helpful Hint

Add Folic Acid to Methotrexate

If you're taking methotrexate, also take 2 to 5 milligrams of the B vitamin folic acid. Methotrexate can block the effects of this vitamin in the body. In fact, many side effects related to methotrexate are due to a lack of usable folic acid. Also increase your intake of foods rich in folic acids, which include enriched breads and grains, cereal, beans, and most fruits and vegetables.

surgery. Numerous procedures are available, including the same surgery performed for carpal tunnel syndrome (described on page 316), joint fusion (in which the ends of two bones are joined together with screws or bone grafts), synovectomy, in which the inflamed tissue lining the affected joint is removed, and joint replacement.

Journal writing. Simply writing about stressful events in a journal can improve your condition, according to a major study published in the *Journal of the American Medical Association*. The reason? Stress reduction. Stress increases your body's production of inflammatory chemicals like cytokines, and journaling is a well-known stress-reduction approach.

Other stress-reduction therapies. In addition to journal writing, other stress-reducing approaches, including relaxation training, biofeedback, and cognitive-behavioral therapy, can improve pain and function, as well as your emotional ability to cope with a chronic disease, according to numerous studies. Ideally, start one of these therapies as soon as possible after your diagnosis; that's when they seem to have the greatest effect.

Exercise. Even though stretching and exercising may be the last thing you want to do when you have RA, you need to do it. Otherwise you

lose muscle strength, and that, in turn, makes your joints less stable and more susceptible to injury. Try light weight training and stretching, as well as some gentle aerobic activity like walking, which studies find can improve mood and help with fatigue, as well as help prevent bone loss.

Acupuncture. Acupuncture has an anti-inflammatory effect in the body, decreasing levels of inflammatory chemicals called cytokines and reducing the pain and inflammation associated with RA. Consider electroacupuncture, shown in at least one study to significantly improve pain and joint stiffness in people with RA—so much so that the study was stopped early so all the participants could get the treatment. Another study using traditional needle acupuncture found no improvement.

Prevention

Load up on brightly colored fruits and vegetables. A large study analyzing the diets of more than 25,000 Europeans found people with low levels of key carotenoids in their diets (antioxidants found in brightly colored fruits and vegetables) were much more likely to develop RA than those with high levels. It doesn't take much. Adding one glass of orange juice a day could help protect against the development of RA and other inflammatory joint diseases, like lupus.

Cut out the red meat. The more red meat in your diet, the greater your risk of developing RA.

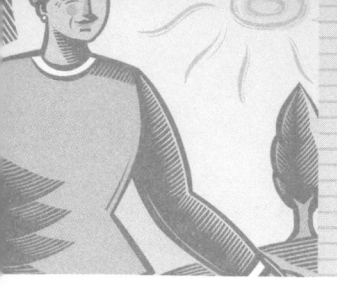

Back Pain

It can come on as suddenly as a summer thunderstorm. One minute you're reaching over to pick up a shopping bag or pluck a weed from the garden, the next you find yourself gripped with pain and unable to straighten up. While this kind of acute back pain responds well to the remedies outlined in Sprains and Strains (page 255) and Muscle Soreness (page 249), if it lasts more than three months, you have chronic back pain, which requires a broader treatment approach.

Chronic low back pain can stem from numerous causes, such as a muscle or ligament strain, disk problems like a herniated disk (in which the rubbery disk that lies between the vertebrae becomes compressed and bulges or breaks through its normal location, pressing on the sensitive nerves along the spine), a fractured or slipping vertebra, or even psychological stress. Osteoporosis (see page 295) can also cause chronic back pain.

The good news is that most back pain improves within six weeks, no matter what you do. The bad news is that once you've had any type of back pain episode, you're likely to have one or more relapses within the year. So prevention is key.

Our Best Advice

For relief of a flare-up, rely on heat or ice (whichever works best for you) and take 750 to 1,000 milligrams Tylenol or 220 milligrams Aleve (for bad pain, take both simultaneously once or twice a day for one to two days). But to help relieve chronic back pain, do the following.

1. Every day, without fail, do the three stretches and three strength moves in "Exercise Therapy for Bad Backs" (page 313).

2. Walk for at least 20 minutes a day, even if you're walking slowly.

3. If you have access to a pool, spend 20 minutes a day walking back and forth in chest-high water in addition to or instead of your walk. As your pain improves, start swimming.

4. Do a posture check at least every hour: Make sure you're standing or sitting up straight.

5. Take a hatha yoga class twice a week.

Why It Works

Exercise is key to reducing back pain. In fact, it's the most important thing you can do. The stretches we recommend increase your flexibility and allow for better nerve and muscle function, which adds up to less pain and fewer muscle spasms and less possibility of pinching small nerves. Move slowly and gently while doing them. The strengthening exercises are just as important; they tone muscles that support the spine.

Swimming is gaining a reputation as one of the best therapies for chronic low back pain. Studies find it not only significantly reduces pain but also

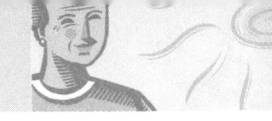

levels of stress hormones. That's important because stress contributes to low back pain. Plus, exercising in water helps prevent further injury because your back doesn't have to bear any weight.

Checking—and straightening—your posture regularly is important because bad posture contributes more significantly to low back pain than you probably realize, putting increased strain on the lower back.

Finally, yoga, with its gentle stretching and core strengthening exercises, improved chronic back pain in several studies. We recommend hatha yoga because it pays special attention to posture to prevent injury, and uses props like belts, blocks, mats, and small pillows to help you get the full benefit of poses even before you're fully flexible.

Other Medicines
Herbs and Supplements

Devil's claw. This bitter-tasting African herb is often used to reduce inflammation. A review of 12 clinical trials found that a liquid formulation standardized to 100 milligrams harpagosides (the active ingredient) or a powder standardized to 60 milligrams harpagosides worked well in alleviating flares of chronic back pain. Follow the package directions.

Capsaicin patch. Capsaicin is the ingredient that gives hot peppers their heat. It works by depleting a chemical called substance P (P is for *pain*) from the nerves in the skin, short-circuiting the transmission of pain signals from those nerves to the brain. Use as directed, because keeping the patch on too long could cause skin irritation.

Vitamin B_{12}. We've found good results with one B_{12} shot every other week for six weeks (a total of three shots). If that provides relief, then talk to your doctor about an oral B_{12} vitamin you dissolve under your tongue. In one study, 60 people who had severe low back pain for six months to five years received either the B_{12} shot or a placebo. While both groups reported a sharp decrease in pain (the placebo effect is generally high in chronic pain studies), the group receiving the B_{12} shots had less pain and took far fewer pain relievers than the placebo group. We're not entirely sure how it works, but we do know that B_{12} affects nerves and the transmission of signals along those nerves.

Prescription Drugs

Muscle relaxants. These drugs include benzodiazepines like Valium, sedatives, certain antihistamines (which can be very sedating), and other medications that act on the central nervous system. They're often prescribed after an acute injury, but haven't been studied for chronic back

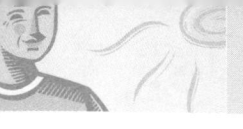

pain. However, their relaxing effects may help, particularly if anxiety or tension makes your pain worse. Don't take for more than four weeks, however, because they can be addictive.

Antidepressants. Generally, low doses of tricyclic antidepressants like Elavil (amitriptyline) help with sleep and pain management, probably because the perception of pain occurs in the brain, not at the site of the pain itself, and antidepressants alter levels of neurotransmitters, chemicals in the brain that relay signals between brain cells.

Other Approaches

Injections. Your doctor can inject medication into the spaces between the vertebrae in the back (epidural injections), certain muscles (trigger point injections), or into the joints between the vertebrae (facet injections). Medications include steroids to reduce inflammation and anesthetics to deaden pain. Benefits depend on the reason behind the pain. For instance, epidural steroid injections work very well to alleviate pain from compressed nerves, while facet injections work best if the pain is related to the vertebral joint.

Acupuncture. The evidence is mixed on acupuncture's benefits for low back pain, but it can have good results in some people, possibly by increasing the release of feel-good hormones called endorphins. We recommend trigger point acupuncture, in which the acupuncture needles are inserted deep into the muscles triggering the pain. (This may be a little painful, depending on the point and the skill of the operator.) One study found it relieved pain better than standard acupuncture or superficial trigger acupuncture.

Chemical enucleation (chemonucleolysis). In this procedure the doctor injects an enzyme such as papain (from the papaya) into the disk. The enzyme "digests" the disk material, reducing the disk bulge. One published report on its use in

3,000 patients found an 85 percent success rate, with much higher benefits in those who complained of leg pain in addition to low back pain. Other long-term studies find similar results to back surgery. If your back pain gets worse when you sit and try to lift your legs, talk to your doctor about this procedure.

Surgery. The primary surgery for chronic low back pain is fusion surgery, in which bone grafts are inserted between vertebrae so the vertebrae grow together. This limits movement in that part of the spine, however, and there's little evidence that it's effective for any kind of back pain beyond that caused by isthmic spondylolisthesis, in which one cracked vertebra slides over another. This condition occurs in only about 5 or 10 percent of people with back pain.

Chiropractic. As with many therapies for chronic low back pain, the evidence on chiropractic is mixed. It does seem to help with acute low back pain, but how much it really helps chronic back pain is less clear. One large review of 69 clinical trials found that it had an effect similar to prescription NSAIDs, and was more effective in the long term than physical therapy. Bottom line: It's worth a try. You should feel some relief within five sessions; if not, move on to something else.

Mind-body therapies. Relaxation therapy (such as deep breathing and visualization), biofeedback, cognitive-behavioral therapy, and progressive muscle relaxation all help with chronic low back pain, probably because of the strong connection between your emotional and physical states. We describe each of these therapies in depth beginning on page 24. If one doesn't work for you, try another.

McKenzie therapy. This form of physical therapy combines exercises with posture changes. An article that pooled the results of studies comparing the therapy to massage, strength training, general exercises, and NSAIDs found more pain

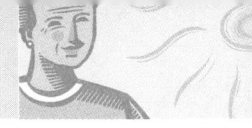

Exercise Therapy for Bad Backs

Do these every day. If a move hurts, stop. Once these exercises become easy, ask a physical therapist for more advanced exercises.

Stretches

Pelvic tilt. Lie on your back with your knees bent but touching, and your feet flat on the floor. Flatten your lower back against the floor, tilting your pelvis down. Hold for 20 to 40 seconds while breathing slowly and deeply, then release. Repeat twice.

Lumbar stretch. Sit up tall on a chair and slowly, one vertebra at a time, roll your head, neck, chest, and low back forward until your head is between your knees (or as far as you can comfortably go). Hold for three deep breaths, then slowly roll back up to a sitting position. Repeat twice.

Cat. Kneel on all fours with your knees hip-width apart. Keeping your stomach muscles tensed, arch your back like a cat and hold for five seconds, then release. Repeat. Now let your stomach drop a bit toward the floor. Hold for five seconds, then repeat. Finally, sit back on your heels and reach your arms in front of you on the floor and hold.

Strength Moves

Curl-ups. Lie on your back with your knees bent and your feet flat on the floor. Place your hands behind your head. Tense your stomach muscles, then lift your head and shoulders and upper back off the floor. Don't pull with your hands. Repeat 10 times if you can.

Dry swimming. Lie on your stomach with a rolled-up towel under your belly for back support. Tighten your buttocks and simultaneously raise one arm and the opposite leg, then switch. Repeat for up to two minutes.

Leg lift. Lie on your back with your knees bent and your feet flat on the floor. Press your lower back into the floor. Now straighten one leg, keeping your knees aligned. Bend your leg to return to starting position, then repeat on the opposite side. Repeat 10 times if you can.

---

relief and less disability in the short term than with the other standard therapies.

Massage. Several reviews of studies found that massage probably works for chronic low back pain, but the effects don't last long. If you can afford it and/or your insurance will pay for it, we still recommend it, both for the pain relief and the stress reduction it provides. Ask for deep tissue, myofascial release, or acupressure massage, which studies find are best at increasing function and mobility.

Prevention

Lift with your legs, not your back. To lift something heavy, stand near the object, bend your knees, grasp the object, then lift by straightening your legs.

Take a Pilates class. Pilates is ideal for strengthening and stretching the muscles that support the back. One case report on a woman with curvature of the spine who couldn't even carry her child found she improved substantially after a series of Pilates classes.

Make sure your workstation is ergonomically correct. That means an adjustable chair that provides adequate lumbar (lower back) support and has armrests, a computer monitor with the top of the screen at eye level, and a wrist rest in front of your keyboard. Your knees and elbows should be bent at 90-degree angles.

Bursitis and Tendinitis

Think of bursitis and its cousin, tendinitis, as your body's way of telling you to take it easy. Both conditions are the result of too much repeated motion, and both are more common as we age.

Bursitis occurs when sacs called bursa become inflamed and filled with fluid. These sacs act like a felt pad that reduces friction between muscles, tendons, ligaments, and bone. Tendinitis occurs when the tendons become inflamed. Tendons are tough cords of tissue that connect muscles to bone. Both conditions are most likely to occur in the elbow, shoulder, hip, knee, ankle, or heel.

There's no magic medicine for either problem, just rest and an integrative approach to reducing inflammation while the body heals itself.

Do This Now

First and foremost, you need to rest the affected part of your body, or you're guaranteed to remain in pain and maybe even make the damage worse. We also recommend you do the following.

1. Apply an ice pack for 15 to 30 minutes four to eight times a day. If the area of the skin is too big or oddly shaped for a conventional ice pack, use a large bag of frozen corn or peas. You can also make a slushy ice pack by mixing two parts water to one part alcohol in a plastic bag, sealing, and freezing. The alcohol acts like antifreeze so the mixture gets very cold and slushy but doesn't freeze hard, making it perfect for awkwardly shaped body parts like shoulders.

2. After the ice, apply a hot compress to the area for three to five minutes.

3. After each treatment with ice and heat, massage Traumeel ointment or gel into the aching area.

4. Take oral arnica 30C every 15 to 30 minutes (follow package directions) for four hours, then four times a day for the first 48 hours.

5. Take 400 to 600 milligrams ibuprofen (Advil) or 225 milligrams Aleve every four hours for up to two days.

Why It Works

Cold and heat give your pain a one-two punch. The cold compress reduces swelling and pain by shrinking blood vessels and, studies find, sealing off leaky blood vessels, which helps reduce inflammation. The warm compress brings more blood and healing nutrients to the area, aiding in repair.

Traumeel cream is a homeopathic product containing arnica, calendula, belladonna, and many other herbs known to reduce pain and swelling and speed healing. Although there aren't any studies in humans, one study in rats found the cream resulted in less swelling and faster healing. Experience in patients also tells us Traumeel cream works.

Arnica, one of the ingredients in the cream, also works well if you take it internally. We recommend it for lots of injuries that cause inflammation, including these two.

Advil and Aleve bring down inflammation, which is why they're called nonsteroidal anti-inflammatory drugs (NSAIDs).

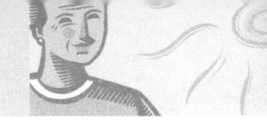

Other Medicines
Herbs and Supplements

Comfrey root salve or ointment. Like arnica, comfrey is popular for injuries that cause inflammation. Although it hasn't been studied specifically in bursitis or tendinitis, a German study using this salve for sprains found it significantly reduced swelling and pain. (Unlike arnica, it should never be used internally.)

Vitamin C with flavonoids. These antioxidants strengthen tiny blood vessels, reducing the leaking that can increase swelling and inflammation. Take 500 milligrams twice a day.

Bromelain. This pineapple-derived enzyme reduces swelling, pain, and tenderness. Take 500 milligrams when you first notice the pain, then twice a day for three more days. Make sure the supplement contains at least 2,000 MCU (milk clotting units) or 1,200 GDU (gelatin dissolving units), and wait at least an hour after a meal before taking it.

Other Approaches

Splinting. If your pain is in the ankle, hand, or arm, a drugstore splint can help by keeping the area immobilized, forcing you to rest it.

Ultrasound. For chronic pain from bursitis or tendinitis, ask your doctor to refer you to a physical therapist for treatment with ultrasound. Sound waves penetrate beneath the skin, increasing blood flow to the injured area and softening the scar tissue that forms as part of the repetitive injury.

Prevention

Warm up and stretch before beginning any strenuous activity. And don't push too hard.

Rest frequently when engaging in repetitive motions. Better still, avoid repetitive motions altogether. And make sure you're using proper technique and equipment when playing sports like tennis.

Carpal Tunnel Syndrome

Our hands were just not designed for the kind of repetitive work we do these days, especially the hours we spend typing. (Sewing, knitting, and guitar playing are other culprits.) And so we have an explosion of carpal tunnel syndrome, a painful wrist and hand condition.

The condition is a form of nerve damage rather than a muscle, ligament, or joint problem. Picture a strand of cooked thin spaghetti. Now imagine threading that spaghetti through a rubber tube—and then squeezing the tube. The result: squished spaghetti. In carpal tunnel syndrome, the spaghetti is the median nerve, one of two nerves that transmit feeling in the hand. The tube is the carpal tunnel, a channel at the front of the wrist. The bottom of the channel is composed of the bones of the wrist, while the "roof" is composed of the carpal ligament.

Anything that squeezes or inflames the carpal tunnel—ranging from injury to medical conditions like rheumatoid arthritis—puts pressure on the nerve, causing pain, numbness, or tingling. Medical conditions that lead to fluid buildup, like pregnancy, hypothyroidism, and diabetes, increase pressure on the nerve from inside the tunnel.

Luckily, about 80 percent of carpal tunnel syndrome cases improve with nonsurgical methods like those described below. The rest, however, may need surgery.

Do This Now

To alleviate the pain of carpal tunnel syndrome, do the following.

1. Give yourself an ice massage. Freeze a couple of inches of water in a Styrofoam cup and peel off the top of the cup, exposing the edge of the ice but leaving the bottom of the ice covered so you can hold it. Grasp the bottom part of the cup and rub the exposed ice over your wrist. Massage for 10 minutes several times a day during flares.

2. After icing, perform the range-of-motion exercises described in "Stretches for Carpal Tunnel Syndrome" (page 319) to stretch your hand and wrist.

3. When performing repetitive actions (like using a computer mouse), set an alarm to beep every 15 minutes. Get up, stretch, flex your hands and wrists, ball up your hands and squeeze tightly, then release. Repeat several times before resuming your activity.

4. Wear a wrist splint at night to keep your wrist in a neutral position.

GETTING TESTED

Although our remedies may improve your carpal tunnel completely, if it continues for more than three months you should see a doctor for a complete evaluation. Continued pressure could permanently damage the nerve to the point that even surgery won't completely restore function. Also see your doctor if:

- you develop sudden weakness or loss of feeling in your hand or arm;

- you can't grasp things, or you drop things when you try to hold them;

- your thumb isn't as strong or mobile as it should be.

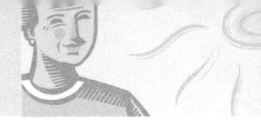

Anti-inflammatory Drugs?

If your first reaction to the pain of carpal tunnel is to reach for the Advil, don't bother. A large review of several studies found that nonsteroidal anti-inflammatories (NSAIDs) like ibuprofen are no more effective than placebo in reducing swelling and improving function, although they may provide some short-term pain relief for some people. That's because most of the pain you feel from carpal tunnel is nerve pain, and NSAIDs are useless against this type of nerve pain, as well as the inflammation that causes it.

5. Take 500 milligrams bromelain. Make sure the strength is at least 2,000 milk clotting units (MCU) or 1,200 gelatin dissolving units (GDU) per 500-milligram dose. Then take the same dose twice a day for three more days. Take it between meals, not with food, or the enzyme will spend itself dissolving your food.

Why It Works

Ice reduces the swelling that squishes the median nerve. The stretching exercises mobilize the tissue lining the carpal tunnel so the nerve slides more freely and blood flows better, which improves toxin removal and nutrient delivery.

Taking frequent breaks can help prevent further inflammation. If you have a bad case of carpal tunnel syndrome, you may need to stop the offending activity altogether for a couple of weeks.

The splints, available in drugstores or medical supply stores, are designed to keep the wrist in a neutral position, that is, not bent or turned in one direction or another. This relieves pressure on the carpal tunnel and, in turn, on the median nerve. Splinting works best when started within the first three months of symptoms.

If you have severe carpal tunnel syndrome, you may need an individually molded splint that's easier to wear during the day. Don't wear it for more than three hours at a time during the day, however, without taking an hour break, or you could permanently damage function in your fingers or other parts of your wrist.

Bromelain, a protein-digesting enzyme derived from pineapple, combats inflammation in the carpal tunnel from inside your body. Use it during an acute flare to reduce pain and swelling.

Other Medicines
Herbs and Supplements

Fish oil. Although there are no studies on the use of fish oil for carpal tunnel syndrome, we recommend it because of its strong anti-inflammatory effects. Also, since it's fat soluble, it can penetrate nerve tissue well (nerve tissue contains a lot of fat). Take 1,500 to 3,000 milligrams fish oil daily. It's also good for your heart.

Willow bark extract. A supplement derived from the original source for aspirin, willow bark extract can reduce carpal tunnel pain if used regularly (unlike aspirin, it doesn't pose a risk of stomach upset, so you can use it longer-term). Use a standardized extract like Asalixx (available online at bionoricausa.com or by calling 800-264-2325) and take one or two pills twice a day.

Pyridoxine. Although the evidence is mixed on its benefits, our clinical experience shows good results with high doses of vitamin B_6, which is important for nerve function. We find it can improve pain after movement, although it doesn't work well at improving pain at night. Start with 50 milligrams a day as part of a B complex, increasing to 100 milligrams of B_6 a day if you don't see any improvement after four weeks. Don't exceed 200 milligrams a day.

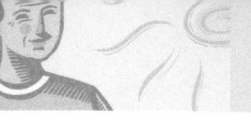

Over-the-Counter Drugs

Capsaicin cream. This cream contains the same compound that gives hot peppers their heat. It interferes with the transmission of pain signals. Use the 0.025% concentration (the lowest) because the skin on the inside of the wrist is so thin and sensitive.

Other Approaches

Anti-inflammatory diet. Follow the anti-inflammatory diet described on pages 42-43 to reduce the inflammation that contributes to pressure of the carpal tunnel on the median nerve.

Ultrasound therapy. This treatment, in which sound waves are directed to the carpal tunnel, can significantly improve symptoms when given daily for at least two weeks.

Surgery. Surgery for carpal tunnel syndrome is recommended only for people who don't improve with the other treatments available, have persistent severe symptoms, or show evidence that the median nerve is significantly impaired, affecting their ability to use their hand.

Typically, the surgeon removes the carpal tendon, releasing pressure on the nerve. This can be done with an open incision, or endoscopically, using a small instrument inserted through a small puncture in the wrist. Which procedure is best is controversial, with most reviews finding the endoscopic form is worse when it comes to reversing nerve damage but better at improving grip strength. Plus, it results in less scarring. Another review found no difference in benefits between the two. Bottom line: Discuss with your surgeon which procedure is best for you.

Acupuncture. The 1997 National Institutes of Health Consensus panel on acupuncture agreed that available evidence at the time suggested acupuncture might be a good treatment for carpal tunnel syndrome. More recently, a small study found that laser acupuncture (using lasers instead of needles on pressure points) along with transcutaneous electric nerve stimulation (TENS), which emits low electrical pulses through the skin onto the nerve, resulted in less pain and greater improvement than a sham treatment. In fact, a computer typist and handyman who hadn't been able to work returned to work and remained in good condition for a year or longer.

Arnica ointment. Although there are no trials on its use for carpal tunnel syndrome, our experience finds that massaging this homeopathic ointment or gel onto the wrist before attempting difficult activities and at night helps with pain.

Yoga. You might not think of yoga when it comes to your wrists, but one study published in the *Journal of the American Medical Association* found eight weeks of twice-weekly yoga classes and relaxation therapy worked better than splinting or no treatment in improving carpal tunnel syndrome. The participants performed 11 poses designed to strengthen, stretch, and balance each joint in their upper body. Tell your teacher about your condition, and ask her to provide you with exercises appropriate for you.

GETTING TESTED

To diagnose carpal tunnel syndrome, your doctor may perform the following tests:

- **Tinel's test,** in which tapping on the middle nerve of the wrist creates a tingling in the middle fingers.
- **Phalen's test,** in which flexing your wrist produces tingling in the fingers associated with the median nerve within 60 seconds.
- **Nerve conduction studies,** in which bursts of electricity are transmitted to the median nerve to measure how well it transmits the signals to the wrist and fingers.

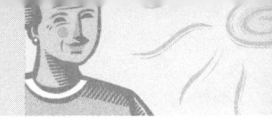

Prescription Drugs

Steroids. Both oral and injectable steroids are used in the short term to reduce swelling and pain in carpal tunnel syndrome. Prednisone is the most commonly prescribed oral steroid. It usually works within four weeks. You may also receive steroid injections into the opening of the carpal tunnel, with or without an anesthetic like lidocaine, which provides temporary relief. Injections seem to work best if you splint the wrist for several days afterward. Neither injections nor oral steroids should be used for long-term relief, however, because of potentially serious side effects.

Prevention

Watch your weight. Because carpal tunnel syndrome is associated with obesity and diabetes, maintaining a healthy weight can reduce your risk.

Take frequent breaks from repetitive motions like typing or using a computer mouse (the mouse is actually more dangerous to the carpal tunnel than the keyboard). You can even get computer programs that remind you to do this.

Squeeze a small ball several times a day with each hand. This helps maintain strength and flexibility in the arms and hands.

Stretches for Carpal Tunnel Syndrome

1. Hold your left arm in front of you and bend your wrist up. Then put the fingers of your right hand against the palm of your left and gently pull back. Count to 10, then switch hands.

2. Hold your left arm in front of you and make a fist. Then fold your right hand over the top of the fist and pull gently. Count to 10, then switch hands.

3. Hold your left arm in front of you, palm up, then bend your wrist down. With your right hand on the knuckles of your left, pull the hand gently toward you. Count to 10, then switch hands.

4. Put a rubber band around your fingers, then slowly open them wide enough to stretch the band. Now slowly close them, maintaining a steady resistance against the band. Repeat 10 times.

Chronic Fatigue Syndrome

Despite how family, friends—and possibly even your own doctor—may make you feel, chronic fatigue syndrome (CFS) is *not* all in your head. This is a systemic disorder that affects hormonal levels, the immune system, and the brain itself. Studies find lesions on the white matter in the brains of people with CFS, as well as poor blood flow to the brain, elevated levels of inflammatory immune cells like T-lymphocytes and cytokines, and low levels of other immune cells, like natural killer cells and immunoglobulin, in the blood.

No one knows for sure what causes the disorder. Some researchers theorize a virus triggers it, but no particular virus has been pinpointed as the culprit. As with many syndromes, there is no definitive diagnostic test for the condition (See "Getting Tested" on page 322).

Although there is no cure for CFS, researchers have uncovered some promising therapies. Just as symptoms differ from patient to patient, however, so will effective treatments. Be patient as you work to find the right ones for you.

Do This Now

Chronic fatigue syndrome is a complex disorder with no simple cure. Although this three-step process will temporarily help relieve fatigue and pain, you must use many of the strategies in this chapter over the long term to experience an effective and sustained improvement.

1. Take 200 milligrams Aleve (naproxen) up to three times a day for two days.

2. When the pain hits, lie comfortably on the floor, and begin breathing deeply. Tense and relax the muscles of your body systematically, starting with your feet and moving up toward your head.

3. Take 600 to 900 milligrams of a valerian extract standardized to 0.4% valerinic acids an hour before bed.

Why It Works

The naproxen reduces joint and muscle pain by stemming inflammation. The deep breathing and muscle-tensing exercise (known as progressive muscle relaxation) helps you enter a state of deep relaxation, providing a short mental and physical "time out." We want you to do it on the floor so you don't fall asleep. (If you have time for a nap, go ahead and do it in bed).

Finally, the valerian helps you get a good night's sleep, which also helps fight fatigue. Take the herb nightly for at least two months.

Other Medicines
Herbs and Supplements

Green supplements. Products such as Emerald Green, Synergy, Barley Green, and Greens+ contain powdered greens, usually in the form of grasses (such as wheat or barley grass) and green vegetables such as spinach. Many of these supplements contain the antioxidant equivalent of six or more servings of fruits and vegetables. Although researchers haven't studied their use in people with CFS, we find they help support the immune system and protect against the antioxidant damage that often contributes to muscle pain in people with CFS. Take one to

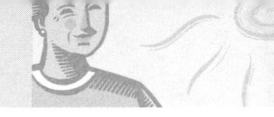

three tablets a day or a rounded teaspoon of powdered product mixed into juice or a shake for at least three months.

Licorice extract. Some people with CFS tend to have abnormally low blood pressure. If you are one of them, and your symptoms include mostly fatigue—not pain—this supplement may help with energy levels. The herb contains an anti-inflammatory compound that increases sodium levels in the blood, which usually leads to higher blood pressure. Take 500 milligrams, two to three times a day, but no more than 3,000 grams a day.

Siberian ginseng. Ginseng, considered a "tonic" herb, may help with your fatigue, especially if it's mild. In one study, CFS patients with mild fatigue who took Siberian ginseng daily for four months reported less fatigue that improved faster than those who took a placebo. Those with severe fatigue, however, showed no improvement in fatigue, although they did report less depression. Take 400 to 500 milligrams of standardized extract containing 2.24 milligrams of combined eleutherosides B and E daily.

Ginkgo. This herb may improve concentration and alertness by boosting blood flow to the brain. Because it's an antioxidant, it may also help protect muscles from oxidative damage that contributes to muscle pain in CFS. Take 80 to 120 milligrams twice a day of a product standardized to 24% flavonoids and 6% to 7% terpene lactones.

Coenzyme Q_{10}. People with CFS may not produce enough adenosine triphosphate (ATP), the energy currency of the cells of the body. When levels of ATP drop too low, you feel bone-tired. Coenzyme Q_{10} helps your body produce more ATP. It's also an antioxidant, so it may boost your immunity and help your muscle pain. In one study of 155 people with CFS, this supplement increased their ability to exercise—a sign they had more energy. Sixty-nine percent of those who took the supplement also reported improvements

in a host of other symptoms during the six months they took it. Take 100 milligrams daily or 60 milligrams twice a day.

Essential fatty acids. People with CFS tend to have low levels of essential fatty acids, which are important for reducing inflammation and boosting immunity. In one study, people who supplemented with essential fatty acids experienced fewer symptoms after 8 to 12 weeks. Take either 2 grams fish oil and 2 grams flax oil or 4 grams of a combination of evening primrose oil and fish oil.

Melatonin. To help you sleep at night, take 1 to 3 milligrams melatonin an hour before bed in lieu of or in addition to the valerian. Although there are no studies on its use for CFS, other research finds that this supplement can improve sleep-wake cycles and energy levels in shift workers and people suffering from jet lag.

Prescription Drugs

Antidepressants. If you are one of the two-thirds of patients with CFS who are also depressed, an antidepressant—either a selective serotonin reuptake inhibitor (SSRI) or a tricyclic antidepressant—may help by improving your mood and sleep quality.

Other Approaches

Gluten-free diet. Some people with CFS also have celiac disease, a genetic disorder that prevents their bodies from digesting gluten, the protein found in wheat, rye, and barley. If they eat these grains, they develop diarrhea, weight loss, and malnutrition. If you suspect you have celiac disease, eliminate all gluten products from your diet for at least one month. If your symptoms subside, continue this diet. If not, you can add the foods back.

Cognitive-behavioral therapy. In addition to boosting your mood and improving sleep, this

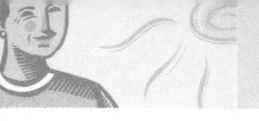
type of therapy, which teaches positive thinking strategies and coping skills, can ease symptoms and help you adopt habits, such as exercise, that could benefit your symptoms.

In one study of 171 people with CFS, this form of therapy worked better than a support group (or no treatment) in alleviating symptoms over eight months. In a separate study of 53 patients, 68 percent rated themselves as either "much improved" or "very much improved" as many as five years after completing the therapy. They were also significantly more likely to meet the criteria for complete recovery from CFS compared to patients who learned a form of relaxation therapy.

Look for a social worker or psychologist trained in CBT, preferably one who's had experience working with people with CFS.

Graded exercise. If you're exhausted from CFS and you don't exercise, you'll become very out of shape. Your heart, lungs, and muscles will become weak—which would make anyone easily fatigued. Graded exercise, in which you slowly and incrementally increase your level of physical activity, helps reverse this vicious cycle. Many studies find it reduces fatigue.

If you decide to try graded exercise, meet with a physical therapist trained in the technique. Your therapist can help you start a program at a manageable level and slowly increase your duration over time. You'll also work on reintroducing daily tasks into your life that you have been avoiding because of CFS.

Magnesium injections. Low levels of the mineral magnesium in people with CFS can lead to low mood and energy. To jump-start a magnesium increase, have your doctor give you magnesium injections once weekly for six weeks. If your symptoms don't improve within that time, stop the shots. If they do improve,

GETTING TESTED

No single lab test will tell you whether you have chronic fatigue syndrome (CFS). To make a diagnosis, your doctor must run a series of tests and evaluations to rule out other diseases that cause similar symptoms. Even side effects from obesity, substance abuse, and some prescription drugs can mimic CFS symptoms. So your doctor should:

- Ask you a series of questions to determine your level and duration of fatigue and to rule out mental illness.

- Perform a series of blood, urine, and other lab tests to screen for conditions that cause symptoms similar to those of CFS. These tests will assess your levels of protein, glucose, electrolytes, iron, and other biological markers.

- Determine whether you have four or more of the following symptoms: muscle pain, joint pain, sore throat, lymphadenopathy (abnormal lymph nodes), headaches, post-exercise fatigue, impaired memory, and impaired concentration.

your doctor should slowly taper off the shots, transitioning you to magnesium supplements. Eventually you'll take 300 to 600 milligrams of magnesium two to three times a day.

Self-hypnosis. This technique elicits a deep relaxation response, which helps turn off inhibitions, fear, pain, and stress. There are no clinical studies on this therapy for CFS, although one case study that was published in a medical journal reported good results (less fatigue and confusion) in one patient.

Friendships. Use some of your energy to keep up with your friends—it may make you feel better in more ways than one. In one study, lack of social support was linked with more severe CFS symptoms.

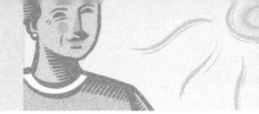

Fibromyalgia

No one knows what causes fibromyalgia, which brings with it difficult symptoms such as muscle soreness, fatigue, disturbed sleep, and "tender points" on the body. But there are several theories. One theory is that people with fibromyalgia (most of whom are women) don't process pain signals properly, making their pain threshold lower. What might feel like a light touch to some people causes significant discomfort to someone with fibromyalgia. The root cause may be imbalances of certain hormones and neurotransmitters (chemicals that transmit messages between brain cells) like serotonin, which play a role in pain perception and mood.

There's no cure for fibromyalgia, but take heart—there is relief to be found. Studies find that a multi-pronged approach, integrating conventional medicine with exercise therapy, stress management, dietary changes, and alternative therapies such as massage, is best at reducing pain intensity, boosting mood, and improving quality of life.

Interestingly, there is no evidence that fibromyalgia is related to inflammation. However, we still find good results with certain anti-inflammatory pain relievers, herbs, and nutritional supplements.

Don't get frustrated if certain approaches don't work for you; nothing works for everyone. Try different approaches for a few weeks or even a few months. If you don't notice any improvement, try something else. Eventually you'll find the right combination of remedies for you.

Do This Now

Like many chronic conditions, fibromyalgia waxes and wanes. Here's what we recommend during a flare to reduce the pain.

1. Take 700 to 1,000 milligrams Tylenol and 200 milligrams Aleve up to three times a day for two days.

2. Give yourself an ice massage. Freeze a couple of inches of water in a Styrofoam cup and peel off the top of the cup, exposing the edge of the ice but leaving the bottom covered. Rub the exposed ice over the painful areas for 10 minutes several times a day.

3. Do a few minutes of gentle stretching.

4. Massage a sports cream like Ben Gay or a natural product like Tiger Balm or White Flower oil (available at health food stores) into the sore areas.

5. Go for a short (10- to 15-minute) walk.

6. Begin taking 400 milligrams SAMe (S-adenosyl-L-methionine) daily. Increase to 400 milligrams twice a day after five days. If you don't see any improvement after two weeks, add another 200 milligrams twice a day, for a total of 1,200 milligrams.

7. Make an appointment with your doctor for an injection of 1 to 2 cubic centimeters of a 50% magnesium sulfate solution, then start taking 300 to 600 milligrams oral magnesium along with 1,200 to 2,400 milligrams malic acid (available in a product called Super Malic).

Why It Works

Take the pain relievers first so they can begin working immediately while you pursue these other approaches. The ice numbs nerve endings, while the gentle massaging and stretching helps

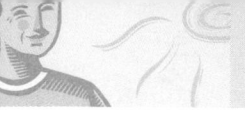

with muscle pain. The salves contain aromatic oils that create a sensation of heat or coolness depending on the oil used, distracting you from the underlying pain. Some salves also contain topical pain relievers or muscle relaxants.

Exercise is probably the best thing you can do over the short and long term for fibromyalgia, although you need to start slow, which is why we recommend gentle stretching and a brief walk. Studies dating back 20 years attest to exercise's benefits for fibromyalgia. It increases pain thresholds and improves overall symptoms. One major study found these positive results held for at least 12 months after participants completed 23 weeks of land-based and water-based exercises.

Swimming in a warm-water pool seems to be one of the best tolerated and most helpful forms of exercise, probably because of the added benefits of warm water on muscle pain. One preliminary study also found good results with a weekly hour of t'ai chi. Your exercise program should begin gradually (talk to your doctor about an ideal amount) and increase over time.

The remaining recommendations will take a while to work, but we want you to start on them now. SAMe is a natural antidepressant that works by increasing levels of important neurotransmitters in the brain, including serotonin. In one study, people who took 800 milligrams SAMe daily for six weeks had less pain, fatigue, and morning stiffness than people who took a placebo, and their mood improved. If you reach the highest dose recommended and don't see any benefit in eight weeks, though, taper down the dose the same way you increased it until you're off it. Don't stop it all at once.

The evidence on the magnesium and malic acid (a fruit acid) is thin, but we've seen excellent results in patients. The theory behind using them is that they are required to generate adenosine triphosphate (ATP), a chemical that provides energy for cells. What's more, magnesium is often used as a natural muscle relaxant, which is why we recommend starting with the high-dose injection.

Other Medicines
Herbs and Supplements

Licorice. If you have low blood pressure (very common in people with fibromyalgia) and more fatigue than pain, we recommend glycyrrhizic acid licorice. This herb is often used to treat low blood pressure (which is why you shouldn't use it in this form if you have high blood pressure). Take 500 milligrams two or three times a day, no more than 3,000 milligrams a day.

St. John's wort. People with fibromyalgia are often depressed. Which problem contributes to which is up for debate, but either way, this herb may help by increasing serotonin levels. Take 300 milligrams three times a day of an extract standardized to 0.3% hypericin or 2% to 5% hyperforin. Check with your doctor or pharmacist first if you're taking other drugs, since this herb can interact with various medicines.

Valerian. Most people with fibromyalgia have disturbed sleep—primarily problems reaching deep, restorative sleep. As with depression, we don't know whether the disease contributes to the sleep problem or vice versa. We do know that valerian can help you get a better night's sleep if you use it regularly. Take 600 to 900 milligrams of an extract standardized to 0.4% valerinic acids nightly for at least four weeks.

Adaptogenic herbs. These herbs, which include Panax ginseng, American ginseng, astragalus, and ashwagandha, are used to increase energy, often a problem for people with fibromyalgia. Pick one (you'll see these herbs recommended for other conditions throughout *Best Remedies,* so pick the one that could help with other conditions you have). Dosages are: Panax

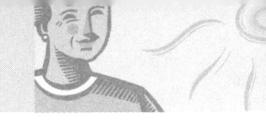

or American ginseng, 300 to 500 milligrams twice a day; astragalus, 500 to 1,000 milligrams twice a day; ashwagandha, 500 milligrams two to three times a day. These are relatively low starting doses and can be gradually increased over time.

Ginkgo and coenzyme Q$_{10}$. One small study found that these two supplements taken together improved fibromyalgia symptoms, although there was no comparison to a placebo. Take 200 milligrams ginkgo extract along with 200 milligrams CoQ$_{10}$ daily.

5-hydroxytryptophan (5-HTP). This amino acid is a building block for serotonin. It works similarly to SAMe, which is what we recommend trying first; but if SAMe doesn't work for you, or is too expensive, try 5-HTP for help with sleep, pain, and mood. Take 50 to 100 milligrams twice a day, taking the second dose an hour before bed. Take this supplement only under your doctor's supervision.

Chlorella. Although it will take a while to have an effect, we've had very good experience with this freshwater green algae, which is rich in proteins, vitamins, and minerals. A couple of small studies suggest a dose of 10 grams a day in tablet form, along with 100 milliliters of a liquid extract daily for two or three months, can significantly improve symptoms. We find chlorella helps increase energy as well as decrease pain. You can use the powdered form in shakes or added to juice, or take oral supplements. Follow package directions for the dosage.

Over-the-Counter Drugs

Capsaicin cream. With daily use, this cream depletes substance P in nerve endings, a chemical critical for transporting pain messages to the brain. Use an ointment, cream, or stick, either 0.25% (low dose) or 0.75% (high dose) three or four times a day. Give it two weeks or more to work.

Prescription Drugs

Ultram (tramadol). This narcotic drug (with or without acetaminophen) is often the first drug prescribed for fibromyalgia. The few studies evaluating its use in fibromyalgia found good results, possibly because it works to increase the amount of available serotonin and norepinephrine (another neurotransmitter often low in people with fibromyalgia).

Antidepressants. Given the link between fibromyalgia, depression, and low levels of brain chemicals that affect mood, it stands to reason that certain antidepressants would improve symptoms, particularly sleep, in some people. As with other chronic pain conditions, the most commonly prescribed antidepressants are the older tricyclics such as Elavil (amitriptyline).

Muscle relaxants. These might be helpful early in the syndrome, particularly if it occurs after some physical trauma that was accompanied by a muscle spasm. We prefer Flexeril (cyclobenzaprine) because it is chemically similar to tricyclic antidepressants and can be used at bedtime without affecting the quality of your sleep. Take the smallest amount possible to provide relief, even cutting low doses in half if you can get by with less.

Other Approaches

Dietary changes. There's some evidence that a plant-based diet might help with fibromyalgia. We don't know why, exactly. Plant-based compounds may help by fighting inflammation, whereas animal-based foods may somehow exacerbate the condition, possibly by lowering levels of the amino acid L-tryptophan, a building block for serotonin.

Also try eliminating wheat and gluten from your diet for a week. Many patients find excellent

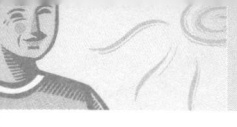

results when they do this, possibly because they're allergic to these foods.

Psychosocial approaches. These include self-help groups (whether over the Internet or in person), meditation and/or guided imagery, and hypnotherapy. All have been found to be helpful in the few, small trials conducted on their use in fibromyalgia. A combination of several of these approaches probably works best.

Massage. Massage may help relieve pain, but ask for light touch, not deep tissue. A deep tissue massage could trigger a flare.

Acupuncture. Several studies have been published on this treatment for fibromyalgia, most showing positive benefits from either needle or electroacupuncture. In one study comparing electroacupuncture to sham treatment, 25 percent of people who received the real thing significantly improved, 50 percent had "satisfactory" relief of symptoms, and 25 percent saw no benefit. Overall, pain threshold improved by 70 percent in the acupuncture group versus 4 percent in the control group.

Chiropractic. We find this therapy helpful, although there's little scientific evidence behind it for fibromyalgia. An initial course of 15 treatments should be enough to see if you're going to have any benefit. If you don't see a large improvement by then, you can stop.

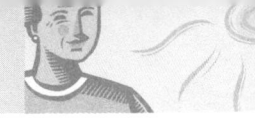

Neck Pain

Given the role the neck has to play—holding up the heaviest part of the body on just seven interlocking bones called the cervical spine—it's a wonder more of us aren't walking around with neck pain. As it is, 7 out of 10 people will experience a bout of neck pain at some time in their lives, often from years of poor posture.

"Neck pain" is a catchall phrase for a variety of conditions that can affect the neck. You could have a pinched nerve (pain or tingling down your arm is one hint), muscle-related pain from poor posture, spinal stenosis (in which the nerve openings in the cervical spine narrow, putting pressure on the nerve), or spinal instability, which occurs when there's increased motion between two vertebrae in your neck. Whiplash, a kind of neck sprain common in car accidents, is another cause.

Your goal is to ease your pain, then strengthen your neck muscles and make certain lifestyle changes to avoid recurrences.

Do This Now

To relieve the pain, follow this advice—and give it some time. Neck pain doesn't usually go away overnight.

1. Take 750 to 1,000 milligrams Tylenol and 220 milligrams Aleve throughout the day, following package directions.

2. Apply ice for 10 minutes at a time to the sore area, then follow with 20 minutes of heat, either a heating pad or moist heat (soak a cloth in hot water and wring out well).

3. Sit up straight in an armless chair. Grab the edge of the chair with your right hand and lean your neck over to the left, trying to place your left ear onto your left shoulder. Hold for 10 seconds, then repeat on the other side. Moving your hand back on the chair seat stretches muscles in the back of the neck; moving it forward stretches muscles in the front.

4. At night, sleep on a water-filled pillow such as the Mediflow WaterBase pillow, available online and from medical supply stores and chiropractic offices.

Why It Works

While the Tylenol works best for the pain itself, the Aleve works best for inflammation. Together the two pack a double whammy. Also talk to your doctor about prescription nonsteroidal anti-inflammatories. There are dozens available; if one doesn't work for you, another might.

Ice and heat, one after the other, are very effective for reducing muscle pain and strain (and may temporarily help with nerve pain). Ice numbs nerve endings in the skin that transmit muscle pain to the brain and reduces inflammation, while heat brings more oxygenated blood to the site, helping to reduce muscle spasms.

Gentle exercise is one of the best things you can do for neck pain. You can start with the stretch we recommend above, but if your pain lasts more than a few days, see a physical therapist for a full set of movements.

Finally, much of neck pain is caused or exacerbated by the way we sleep. Why? The kind of pillow we're sleeping on and our sleeping position. In one five-week study of 41 people with neck

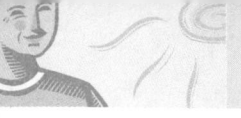

pain, participants slept on a water pillow for two weeks, a roll pillow for two weeks (the kind that looks like a big hot dog), or their usual down or foam pillow for a week. Overall, the water pillow provided the best night's sleep, with the least amount of pain the next morning and throughout the day. Researchers speculate that the water-based pillow just supports neck muscles and other structures better than the other alternatives. Another hint: If your pillow is more than two years old, toss it. It's no longer doing its job properly.

Other Medicines
Herbs and Supplements

Willow bark extract. Aspirin began with the bark of this tree. Although there are no specific studies on the use of the extract for neck pain, several studies show it is very effective at relieving back pain, which is why we recommend it (if you're not also using an NSAID such as aspirin, ibuprofen, or Aleve). The pill form is sold under the name Asalixx, available online at www.bionoricausa.com or by calling 800-264-2325. Follow package directions. Give it time to work; it could take up to six weeks before you see its full benefits.

Devil's claw. This bitter-tasting African herb is often used to reduce inflammation. Although there are no studies on its use in neck pain, there is good evidence it relieves back and arthritis pain, which is why we recommend it for neck pain. Take a liquid formulation standardized to 100 milligrams harpagosides (the active ingredient), or a powder standardized to 60 milligrams harpagosides, once a day.

Capsaicin cream. There are lots of these creams sold over the counter. Capsaicin is the ingredient that gives hot peppers their heat. It works by depleting a chemical called substance P from the nerves in the skin, short-circuiting the transmission of pain signals from those nerves to the brain. Although there's more evidence on its use in back and nerve pain, one study found using the 0.025% cream four times a day for five weeks significantly improved pain in people with chronic neck pain.

Calcium and magnesium. We always make sure people with neck pain supplement with these minerals, since they help with muscle relaxation. Take 1,500 milligrams calcium a day in three or four divided doses and 600 to 800 milligrams of magnesium.

Fish oil. Even though there's no data on the use of fish oil for neck pain, the supplement is such a strong anti-inflammatory that it could help (and it's good for your heart). Take 1 to 2 grams a day.

Prescription Drugs

If your neck pain is bad, your doctor might prescribe any of these. A combination of drugs is usually better than one alone.

Muscle relaxants. These drugs include benzodiazepines like Valium, sedatives, antihistamines, and other medications that act on the central nervous system. Evidence on their use is mixed, but one review of 14 studies found that Flexeril (cyclobenzaprine) was more effective than a placebo in managing neck and back pain. It's our favorite muscle relaxant. The greatest benefit came during the first four days of use. However, the effect was modest and came at the price of side effects, including drowsiness, dry mouth, and dizziness.

Antidepressants. If your doctor prescribes an antidepressant for your back pain, it doesn't mean you're depressed. Low doses of these drugs, particularly tricyclic antidepressants like Elavil (amitriptyline), help with sleep and pain management for a variety of pain conditions.

Anticonvulsants. Once a drug is approved for one condition, doctors are free to prescribe it for others. Anticonvulsants like Klonopin

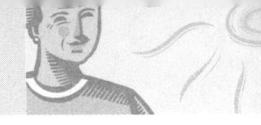

(clonazepam) and Neurontin (gabapentin) are often used to treat nerve-related pain. They probably work by interrupting the transmission of pain signals to the brain.

Other Approaches

Cervical collar. These collars are often used after whiplash. The collar immobilizes the neck just like an Ace bandage immobilizes a sprained ankle, allowing it time to heal without further injury. You can get soft collars in drugstores. Hard collars require a prescription.

Manual therapy. In this form of physical therapy, a therapist moves your neck in various ways to stretch and strengthen the muscles. One study comparing six weeks of weekly manual therapy to twice-a-week physical therapy (in which you move your neck yourself), or standard doctor care found that people who received manual therapy had less pain and greater range of movement than either of the other two groups.

Chiropractic. Spinal manipulation is a good option for acute or chronic neck pain, depending on your individual circumstances (see "Warning", this page). But studies find it works best in combination with rehabilitation exercises (your chiropractor should be able to recommend some).

Surgery. Surgery is a last resort for neck pain, even for a pinched nerve. If everything else fails, however, your doctor may recommend it to remove a disk pressing on a nerve (diskectomy), cut away part or all of a damaged disk or bone spurs (laminectomy), or create more room for your spinal cord (laminoplasty). He may also fuse the vertebrae in your neck together (cervical spine fusion) so they stay in place. Also ask your doctor about artificial disks for the neck. You'll need to join a clinical study, because the disks are still considered experimental.

Acupuncture. Although studies on the use of acupuncture to relieve neck pain are mixed, we've seen good response in patients. Plus, one study on 24 women who had neck and shoulder pain for up to 12 years found that those who received acupuncture 10 times for three or four weeks had much less pain than women who received placebo acupuncture. The benefits lasted up to three years.

Yoga. Yoga can help with neck pain by gently stretching neck muscles and reducing stress. Just make sure you tell your yoga instructor about your neck pain and avoid certain poses like shoulder stands and those that hyperextend the neck.

Prevention

Take frequent breaks from desk work or any other activity in which you bend over or have to maintain your neck in a certain position.

Use a headset or earpiece when talking on the phone.

Sleep on your back or side. Sleeping on your stomach puts too much strain on your neck.

Address emotional issues like unexpressed or unresolved anger with a therapist. Increased tension is often reflected in tense neck muscles.

WARNING

Talk to your doctor first before seeing a chiropractor for neck pain. A study published in the journal *Neurology* found a strong correlation between chiropractic treatment and strokes or mini-strokes in people under 60 who had tiny tears in the blood vessels in their neck. The study found that people who had such strokes were six times more likely to have received cervical manipulation within the past 30 days, suggesting the adjustment led to the tears which, in turn, resulted in the strokes. While the risks are relatively low, avoid chiropractic if you have osteoporosis, rheumatoid arthritis, or signs of nerve damage such as tingling or numbness down your arms.

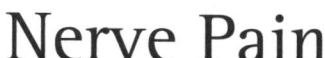

Nerve Pain

Stabbing. Burning. Shooting. This is how people describe nerve pain. The nerve could be damaged and no longer functioning properly, or stuck in the "on" position, continually firing pain signals to the brain even when there's no underlying cause of pain. Culprits include shingles (see page 209), Lyme disease (see page 240), and various autoimmune disorders.

Damage to the peripheral nerves, which link your brain and spinal cord to the rest of your body, is an all-too-common complication of diabetes, especially in people who've had the disease for many years. This nerve damage occurs because not enough blood gets to the feet and legs. It may cause pain or tingling, usually in the feet or lower legs, and could eventually lead to dangerous numbness. Closely controlling your blood sugar will go a long way toward preventing it.

Nerve pain can be difficult to treat. But an integrative approach that includes natural treatments as well as medications your doctor may prescribe should help.

Our Best Advice

We don't have a quick fix for nerve pain, but over time, these steps should bring relief.

1. Add 10 drops geranium, chamomile, or St. John's wort essential oil to 1 ounce massage oil and gently rub into the painful area twice a day.

2. Wait at least an hour, then rub a topical cream containing 0.25% or 0.75% capsaicin, like Zostrix, into the painful area. Repeat four times a day for several weeks until the pain recedes. It will take a couple of weeks before this cream begins to relieve your pain; once the pain recedes, gradually reduce the amount of cream you're using until you reach the minimum amount that still helps.

3. Begin taking 200 milligrams a day of alpha-lipoic acid, gradually increasing the dose until you notice some benefit, up to 800 milligrams a day.

4. Begin taking a daily B50 or B100 supplement. Follow the dosage instructions on the label.

Why It Works

Geranium and chamomile oils fight inflammation. St. John's wort is traditionally used to soothe nerve pain, although we're not sure exactly how it works.

You may need to use capsaicin cream for a few weeks before it reaches its full benefit, but it's a very effective treatment for nerve pain. It works by depleting chemicals that facilitate the transmission of pain signals from the nerve to the brain. The cream will probably cause a bit of tingling or burning the first couple of weeks; after a few weeks, that will disappear. One study found capsaicin worked just as well as a tricyclic antidepressant, often prescribed for nerve pain, with fewer side effects, while other studies find it significantly improves symptoms compared to placebo.

Alpha-lipoic acid is a powerful antioxidant produced by the body. Supplements are approved for the treatment of diabetic neuropathy in Germany. It works by improving blood flow to the nerves, as well as improving nerve function by preventing free-radical damage, which you read about in Part 2. One recent review of 15 clinical trials on short-term treatment with alpha-lipoic

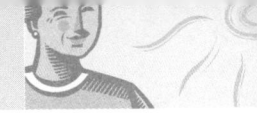

acid concluded it could reduce neuropathy symptoms. Although those studies used an injectable form of the supplement that's not available in the United States, other studies using oral doses of 600 to 1,200 milligrams a day find similar benefits.

Finally, while the B vitamins won't immediately reduce your pain, they do play a large role in nerve health, particularly vitamin B$_{12}$, which is why we recommend the daily supplement.

Other Medicines
Herbs and Supplements

Gotu kola. This herb, a mainstay of Ayurvedic medicine, is known for its ability to revitalize nerve and brain cells, as well as help maintain the health of blood vessels. In one study, participants who took 1 gram of the herb twice a day for six months reported improved symptoms.

Evening primrose oil. This plant oil is a superior source of gamma linolenic acid (GLA), found in the covering of nerve cells and nerve membranes. Besides helping to protect nerves, it also fights inflammation (it's converted in the body to anti-inflammatory substances). Some studies on people with mild to moderate diabetic neuropathy find daily supplements can significantly improve nerve function. Take 1,500 to 3,000 milligrams daily. GLA is also found in black currant and borage oil.

Over-the-Counter Drugs

Pain relievers. All the common over-the-counter pain relievers such as acetaminophen (Tylenol), ibuprofen (Motrin), aspirin, and naproxen (Aleve) can help. They're often prescribed in conjunction with other therapies.

Prescription Drugs

Antiseizure medications. These drugs, including Tegretol (carbamazepine), Neurontin (gabapentin), and Lyrica (pregabalin), work by interfering with pain signals to the brain. Side effects include dizziness and fatigue, although newer drugs, like Lyrica (the only one in its class approved specifically for diabetic neuropathy), may have fewer side effects.

Antidepressants. As we've said elsewhere, antidepressants aren't just for treating depression. Some of them, particularly tricyclic antidepressants like Elavil (amitriptyline), are also used in chronic pain conditions. They work fairly well as pain relievers in some people, although they may not work at all in others. Side effects may include fatigue, weight gain, dry mouth, and headaches.

Clonidine patch. Clonidine is a blood pressure drug that works by controlling nerve impulses along certain nerve pathways. When used as a patch over the painful area, it seeps into the skin to directly affect the problematic nerves, short-circuiting pain signals.

Lidocaine patch. This patch is impregnated with the anesthetic lidocaine. It blocks pain, but it doesn't reverse the cause of the pain.

Other Approaches

Acupuncture. Acupuncture can help ease many types of chronic pain, including nerve pain. A study in 44 people with diabetic neuropathy found 77 percent significantly improved after six acupuncture treatments over 10 weeks. During the next 4 to 12 months, 67 percent were able to stop or significantly reduce the amount of pain medication they were taking. We recommend a treatment trial of 20 sessions over 10 weeks.

Dietary changes. Limit your consumption of alcohol, which depletes vitamin B$_{12}$, critical to nerve health, and caffeine, which may increase your perception of pain. If you're willing, try a vegetarian diet or a vegan diet (which cuts out eggs and milk products as well as meat). One published report suggests that such a diet, coupled with daily walking, may improve peripheral neuropathy in people with diabetes by thinning the blood and making it less likely to clot, thus improving circulation.

Thermal biofeedback. This form of biofeedback teaches you to raise your skin temperature, which means increased blood flow. Studies in people with diabetes find the increased blood flow helps heal leg ulcers, which could also stem nerve damage.

Percutaneous electrical nerve stimulation (PENS). In PENS, needles deliver tiny electric shocks through your skin to the nerve, blocking transmission of more serious pain signals. One study in people with diabetic neuropathy compared PENS to a sham treatment and found it improved pain in the legs, as well as sleep quality and overall sense of well-being. Participants also used less pain medication.

Prevention

Control your blood sugar levels if you have diabetes. See page 276 for more on this, and also review our advice in Part 2 for combating Super Threat #3, insulin resistance—a major risk factor for diabetes.

Take 200 to 400 milligrams magnesium daily if you have diabetes. People with diabetic neuropathy often have low blood levels of this mineral, and studies find that supplements can help with blood sugar management. You may need higher doses, but only take those doses under your doctor's supervision.

Sign up for yoga classes. One study compared 20 people with diabetes who took yoga every day for 40 days to 20 people with diabetes who did light physical exercises like walking. It found that nerve function improved in the yoga group even as it deteriorated in the control group.

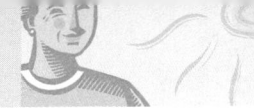

Osteoarthritis

Most people will have some degree of osteoarthritis by the time they hit 70. What causes it? It's not just the simple wear and tear of daily living. The condition stems from microscopic damage in the structure and makeup of cartilage, the soft, slippery tissue that covers the ends of bones in a joint. This damage may be triggered in part, or exacerbated by, oxidation (Super Threat #2 from Part 2 of this book) by free radicals. The damage impairs the ability of cartilage cells to repair and maintain cartilage.

When cartilage is healthy, your bones glide smoothly over one another, the cartilage acting as a kind of shock absorber. But with osteoarthritis, that surface layer of cartilage has worn down, allowing the bones to rub together. The result? Pain, swelling, and loss of motion. Over time, bone spurs called osteophytes might grow on the edges of the joint, and bits of bone or cartilage can even break off and float inside the joint space, increasing the pain.

Inflammation isn't a major player in the development of the disease (unlike in rheumatoid arthritis), but it can contribute to the pain, so many of our Best Remedies are aimed at reducing it.

Do This Now

When your arthritis pain flares, follow this advice for relief.

1. Take 700 to 1,000 milligrams Tylenol and 200 milligrams Aleve three times a day.

2. Begin taking 1,500 milligrams a day of glucosamine, either at one time or in three divided doses. It also comes in a powdered formulation.

3. Massage a sports cream like Ben Gay or a natural product like Tiger Balm or White Flower oil (available at health food stores) into the sore area.

4. If joint stiffness is the main problem, wet a thin towel with very warm water, wring it out, and apply to the affected joint, then cover with plastic wrap and lay a hot water bottle or heating pad atop the wrap for added effect. If the joint seems swollen, however, apply an ice pack instead of heat.

5. Head to your local pool for a gentle water workout.

Why It Works

A large review of numerous studies on the use of acetaminophen (Tylenol) and nonsteroidal anti-inflammatories (like Aleve) for osteoarthritis concluded that while the NSAIDs were slightly better at relieving pain, the acetaminophen did a better a job at restoring function. We recommend taking both during an acute attack (not long term) to get both benefits.

Glucosamine is the most important, noninvasive treatment that is available for osteoarthritis. It provides an important building block for

TIME TO WORRY

If your joint becomes red, hot, swollen, and significantly more painful, see your doctor to make sure you haven't developed gout (in which uric acid crystals collect in the joint, causing inflammation) or an infection.

substances required to maintain and grow healthy cartilage. There is some evidence that it can not only preserve joint function but also reduce the destruction of cartilage. In fact, it is the only oral treatment, conventional or alternative, found to actually alter the course of the disease. Commercial glucosamine is made from shellfish products, so don't use it if you're allergic to shellfish. Give glucosamine up to four weeks to begin working,

The salves we recommend contain aromatic oils that dilate blood vessels and speed the removal of toxins. They also create a sensation of heat or coolness depending on the oil used, which distracts you from the underlying pain. Some of the salves also contain topical pain relievers or muscle relaxants.

Wet heat is wonderful for relaxing the muscle around the joint and bringing more blood to the area. Heat tends to change the perception of pain in the joint (making it hurt less), while the moisture helps the heat penetrate more deeply. The ice numbs the pain by reducing swelling and increasing your pain threshold (so it takes more pain before you feel it). As little as 20 minutes of ice massage five days a week will significantly increase function, according to studies.

Studies find that any type of aerobic and/or resistance exercise improves the pain and disability of osteoarthritis as well as slows the progression of the disease. Exercise helps strengthen muscles, thus taking some load off joints, and increases flexibility, thus reducing strain on joints. It also helps you maintain a healthy weight.

We recommend pool exercises, which many YMCAs and health clubs offer specifically for people with arthritis, because they're gentle on the joints while still giving you and your muscles a workout. One study of 106 people with osteoarthritis of the hip and/or knee found those who exercised in the pool two hours a week for one year significantly improved their physical function and reduced their pain compared to a placebo group. Talk to your doctor before beginning any exercise program.

Other Medicines
Herbs and Supplements

Willow bark extract. Aspirin was first derived from this bark, and the extract is often used as an alternative to aspirin and similar pain relievers in Europe. A handful of studies in people with knee and hip osteoarthritis found it reduced pain much more than a placebo did, although not nearly as well as a prescription drug did. However, unlike most NSAIDs, willow bark is gentle on the stomach and doesn't interfere with blood clotting. The pill form is sold under the name Asalixx, available online at www.bionoricausa.com or by calling 800-264-2325. Give it time to work; it could take up to six weeks before you see its full benefits.

Devil's claw. This bitter-tasting African herb is often used to reduce inflammation.

A study that compared devil's claw to a prescription anti-inflammatory found similar benefits between the two, with fewer side effects from the supplement. Take 2.6 grams a day of an

✍ What About...

Chondroitin?

Glucosamine is often sold packaged together with chondroitin, another substance that contributes to the construction of cartilage. However, there's little evidence that the two together work much better than glucosamine alone—and the combo pills typically cost more. Also, because chondroitin is made from the trachea of animals, there's a tiny risk that prions (small particles that cause mad cow disease) could be transferred into the supplement.

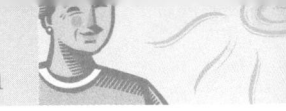

extract standardized to 3% iridoid glycosides in divided dosages.

Boswellia. This traditional Ayurvedic herb has strong anti-inflammatory properties, and thus works well for arthritis pain. In one study involving 30 people with osteoarthritis of the knee, those who took the herb had less pain and greater range of movement and could walk farther than those who took a placebo.

Antioxidants. Because a growing body of evidence links osteoarthritis to damage from oxidation, we recommend supplementing daily with antioxidants to help prevent further damage. Take a supplement that contains 250 milligrams vitamin C, 400 IU or less vitamin E, 2,500 IU beta-carotene, 200 micrograms selenium, and 15 to 25 milligrams zinc. You can add a separate vitamin C supplement for a total of 1,500 milligrams vitamin C supplement daily in divided doses (no more than 500 milligrams at a time).

SAMe (S-adenosyl-L-methionine). This supplement, often used for mild depression, turns out to be very beneficial for osteoarthritis. Studies comparing it to two different NSAIDs found it worked just as well at relieving pain after a month, with fewer side effects. We're not quite sure how it works, but it may play a role in cartilage development. Take 600 to 800 milligrams along with a B50 complex vitamin to increase the amount of SAMe your body absorbs.

Over-the-Counter Drugs

Capsaicin cream. Sold as Zostrix, this cream comes in two strengths, 0.025% and 0.075%. It works by depleting a chemical known as substance P that contributes to pain perception. You need to apply the cream several times a day, and it may take several days before you feel relief. Start with the lower dose, watch out for skin irritation (this stuff has the same ingredients as hot peppers), and wash your hands well after applying it. Some researchers are now experimenting with injecting capsaicin into the joint itself; a single injection has been found to reduce pain for up to two weeks.

Other Approaches

Weight loss. Losing weight is, without a doubt, the best thing you can do to reduce the pain and disability from osteoarthritis (and reduce your risk of developing the disease). Even losing just 5 percent of your body weight can help.

Anti-inflammatory diet. Even though inflammation doesn't contribute to the disease directly, it does contribute to the pain. Following the anti-inflammatory diet described on page 42 can not only help reduce inflammation but also increase your levels of antioxidants and the B vitamin folate, both of which may slow the progression of osteoarthritis, some studies suggest.

Medical equipment. Using a cane or crutches, or putting special inserts in your shoes, can improve shock absorption and take pressure off an arthritic knee or hip.

Acupuncture. There's good evidence for acupuncture's benefits in treating osteoarthritis. In one well-designed study published in a major medical journal, people who received acupuncture 23 times over 26 weeks had significantly less pain and better function than those who received sham treatments.

The Arthritis Self-Management Program. This is a program available through hospitals and local Arthritis Foundation chapters that teaches you how to manage your disease. One study found that after four years in the program, participants had far less pain, made fewer visits to the doctor, and spent fewer days in the hospital than those who weren't in the program.

Surgery. The most common surgical procedures involve cleaning out and/or repairing existing cartilage (arthroscopy) or replacing the entire joint (arthroplasty). They're pretty good at improving function and reducing pain, but, over time, may need to be repeated. However, if your cartilage is completely gone, and bone pain has made it hard for you to exercise or enjoy daily life, then surgery is a good option.

Prescription Drugs

Nonsteroidal anti-inflammatory drugs (NSAIDs). Even though one category of NSAIDs, the COX-2 inhibitors (which included Vioxx), has nearly disappeared from the market, there are dozens of other prescription NSAIDs that work just as well. And despite some marketing claims that the COX-2s were easier on the stomach than other pain relievers, the evidence for that claim is weak. So talk to your doctor about some of the older prescription NSAIDs, like Voltaren, Daypro (oxaprozin), Relafen (nabumetone), Lodine (etodolac), and Indocin (indomethacin).

Steroid or anesthetic injections. With this treatment, the drug is injected directly into the joint. It's only recommended in the case of severe pain and only for the short term, because long-term use can damage the joint. Plus, it's

✲ Helpful Hint

Make Your Pain Reliever Work Better

If you're taking NSAIDs (such as aspirin or ibuprofen) for arthritis pain, try also taking the herb nettle. One study found that adding 50 grams of stewed nettle leaf a day to 50 milligrams of the prescription NSAID Voltaren (diclofenac) provided the same pain relief as taking 85 milligrams of the drug (75 percent more).

dangerous to numb a joint—if you can't feel pain, you could hurt yourself and not know it.

Magnets. One of the few placebo-controlled studies to evaluate the use of magnets on arthritis involved 194 people with osteoarthritis of the hip or knee. Participants wore either a strong magnetic bracelet, a weak magnetic bracelet, or a dummy bracelet for 12 weeks. Those with the magnets (strong or weak) had less pain.

Physical therapy. Physical therapy ranges from the use of ice and heat to exercises designed to improve your joint function and range of movement. You'll need a doctor's prescription and should be prepared to commit several hours a week. Different forms of physical therapy affect different types of arthritis in different ways. For instance, one study found manual therapy (a hands-on approach that includes stretching, therapeutic massage, and joint movement) worked better for people with osteoarthritis of the hip than exercise therapy.

Prevention

Maintain a normal weight. If you're overweight, you can significantly cut your risk of arthritis by slimming down.

Get enough vitamin C. We only have studies in animals to go on, but it appears that maintaining a high vitamin C intake may reduce your risk of developing osteoarthritis. Ideally, get your vitamin C from your diet, in citrus fruits, red and green peppers (sweet or hot), spinach, broccoli, and other fruits and vegetables.

Keep moving. Just as exercise helps reduce osteoarthritic pain and disability by strengthening the muscles around the joint, it can help prevent joint breakdown by keeping muscles strong and taking some of the stress off the joints.

PART 4

Integrative Cancer Care

A New Way to Treat Cancer Patients

"When you receive a diagnosis of cancer, the rug is ripped out from underneath you—the whole foundation for your life is turned upside down," says Cynthia Medeiros, L.S.W., administrative director of the Zakim Center for Integrated Therapies at Dana-Farber Cancer Institute in Boston. "You want—and need—to regain a sense of control, and not just be sliced open or lie down for radiation or passively receive chemotherapy drugs."

The battle against cancer can produce devastating side effects. Doctors fight this ravaging disease with an equally ravaging arsenal of treatments—chemotherapy, radiation, and surgery. And they're often effective. "Cancer treatments are better than ever—the cure rate for cancer is up to 64 percent," says Barrie Cassileth, Ph.D., chief of the Integrative Medicine Service at Memorial Sloan-Kettering Cancer Center in New York City. But the collateral damage can include fatigue, pain, insomnia, nausea, an inability to eat, weakened immunity, low energy, depression, fear, and anxiety.

Once, doctors sent cancer patients home (perhaps with a few drug prescriptions) to deal with it on their own. But the story is changing. Cutting-edge cancer centers across the United States are treating mind, body, and spirit with an array of integrative therapies such as acupuncture, massage, guided imagery, yoga, and art therapy. "These techniques don't cure cancer," says Lorenzo Cohen, Ph.D., director of the Integrative Medicine Program at the University of Texas M. D. Anderson Cancer Center in Houston. But they do help cancer patients stay stronger and healthier during and after treatment. "A more well-balanced body may even respond better to cancer treatment," says Cohen.

In addition, some doctors are beginning to recommend herbs such as ginger to help blunt side effects of chemotherapy. And many other herbs and supplements are being studied for their potential ability to help fight the cancer itself—more on these later.

Integrative Cancer Care Arrives

Until recently, mainstream medicine dismissed *all* unconventional healing techniques for cancer as bogus, dangerous, even fraudulent. And yes, there are still plenty of unscrupulous manufacturers selling worthless cures to desperate patients who don't respond to conventional cancer treatments or don't like the idea of chemotherapy poisons going into their body.

But at the same time, herbs and supplements are being aggressively studied by researchers at the top cancer research institutes in the world because some of them have proved quite promising in preliminary research. For the most part, these substances are not being thought of as cures for cancer, but rather as adjunct therapies to decrease the side effects of conventional cancer treatment or increase the effectiveness (sometimes by reversing the tumor's resistance to chemotherapy). In a few very select cases, they may also slow the rate of progression of disease. You'll read more about some of these substances in the next chapter, but most of them are still experimental, not yet ready for "prime time."

As the research continues at a furious pace into herbs and supplements, other complementary approaches, such as acupuncture and relaxation therapies, are already changing "the cancer experience" for many cancer patients. Surveys in the 1990s showed that over half of all cancer patients were using at least one complementary therapy on their own, a revelation that alarmed some doctors and woke up others. After positive research results on some of these therapies starting pouring in, forward-looking doctors began advocating for integrative cancer care—places where people with cancer could receive safe, effective nurturing therapies alongside heavy-duty cancer treatments.

Today they exist in about a dozen university and medical-center-based integrative cancer centers (see the resources section at the back of the book for a listing), where you can walk down the hall from your oncologist's office to visit the acupuncturist or yoga instructor, and where the menu of

*Cutting-edge cancer centers across the United States are **treating mind, body, and spirit** with an array of integrative therapies.*

add-on services may include sessions with a trained art or music therapist, classes in the traditional Chinese exercise method called qi gong, or lessons in relaxation therapy or meditation.

At the Stanford Cancer Center in Stanford, California, for example, patients can choose from a large menu of integrative therapies, including restorative yoga, guided imagery, and qi gong. At the M. D. Anderson Cancer Center, on-staff massage therapists visit patients in their rooms. At Memorial Sloan-Kettering, pharmacists trained in herbal medicine and other supplements will help evaluate supplements a cancer patient wants to take after treatment.

Finding Integrative Cancer Treatment

In truth, the revolution in cancer care is just beginning. If you happen to live near, or can travel to, one of the nation's integrative cancer centers, you'll find integrative care under one roof, with a doctor or staff members coordinating it. But many oncologists and cancer centers in the United States still do not offer or recommend integrative therapies, simply because they're not very familiar with them. That doesn't cut off your access to these therapies. In this chapter you'll learn about the techniques that can help you or a loved one at any stage in the cancer journey, whether you've just received a diagnosis, are in treatment, or are a cancer survivor, and how to find the right therapy and practitioner for you.

There are plenty of remedies we won't discuss in this chapter, including those that have been dismissed by cancer experts as ineffective or dangerous, and those in the "gray area" because not enough is known about their safety or effectiveness yet. There's plenty of disagreement in the world of oncology about some of these "gray area" therapies, especially in the realms of nutrition, megadose antioxidants, and other supplements. Doctors in cancer clinics not affiliated with major medical schools may recommend them to their patients. But for now, we suggest you avoid them, or at least approach them cautiously. (And always let your oncologist know what you're taking.)

To put together your own integrative cancer care, then, we recommend the following:

Start with your oncologist. "Tell your doctor you want to be treated in a holistic manner," Medeiros says. "See what she can recommend— at this point, doctors are reading about integrative medicine in medical journals and may know more than you realize. She may be able to recommend specific practitioners, or be willing to work with a practitioner you find." Also ask your oncologist or family doctor if she will review all the medications you take to look for potential interactions with supplements you might like to try.

Use your local hospital's resources. "It's absolutely true that most oncologists don't talk about diet and nutrition and supplements," Cassileth says. "There's no way they can be on top of all these fields. But most institutions have dietitians on staff who can help you set up a healthy eating plan."

Contact a national comprehensive or clinical cancer care center. There are 60 of these centers across the United States, one in reach of everyone in the country. Designated by the

Therapies for Cancer-Related Problems

Which therapies can best address your symptoms? Consult our symptom-solver chart, and then turn to the next chapter for details.

Symptom	Treatment
Anxiety, fear, and worry	Creative therapies, meditation, massage
Depression	Massage
Despair	Creative therapies
Dry mouth after radiation therapy	Acupuncture
Fatigue	Acupuncture, exercise, qi gong, massage
Hiccuping caused by radiation therapy	Acupuncture
Hot flashes	Acupuncture
Insomnia	Creative therapies, exercise, yoga, qi gong, massage
Lymphedema	Manual lymph drainage massage
Mouth and throat inflammation	Acupuncture
Nausea and vomiting	Acupuncture, ginger
Pain	Acupuncture, guided imagery, relaxation exercises/meditation, hypnosis
Stress relief	Exercise, yoga, qi gong, meditation, aromatherapy
Comfort for caregivers	Massage, creative therapies

National Cancer Institute (NCI), they offer well-trained staff and a wide variety of resources. You may find advice on locating integrative therapy practitioners, classes, or help designing a diet or evaluating a potential supplement. (Turn to the resource guide for a link to a list of centers.)

Go online. Use the resource guide in this book to find reputable, science-based info online about therapies you'd like to try. Several cancer centers, including Memorial Sloan-Kettering and M. D. Anderson, offer extensive databases packed with information about the safety, usefulness, and potential dangers of dozens of complementary and alternative therapies, foods, and supplements.

Track down expert practitioners. Not just any massage therapist or acupuncturist will do after a cancer diagnosis. Massage in the wrong place, or at the wrong pressure, for instance, could damage skin or threaten bones if you have certain types of cancer or have undergone certain therapies. Inverted yoga positions, where your head is lower than your heart, could pose a potential danger for anyone with brain cancer. And some supplements can interact with medications you're taking. You need someone who's aware of your medical needs and can communicate with your doctor about what to do and what not to do. The resource guide of this book contains contact information to help you find qualified practitioners.

The Integrative Approaches

Nutrition

After the last radiation session, the final round of chemotherapy, or the end of surgery, cancer survivors turn to Sally Scroggs, a registered dietitian at the M. D. Anderson Cancer Center, with one question: "What's going to keep cancer away?"

"They want to know what to eat to protect themselves from a recurrence or an entirely new cancer," says Scroggs. But pinpointing the best post-cancer eating strategy can be tricky. Nutrition researchers are still sorting out the intricate ways in which nutrients in our diets protect against cancer.

At major integrative cancer centers, where food is considered a crucial part of cancer recovery and survivorship, dietitians balance science, safety, and common sense. "I take an 'It might help and it won't hurt' approach," Scroggs says. "We base a lot of our advice on eating patterns shown to prevent cancer in the first place—these strategies could help lower your risk for recurrence, though we need to learn much more about that. I feel confident about this approach because we know the same type of diet also lowers your risk for other health issues that cancer survivors, and anyone else, could encounter over the years such as heart disease and diabetes."

During treatment and recovery, work with a dietitian to eat healthy foods that will keep your body well fueled during the rigors of chemo or radiation. (Your during-treatment eating plan should be individually tailored.) Once you've recovered, aim for lots of vegetables and fruit, more whole grains, fewer refined carbohydrates, a limit on saturated fat (hello, low-fat milk, so-long marbled steak), and an emphasis on "good" fats such as olive and canola oils as well as foods rich in omega-3 fatty acids such as salmon, flaxseed, and walnuts.

What about special "cancer diets"? Consider a middle ground. "No diet can cure cancer. But rather than telling people to avoid diets like macrobiotics after cancer therapy, I like to talk about common themes all healthy diets share," says dietitian Donald Garrity, R.D., C.D.N., a nutrition counselor in the Integrative Medicine Service at the Memorial Sloan-Kettering Cancer Center. "A plant-based diet low in animal fats and refined carbohydrates is the smartest choice. Most of the people I've worked with who've adopted a healthier diet after cancer report that they just feel better."

Eating Strategies for Cancer Patients

No one food can cure cancer, but the right approach to eating can help you live better during and after cancer treatment.

In Search of Cancer-Fighting Foods

Certain foods may offer some protection from cancer or help the body cope with cancer treatments. Here are five to watch.

Green tea

In test tube studies, a powerful compound in green tea called epigallocatechin-3-gallate (EGCG) blocks many processes involved with cancer development and growth. Population studies suggest it may protect against several cancers, including those of the esophagus, stomach, prostate, and breast. Some research has found no benefit for people with cancer. But one Chinese study on women with a certain type of ovarian cancer found that those who drank the most green tea after their diagnosis had higher survival rates than those who drank the least. More research is under way, so stay tuned. Meanwhile, go ahead and drink 2 to 4 cups a day if you enjoy the light flavor of this delicate tea, which is also rich in antioxidants.

Turmeric

Curcumin, the antioxidant that gives this spice its brilliant golden tint, seems to dampen inflammation, protect DNA from damage, and possibly even stop tumors from growing blood vessels. Turmeric protected lab animals against some cancers, but human studies haven't been as convincing. Until we know more, sprinkle away, especially when cooking Indian and Asian dishes. In amounts called for in recipes, it can't hurt, and might help.

Garlic

Garlic supplements are being studied for their potential to help prevent and possibly even slow the growth of certain cancers. Population studies suggest that garlic may help prevent stomach and colorectal cancers. Eating garlic certainly can't hurt, and garlic supplements, possibly combined with small doses of the mineral selenium, might prove useful. Research is ongoing.

Soy

Packed with plant estrogens called isoflavones, this Asian food staple has been shown to lower the risk of breast and endometrial cancers in most population studies. Yet some experts worry that soy's weak estrogens could raise risk of hormone-sensitive cancers (for example, breast, ovarian, and endometrial/uterine). We don't recommend supplements of isoflavones. But for most people, a few helpings of soy per week are perfectly fine. If you have estrogen-receptor positive breast cancer, have no more than 50 milligrams to 85 milligrams of isoflavones a day.

Ginger

This herb, already popular for treating morning sickness and motion sickness, is being studied for delayed nausea and vomiting associated with chemotherapy, a common side effect of cancer treatment and one that can make it difficult to eat. Ginger is thought to affect receptors in the digestive tract for the neurotransmitter serotonin—similar to how antinausea drugs work.

Fill your plate with fruits, veggies, and whole grains. Nutrition experts say that eating at least five servings (one serving is a half-cup of cooked veggies, one cup of raw veggies or chopped fruit, or a medium-sized piece of whole fruit) of produce daily could decrease overall cancer risk by up to 20 percent. Fiber, minerals, vitamins, and plant chemicals (such as antioxidants) in these foods may help prevent the development and growth of various cancers.

Reserve two-thirds of your plate for produce, grains, and beans, one third or less for animal proteins. To get as many beneficial plant chemicals as possible, aim for a rainbow of colors—red tomatoes, orange squash, blueberries, and black raspberries, etc. For convenience, stock up on canned or frozen fruit and veggies, canned beans (rinse thoroughly to remove sodium), quick-cooking versions of brown rice, and plain oatmeal.

Cut back on fat. Eating lean—by getting only 15 percent of your daily calories from fat—cut risk of cancer recurrence by up to 42 percent for women with a common form of breast cancer, according to a recent study of 2,500 breast cancer survivors. Women in the study lowered their fat intake by making simple switches, such as eating plain popcorn instead of potato chips and breakfast cereal instead of a sweet roll.

Since eating less fat can help everyone control weight, a lean diet is recommended by the American Institute for Cancer Research for all cancer survivors. Another smart idea: Switch from foods rich in saturated fats, such as cheese and fatty meats, to those rich in "good" (unsaturated) fats, such as fish, flaxseed, avocados, and nuts. (Talk with your doctor about fish oil capsules too.) And replace cooking oils high in omega-6 fatty acids, such as safflower, corn, and sunflower oils, with olive and canola oil, which are high in omega-3 fatty acids (you may recall reading about these anti-inflammatory fatty acids in Part 2). Lab studies suggest that omega-3s could slow tumor growth.

Eating at least five servings of produce daily could *decrease overall cancer risk* by up to 20 percent.

In studies, cutting fat protected women with estrogen-receptor negative breast cancer, the type that will ultimately affect one in three postmenopausal women according to the American Cancer Society. Other research shows that cutting back on red meat could cut the risk of colon cancer by up to 70 percent.

Eat in moderation. Being overweight may decrease your odds of survival after breast cancer according to University of California-San Diego scientists. And a huge American Cancer Society study of 900,000 cancer patients found that death rates were 52 percent higher for the heaviest men and 62 percent higher for the heaviest women, compared to mortality rates for normal-weight people. We also know that being overweight appears to increase the risk for developing certain cancers—including postmenopausal breast cancer as well as cancers of the colon, pancreas, uterus, prostate, kidney, and ovary.

Once you've recovered from cancer therapy, use smart food choices, portion control, and moderate exercise to control your weight—and if needed, slowly nudge it toward a healthier range.

Shun refined carbohydrates. You might remember from Part 2, especially the chapter on Super Threat #3, insulin resistance, that eating foods high in refined carbohydrates, like sugar and white flour, can raise your blood sugar and insulin levels. In turn, high insulin levels could raise your risk for a quick recurrence of breast cancer, say researchers from Mount Sinai Hospital in Toronto. They may also set the stage for prostate cancer. Researchers have a hunch that insulin acts like a growth factor; too much might stimulate the growth of tumors.

Lower your blood insulin levels by controlling your weight (especially belly fat), exercising regularly, and eating a diet low in refined carbohydrates. That means choosing oatmeal and fresh fruit instead of pancakes and syrup, whole-wheat bread instead of white bread, and water or unsweetened tea or coffee in place of sodas and sweetened soft drinks. (This strategy may also make it easier to lose weight.)

Grill cautiously. Cooking meat, poultry, and fish at very high temperatures, especially over an open flame, can promote the formation of cancer-promoting compounds.

These techniques can make grilling safer: Add lemon juice or vinegar to meat marinades, remove all visible fat from meats before cooking, flip meats frequently during grilling, put foil on the grill and cook on that, grill vegetables (or veggie burgers) instead of meat, and microwave or bake meat until it's almost done, then finish it on the grill for a smoky flavor.

Herbs, Vitamins, and Other Supplements

We've already hinted about the research under way into supplements that could help tame the side effects of conventional cancer treatments or even make those treatments work better. Researchers at the National Cancer Institute and elsewhere are looking for ways to appropriately use these substances—and in some cases doctors are already using them. For instance, some doctors recommend that men with prostate cancer, which is sometimes treated with a "watchful waiting" approach, take lycopene, the antioxidant abundant in tomatoes that has been shown to reduce the risk of the cancer. Other substances are still under more preliminary investigation.

For example, coenzyme Q_{10}, a substance found in the body that has generated excitement for its heart benefits, is now being examined as a possible therapy for preventing heart problems related to chemotherapy. A natural substance called PSK, already popular in Japan, is being studied as a way to increase survival rates in chemotherapy patients. And herbs such as ginseng are being studied for their potential ability to bolster the body's resilience and possibly inhibit tumor growth.

That doesn't necessarily mean you should go out and stock up on any of these at the drugstore. While some of these herbs may work for people who don't have cancer, they haven't yet been studied in big, controlled research projects for cancer patients. Five or ten years from now, oncologists may recommend some of them as part of conventional cancer therapy. But for now, they're still experimental. In studies, some supplements may have actually increased risk to patients. If you do decide to try any supplement when you have cancer, we strongly advise you to work with an integrative cancer physician, who can give you expert guidance for your particular situation based on the most recent research available.

And we should mention here that we don't recommend that you use any natural product instead of conventional cancer treatment. Again, most of the herbs and supplements being studied by legitimate researchers are intended as *adjunct* therapies—to *improve* cancer treatment, not replace it.

If the supplements we mentioned aren't ready for "prime time," what about multivitamins, antioxidants, and supplements extracted from everyday foods such as green tea, garlic, and fish oil capsules? Surely these could only help?

Maybe, maybe not. Over half of all cancer patients take supplements in hopes of boosting immunity, battling cancer side effects, or warding off recurrence. And while many supplements show cancer-fighting promise in test tube studies, we're not sure yet which ones work in people, or in what doses. Remember that cancers take decades to develop; substances that might protect you by stopping the disease at its earliest stages, such as by protecting cells against genetic damage, probably can't work their magic once the disease is full-blown.

Some vitamin and food-based supplements do show promise. We told you about the benefits of lycopene for prostate cancer a minute ago. In addition, vitamin E may help protect nerves from damage caused by certain chemotherapy drugs (see "Antioxidants and Cancer," below). Probiotics, or "friendly bacteria," may help to prevent infections in cancer patients with low white blood cell counts. A component of green tea has been studied in test tubes for reducing cancer cells' resistance to chemotherapy drugs; in another test tube study, the green tea compound EGCG was

Antioxidants and Cancer

Antioxidants—the cell-protecting compounds that give fruits and veggies their vibrant colors and flavors—seem like they'd help against cancer. As you read in Part 2, where we talked about oxidative stress as Super Threat #2, these substances disarm free radicals, the rogue molecules that can damage your DNA and contribute to cancer's development.

The story's anything but simple, though. In fact, antioxidants are at the center of one of the hottest debates in oncology. While as many as 60 percent of cancer patients may be taking antioxidants such as vitamins A, C, E, and selenium during treatment, most cancer doctors warn that this practice could actually make cancer treatments less effective. That's essentially because the antioxidants may protect the cancer cells as well as the healthy ones from the toxic effects of chemotherapy and radiation.

Some alternative-minded physicians, however, believe that supplementing with the right doses of the right antioxidant supplements at the right time may enhance the effects of cancer treatments, or decrease the side effects, at least in certain cancer patients, and researchers are conducting studies to find out more.

In one study, patients experienced less neurotoxicity (nerve tissue poisoning) when they received supplements of vitamin E along with chemotherapy drugs. In another study, vitamin E helped reduce the risk of mucositis (mouth inflammation) in patients undergoing radiation for head and neck cancer.

Studies are being conducted to investigate which antioxidants, at which doses, could help. For now, no one has definitive answers. If you feel strongly about taking antioxidant supplements during cancer treatment, discuss the issue frankly with your doctor. And proceed with caution. In one breast cancer study, megadoses of antioxidants actually reduced survival rates.

If you're looking to antioxidants to help you *prevent* cancer, look to food, especially fruits and vegetables. Men may want to get extra selenium, since research suggests that getting 200 micrograms a day from all sources (food sources include Brazil nuts, seafood, oats, and wheat germ) can lower prostate cancer risk. This is more of the mineral than you'll get in your multivitamin, so the American Cancer Society recommends using a selenium-fortified brewer's yeast, sold in health food stores.

Certainly don't go overboard on taking antioxidant supplements; several studies show that high-dose antioxidant supplements might actually raise your risk.

shown to inhibit the growth of oral cancer cells; and in a third study, green tea extracts in the form of capsules or ointments helped heal precancerous cervical lesions.

But not enough is known yet about the effects of herbs and antioxidants during cancer therapies such as chemotherapy and radiation. It's possible they could make the therapies less effective, says K. Simon Yeung, R.Ph., Lac., research pharmacist and manager of the herb/drug information center at the Memorial Sloan-Kettering Cancer Center. For instance, at certain dosages some herbs may speed up or slow down the speed at which the body metabolizes drugs, raise blood pressure, or increase the time it takes blood to clot.

Using Supplements Wisely

If you're diagnosed with cancer, we recommend that you:

Start with your oncologist, not the health food store. Never delay oncology appointments in order to give supplements a try first. Putting off conventional cancer care only gives the disease time to grow and spread, closing an important window of opportunity for early, effective treatment.

Tell your doctor about everything you're taking. Make a list or, better yet, toss all vitamins, minerals, herbs, and other supplements you take (plus prescription drugs and over-the-counter remedies) into a bag to take to your next appointment. Then follow your doctor's advice for what to stop, what to continue, and what you can resume after treatment.

Use foods to help prevent a recurrence. Fruits, veggies, whole grains, and healthy fats deliver thousands of micronutrients that work together to promote good health—something no pill can do. Research consistently shows that foods are a more effective source of potentially cancer-fighting nutrients than supplements. Of course,

salads and brown rice may not be very appealing or easy to eat in the weeks or months after radiation or chemotherapy. Talk with your doctor about the best supplement strategy for times when you can't manage to eat as well as you should.

After treatment, seek out personalized supplement advice. If you're determined to add herbs or other supplements to your healing regimen, talk first with your oncologist and family doctor. If they cannot make recommendations (conventional physicians often aren't trained very extensively in the use of supplements), schedule an appointment with a physician trained in natural medicine. Don't just wander into the health food store or shop online for stuff that sounds good. The best choices for you will depend entirely on your health status, your diet, and the type of cancer you had. And don't go overboard. We suggest taking no more than five to six different supplements, including a multivitamin.

Stay alert for side effects. Like drugs and other remedies, herbs and supplements can cause unexpected reactions. Gastrointestinal complaints are usually the earliest symptoms reported. If you have a negative reaction to a supplement, stop taking it and tell your doctor.

Acupuncture

In the high-tech hush of a Manhattan medical laboratory, 21st-century researchers are discovering that this ancient healing art can offer new hope for cancer patients.

"What we're learning about acupuncture is very striking," says Barrie Cassileth of Memorial Sloan-Kettering, where a handful of acupuncture studies are under way. "Cancer patients experience problems such as chronic pain, fatigue, extreme dry mouth, and even hot flashes, that can't be effectively and completely treated in other ways. Acupuncture has benefits that are extremely important."

Acupuncture is the practice of piercing specific points on the body with disposable hair-thin needles (the process is nearly painless) to unblock "energy," called qi or chi (pronounced "chee") and ease discomfort or pain. Most treatments require the shallow insertion of needles in 10 or 12 points on the body, face or ears, though over 1,000 acupuncture points are recognized. Needles may be twirled or heated; mild electrical stimulation may be added; or the needles may be replaced entirely by laser beams or sound waves.

While acupuncture cannot cure cancer, it shows great promise for relieving side effects caused by the disease and by chemotherapy, radiation, and surgery, especially when pain relievers, antinausea drugs, and other medicines fall short or fail. Cutting-edge integrative cancer centers now have acupuncturists on staff. And the federal government is spending millions of dollars to fund studies looking at how, and why, it works.

One clue: "It's not magic," Cassileth says. "It's not what people used to think three thousand years ago. Functional MRI studies of people's brains during acupuncture show that it works through the nervous system to stimulate the release of beneficial hormones such as endorphins." Acupuncture and its cousin, acupressure (which uses hand pressure, not needles), may also trigger the release of chemicals called opioids that control pain and improve blood flow.

How It Can Help

There's still more to learn, but the results are clear: This ancient healing art can help cancer patients in a variety of ways.

More pain relief. Up to half of all cancer patients in treatment and up to 90 percent of those with advanced cancers endure chronic pain, often the result of damage to nerves, organs, bone, or skin by the cancer itself or by cancer

While it cannot cure cancer, *acupuncture shows great promise* for relieving side effects caused by the disease and by chemotherapy, radiation, and surgery.

treatments. Sometimes painkillers aren't enough, or they produce side effects from drowsiness to dizziness to nausea that are difficult to live with. In those cases, integrative medicine experts recommend adding acupuncture.

When French anesthesiologists inserted tiny needles at key points on the ears of people with advanced cancer, cancer-related pain decreased by 36 percent, and the relief lasted for at least two months. Researchers used tiny, thumbtack-like needles that are left in place for weeks at a time, a practice now under study in the United States

Pain in cancers of the head, neck, and lungs can also been eased by acupuncture. "Lung cancer surgery can produce pain that's about as bad as it gets—it cuts through nerves and bone," Cassileth says. "This pain can go on for many years if it's not well controlled early. Acupuncture, along with pain medications, seems to control it."

Best strategy: Use acupuncture for intractable pain or breakthrough pain not completely relieved by medications such as NSAIDS and narcotics. If you're bothered by pain-pill side effects, adding acupuncture may allow you to lower your dose.

Less nausea and vomiting. Until recently, severe stomach upset was commonplace during and after chemotherapy. Today new antinausea drugs have put a lid on this dreaded side effect. But if they don't provide sufficient relief, consider electroacupuncture, mild electrical stimulation of key acupuncture points.

National Institutes of Health researchers recently reported that among women who underwent high-dose, multiple-drug chemotherapy for breast cancer, those who received antinausea medicines plus daily electroacupuncture for five days had less vomiting than those who only took anti-emetic drugs. Electroacupuncture may also relieve stomach reactions to general anesthesia for breast cancer surgery—and do it more effectively than antinausea drugs, suggests a Duke University study.

Fewer hot flashes after breast and prostate cancer treatment. Seventy-five percent of men undergoing hormone-deprivation therapy for prostate cancer and 66 percent of women who've survived breast cancer live with moderate to severe hot flashes, the result of hormonal changes that knock the body's thermostat out of whack. In one small study, acupuncture chilled hot flashes by 50 to 70 percent for men with prostate cancer. Studies under way at Memorial Sloan-Kettering suggest this technique works for both prostate and breast cancer.

Less fatigue. Stubborn exhaustion, the type that leaves you so tired it's tough to hold a job, maintain a friendship, or be the kind of spouse or parent you want to be, is a frustrating fact of life for many people with cancer. If your doctor has ruled out anemia, she may suggest rest, exercise, caffeine, or even an energy-boosting prescription drug. To this list, we would add acupuncture.

Studies show that regular acupuncture sessions (either twice a week for a month or once a week for 6 weeks) cut fatigue levels 31 percent for cancer patients who'd undergone chemotherapy. The researchers suspect that activating key acupuncture points normalizes levels of serotonin, a feel-good brain chemical often out of balance in people with cancer and in people with chronic fatigue syndrome.

What You Should Know

ABOUT ACUPUNCTURE

- **Expect significant relief** of your symptoms within six visits (often, symptoms ease after one to two). Sessions can last 20 minutes to 1 hour. Most treatments require 6 to 10 sessions.

- **Be ready to pay out-of-pocket.** Costs can vary from $50 to over $100 per session and only about half of American HMOs and conventional insurance plans cover acupuncture and acupressure. Some insurance plans offer discounts if you use pre-approved practitioners—but be careful, many are not trained to work with cancer patients. Medical spending accounts, offered by many employers and funded with your own pretax dollars, usually reimburse for acupuncture treatment.

- **Acupuncture is generally safe,** in the hands of trained practitioners. European and Japanese reviews show that less than 2 in 1,000 patients had an adverse side effect such as bleeding, dizziness, pain, or infection.

- **Talk with your oncologist before signing up for acupuncture.** Due to the slight risk for infection and bleeding, some experts advise against it if you're receiving a heavy dose of chemotherapy, a bone marrow transplant, or flap reconstruction (such as after mastectomy), if you have a low white blood cell count (neutropenia) or low blood platelets (thrombocytopenia), or if you already have a fever, infection, or a tendency to bleed heavily. If you have lymphedema (a swelling of the arms or legs) after cancer treatment, do not have acupuncture performed on that limb.

- **Make sure your acupuncturist cleans your skin** with Betadine or alcohol before starting and always uses sterile needles.

More saliva production. Radiation beamed at cancer cells in the mouth, head, or neck can damage the salivary glands, drying up production of the saliva that helps you taste and swallow food, keep your teeth clean, and moisturize your mouth. The result: a burning, painful mouth, tooth decay, and difficulty eating.

When 50 cancer patients with xerostomia received acupuncture treatments, 70 percent reported that their symptoms improved. Eight needles (three in each ear and one in the middle finger of each hand) were used. Sessions lasted a half-hour to an hour. Participants had an average of five sessions; for some, relief lasted for more than a month after acupuncture ended. The researchers, from the Naval Medical Center in San Diego and the University of California-San Diego, suggest three to four weekly treatments, then monthly treatments after that for best results.

Less mouth inflammation and hiccuping. Scientists are also discovering that acupuncture can relieve the pain of mucositis, an inflammation of the lining of the mouth and throat caused by high-dose chemotherapy. It also seems to relieve hiccuping caused by radiation.

Finding a Qualified Practitioner

State-of-the-art integrative cancer centers such as Memorial Sloan-Kettering and the M.D. Anderson Cancer Center have on-staff acupuncturists. If you're not being treated at one of these centers, ask your oncologist if she works with a certified acupuncturist or can recommend one. The best ways to find a trained acupuncturist on your own is to contact the National Certification Commission for Acupuncture and Oriental Medicine. You can also locate physicians trained to perform acupuncture by contacting the American Academy of Medical Acupuncture. (For contact information, see the resource guide starting on page 361.)

Your acupuncturist should have experience working with cancer patients. Bring treatment notes from your doctor to your first session, and ask the practitioner to contact your doctor before inserting any needles.

Creative Therapies

A man with leukemia swirls a brush in paint and begins to recount a long and difficult cancer journey. "I'll never forget this man," says Karen Hammelef, R.N., M.S., director of patient support services of the University of Michigan Comprehensive Cancer Center. "He was an accountant, a very concrete thinker. But after his diagnosis, he asked for watercolors and illustrated everything that happened to him—his hospital room, the treatments, even the bathroom. Art kept him going and helped him find meaning."

Creative therapies—art, music, expressive writing, even dance—help people with cancer (and their families) express hidden emotions, ease stress, fear, and anxiety, and sometimes, simply provide a much needed distraction during cancer therapy. Available at many integrative cancer centers, this approach is especially good at helping people with cancer uncover difficult feelings, thoughts, or memories related to the cancer experience, stuff they may have been pushing aside in order to get through a tough time. Some research suggests that

Creative therapies—art, music, expressive writing, even dance—help people with cancer *express hidden emotions,* ease stress, fear, and anxiety, and provide distraction.

these techniques may have physical benefits as well, including better sleep and less pain.

What counts are your emotions, not the painting, the poem, or the song you ultimately produce. "It's never about the final product," Hammelef says. "What's important is the process, because that's when you learn what it is you're feeling. And if you're working with a trained creative-arts therapist, such as an art therapist or music therapist with a background in mental health and psychotherapy, you'll get support and learn how to understand and cope with profound feelings."

How It Can Help

During and after cancer treatment, creative therapies can help restore health to mind and body.

Better sleep. Writing about deep feelings helped 21 people with advanced kidney cancer sleep longer and more soundly, report researchers at the M. D. Anderson Cancer Center. In contrast, another 21 people with the same cancer who wrote about good health habits got no benefits.

Less despair. People with cancers of the blood who were hospitalized for stem cell transplants felt significantly less depressed if they also participated in music therapy, say researchers at Memorial Sloan-Kettering Cancer Center.

Acceptance of enormous changes. Women with recurrent breast cancer who wrote letters to their own bodies moved more easily through the process of grief and acceptance of a new body image after breast reconstruction, report nurses at the Arthur G. James Cancer Hospital in Columbus, Ohio.

A quiet way to think about big questions. Art therapy offers a private, nonverbal way to deal with strong emotions and thoughts about life and death, Memorial Sloan-Kettering researchers say.

Distraction during treatment. Keeping your mind and hands busy by making something—a

poem, a sculpture, a crayon drawing—can break through worry and fear during chemotherapy and radiation. "Anxiety alone can make you feel nauseated before treatment," Hammelef says. "Art therapy can keep you busy, so you don't create associations between feeling sick and seeing a certain room or person or piece of equipment. You feel better, and are less likely to have an anxious reaction the next time."

Greater physical well-being. Dance therapy may increase levels of the feel-good brain chemicals called endorphins. Art therapy may alter brain waves so you feel more relaxed. Music therapy can slow down your heartbeat and breathing.

Exercise and Movement

On a glorious summer day in 2003, cancer surgeon Carolyn Kaelin, M.D., then 42, noticed a slight puckering of the skin on her right breast. Scans soon revealed that Kaelin, a mother of two and director of the Comprehensive Breast Health Center at Brigham and Women's Hospital in Boston, Massachusetts, had, of all things, breast cancer.

Early in her treatment—a drawn-out regimen that ultimately included five surgeries, a mastectomy, chemotherapy, and breast reconstruction—she cycled 75 miles of the Pan-Mass Challenge, a popular Massachusetts bike ride that raises funds for cancer research. And throughout her therapy, she made it a point to hit the gym despite fatigue, stress, and worry, she recounts in her book *Living Through Breast Cancer.* "It's the one thing that I can do for myself that I know is beneficial," Kaelin told an interviewer a year after her diagnosis.

Once, oncologists advised cancer patients to go home and take it easy after surgery, radiation, and/or chemotherapy. But that's old thinking. A compelling body of research now demonstrates that staying active can help relieve fatigue and anxiety, lift pain and nausea, boost energy, preserve muscle strength and flexibility, protect bones, make it easier to perform day-to-day activities and work outside the home, and support healthy self-esteem. You can reap benefits at any activity level, whether you're biking up mountain roads like prostate cancer survivor Lance Armstrong did during his cancer recovery or simply walking up and down your driveway.

"Cancer treatments can go on for many months, maybe years," says Kerry S. Cournyea, Ph.D., one of the authors of the American Cancer Society's physical activity guidelines and a professor of physical education at the University of Alberta in Edmonton, Canada. "And if you stop being physically active, the amount of de-conditioning and muscle wasting that goes on is phenomenal. You get into this cycle of not feeling well and remaining inactive that's hard to break out of."

And yet it's quite likely your doctor hasn't encouraged you to get out and get moving. In one recent Duke University Medical Center survey of 281 Canadian oncologists, just 43 percent said they recommend exercise to patients they feel are able to be physically active. If yours hasn't, we suggest setting up your own safe, gentle routine.

Finding the Right Type of Exercise

"There are many forms of movement and exercise that can really benefit people with cancer," says Lorenzo Cohen of the M. D. Anderson Cancer Center. "And that's good, because one person might not enjoy yoga or walking with a group of people, but may prefer a Pilates class or resistance training with light weights. And depending on the type of cancer you have, you may not be able to do certain types."

Talk with your doctor to find out what types and intensity of exercise are okay for you. Among the movement and exercise "styles" available at top academic integrative cancer centers (and that you can probably find in your own community):

Traditional phys ed, at a gentler pace. This involves stretching, light aerobic activities, and strength training with light weights, elastic bands, or your own body weight for resistance.

Yoga. For cancer patients, the best bets are easygoing yoga styles such as restorative yoga (quiet, restful poses that nurture the body by releasing tension) and gentle hatha yoga. "If you put your body in the right position, your physical response for relaxation is stimulated," notes certified yoga instructor Jane Verdurmen Peart, C.Y.T., who leads a restorative yoga class at the Stanford Cancer Center. "People come to my yoga class who are recovering from surgery or who are in the midst of chemotherapy and they look tired. Their complexions are pale, almost gray. They leave the class with rosy cheeks and a smile." According to Peart, restorative yoga is especially helpful after cancer surgery involving the abdomen or chest, which leads to muscle weakness and scar tissue that contracts your muscles, prompting you to hunch over to protect yourself. "Gentle yoga can enhance flexibility, improve range of motion, and counteract that contraction."

Qi gong (pronounced "chee gung"). This is a series of flowing, dancelike movements that combine breathing, meditation, and specific postures to strengthen your life force, or qi. In the hands of a trained qi gong instructor, these moves can be modified for people who are bedridden or who must remain seated, says medical qi gong expert Arnold Tayam, D.M.Q., who teaches a 12-week qi gong class at the Stanford Cancer Center's Supportive Care Program. "Qi gong is a way of remembering your own wholeness," Tayam says. "It allows people to bring themselves back to a state of balance."

What You Should Know

ABOUT EXERCISE AND MOVEMENT THERAPIES

General Exercise

• **Don't exercise if your blood counts are low** and you are at risk for infection, anemia, and bleeding, or if the level of minerals in your blood, such as sodium and potassium, is not normal. This can happen if you have had a lot of vomiting or diarrhea. Also check with your doctor first if you're receiving treatments that affect your lungs (such as bleomycin or radiation to the chest) or your heart (such as doxorubicin, epirubicin, or Cerubidine) or if you're at risk for lung or heart disease or have high blood pressure.

• **If you're in cancer therapy, ask the hospital physical therapists to help you design a gentle program** that includes low-intensity aerobic activity (such as walking) and resistance moves to maintain muscle strength and bone density.

• **Stick with a mild- to moderate-intensity routine** unless your physician okays a more intense program. If you can only be active for short periods, start with 5 to 10 minutes of walking or chair exercises one to three times a day.

• **To avoid injury, don't exercise on uneven surfaces or with heavy weights** that could make you fall or hurt yourself. If you have cancer in your bones, it may not be appropriate to do weight-bearing balancing exercises.

Qi Gong

• **Sessions can last from 15 minutes** to an hour or more.

• **You can learn gentle qi gong moves from a book or video,** but it's smart to have a few sessions with a qi gong master who can guide you safely through the routines.

• **If you have balance problems, definitely work with a teacher**—and ask about moves and breathing techniques that can be performed sitting down or while leaning against a wall for support.

Yoga

• **Practicing several times a week for 10 to 30 minutes is recommended,** but even once-a-week sessions can be helpful.

• **Avoid strenuous yoga styles,** such as Bikram or Ashtanga yoga, during and after cancer treatment.

• **You can find a class at a local hospital, gym, or through an adult-education program** in your community. Start slowly and gently—learning with a certified instructor will help keep your practice safe and effective. Look for someone who's worked in a hospital setting who will understand your needs.

How It Can Help

During and after a battle with cancer, exercise is powerful medicine. It offers:

A sense of well-being and better sleep. In an informal survey among cancer patients at Stanford who took Tayam's 12-week qi gong class, 94 percent said their general well-being was enhanced, 79 percent reported less stress, 56 percent had more energy, and 43 percent said sleep improved. Yoga helps too. An M. D. Anderson study of Tibetan yoga, a form that emphasizes controlled breathing and visualization, found that it eased sleep disturbances. "This form of yoga may be particularly useful for patients undergoing and recovering from chemotherapy," says Cohen.

Stronger immunity. Natural killer cell activity increased for 52 breast cancer survivors who rode exercise bikes three times a week for 15 weeks in a University of Alberta study.

Bone density protection. Men who receive androgen-deprivation therapy for prostate cancer and premenopausal women who use chemotherapy and tamoxifen for breast cancer are at risk for thinning bones and debilitating fractures. Weight-bearing exercise can help maintain bone density (though you may also need a bone-protecting medication).

Easier recovery from bone marrow transplant. Fitness and physical well-being improved, while fatigue dropped for 17 bone marrow transplant recipients who worked out at home for 20 to 40 minutes a day, 3 to 5 days a week in a 12-week-long study from the University of South Florida College of Medicine. Study volunteers had finished treatment six months earlier, and received careful instructions before beginning their routines.

Less fatigue during radiation therapy. Moderate-intensity walking during four weeks of radiation therapy kept energy levels steady for 33 men with prostate cancer in a recent Scottish study; a control group of 33 prostate cancer patients who didn't exercise during their treatment weeks had a tougher time. "Men who followed advice to rest and take things easy if they became fatigued demonstrated a slight deterioration in physical functioning and a significant increase in fatigue at the end of radiotherapy," the researchers report.

More energy. Fatigue is one of the top reasons cancer patients don't get more physical activity, University of Alberta scientists say. But not exercising just leads to more fatigue, as well as weight gain. Worried exercise will make you feel more tired? A British review of 33 studies of exercise for cancer patients found that fatigue decreased with activity.

Better long-term health. When researchers at the University of Southern California checked back with 374 breast cancer survivors an average of 13 years after their diagnosis, those who were exercising regularly scored highest for all-round physical health.

Researchers aren't certain exercise can reduce risk of cancer recurrence. But exercise does help control weight—and maintaining a healthy weight may cut the risk of recurrence for some forms of cancer. Exercise can also keep insulin levels lower and healthier. That's good news for breast cancer survivors, since early evidence suggests that high insulin levels increase recurrence risk and lower survival odds.

Exercise also guards against America's top killer, heart disease. And since many people who survive cancer ultimately die from cardiovascular disease, this is no small deal.

Massage and Bodywork

The most soothing and spa-like of all complementary cancer care services, massage was until recently considered off-limits for cancer patients due to unfounded fears that it could spread malignant cells. Today it's a mainstay at integrative cancer centers, where massage therapists trained to work with cancer patients provide everything from full-body rubdowns to simple foot and hand massages. In fact, massage for cancer survivors has become an official spa treatment. At the Elizabeth Arden Red Door Salon & Spa in New York City, breast cancer survivors can be pampered and soothed with a massage designed especially for women who've undergone breast surgery.

Available in many hospitals, or privately through licensed practitioners, massage brings pleasure and a sense of reconnection with your own body, as well as much needed relaxation and relief from worry, pain, nausea, and depression. For breast cancer patients, a type of massage called manual lymph drainage—gentle, rhythmic, pumping techniques usually performed by a physical therapist—can even reduce painful swelling in the arms.

After Memorial Sloan-Kettering Cancer Center researchers conducted the nation's largest, longest-running study of massage, their report was very enthusiastic: "Massage therapy appears to be an uncommonly noninvasive and inexpensive means of symptom control." In reviewing the benefits of 1,290 massages given to cancer patients over three years, the researchers found that anxiety fell 52 percent, pain dropped 40 percent, fatigue eased 41 percent, depression lifted 31 percent, and nausea lessened 21 percent.

Types of Massage and Bodywork

Among the types of bodywork offered at major integrative cancer centers:

Light-touch massage. Massage therapy during the weeks or months you're undergoing cancer treatment, or in the recovery phase after treatment ends, must be very gentle, of course. Trained therapists recommend a mix of light-

> ## The Art and Science of Scent
>
> Relaxing lavender. Invigorating lemon and peppermint. Scent has a powerful effect on our emotions and our stress and energy levels. It can even help distract our minds from pain. That's why aromatherapy—the therapeutic use of fragrant natural plant oils—can potentially help cancer patients. Scents can even change the hospital environment for the patient, making it seem less, well, hospital-like.
>
> Aromatherapy oils may be wafted through the room via an infuser (a device like a small humidifier), added to a warm bath or foot soak, or even added to massage oil. But a few cautions are in order. Strong odors can be challenging if patients are nauseated, so start with diluted oils. Essential oils may be toxic if ingested, so only use them externally. And if you have asthma, talk with your doctor before using essential oils.

touch massage and light Swedish massage. Some may also use techniques from Oriental, shiatsu, and/or Thai massage. "Deep-tissue massage and anything that could bruise or damage skin should be avoided," says Curtiss Beinhorn, a massage therapist at the M. D. Anderson Cancer Center's Place ... of Wellness.

During massage, blood vessels dilate, boosting the flow of oxygenated blood to nerves and muscles. Muscles relax. The circulation of lymph increases. Some massage therapists believe that massage even stimulates greater blood flow to internal organs.

Reflexology. In reflexology, the foot is viewed as a "map" of the body. By applying pressure to specific areas of the foot, practitioners believe they can influence the flow of energy through the body. Others think this gentle technique simply works the way massage does—by loosening muscles and improving blood flow. It is especially appreciated by and appropriate for frail or very ill patients.

Reiki and therapeutic touch. Both of these "touch free" techniques involve using specific sweeping movements and hand positions to improve the flow of energy in the body. There's no physical contact during a session, and the recipient remains clothed. Advocates call these therapies "energy healing." Others, including the American Cancer Society, suggest that it's the simple presence of a concerned human being that provides the comfort. Research suggests that both techniques are very soothing.

Bodywork. Many centers offer bodywork classes to help people with cancer gain more flexibility, feel physically connected with their bodies, and improve their sense of wellness. Unlike massage, where you're the passive recipient, in bodywork classes you learn to use specific movements and positions. Two widely used styles are the Feldenkrais Method, which uses slow, gentle movements to improve body awareness, and the Alexander Technique, aimed at moving the head, neck, torso, and spine into proper alignment.

How It Can Help

"When you're diagnosed with cancer," says Beinhorn, "every level of your being seems to be under

"Massage is comforting and nurturing. *It brings you back to yourself—* and there are no needles, no catheters, no tubes. It's all good."

attack. You start associating your whole body with your tumor and you can forget who you are. All the focus is on the disease. Massage is comforting and nurturing. It brings you back to yourself—and there are no needles, no catheters, no tubes. It's all good." Some of its benefits:

Less depression and pain, more vigor. When women with breast cancer received massage three times a week for five weeks, they reported feeling happier, more energetic, and less angry. The massage focused on the head, arms, legs, feet, and back. In contrast, women in a no-massage control group felt more angry and depressed. In a University of Alberta study, cancer patients who received Reiki massage plus painkilling opioid drugs felt better than those who simply rested quietly after taking pain meds.

Relief from arm lymphedema. Manual lymph drainage reduced arm swelling and improved sleep in a French study of 31 breast cancer survivors.

Easier experiences with chemotherapy and radiation. A light Swedish massage three times a week improved sleep and eased discomfort for hospitalized cancer patients in one study.

A drop in anxiety. In a recent British survey of 35 cancer patients, therapeutic touch cut discomfort and tension and boosted relaxation.

Comfort for caregivers. Stress dropped and moods brightened when the spouses of people with cancer got a series of short back massages, report researchers from the Duquesne University School of Nursing in Pittsburgh. "Often patients will ask me to give their spouse a massage," Beinhorn notes. "It's comforting for them to see their caregiver being cared for too."

Finding a Qualified Practitioner

Use a licensed massage therapist. Check with your hospital or even better, the nearest NCI-designated cancer care center, for names. More and more massage therapists receive extra training in order to work with cancer patients (Memorial Sloan-Kettering and M. D. Anderson offer training programs). A cancer center may be able to refer you to one of these therapists.

Mind-Body Medicine

Imagine biting into a slice of fresh lemon—just *thinking* about its acidic tang probably made your mouth water. Now picture yourself receiving a neck massage; we bet your muscles relaxed. At their core, the techniques of mind-body medicine—including guided imagery, hypnosis, and meditation—are powered by the simple "change your mind, your body will follow" principle you just experienced.

Used since ancient times, mind-body medicine today is helping people with cancer better withstand physically demanding treatments, avoid nausea and vomiting, manage pain, enjoy deeper sleep, boost their immunity, and feel more connected with their bodies and inner selves despite the fears and stresses raised by a cancer diagnosis and treatment. (Benefits may go further too: Studies are under way to see if hypnosis reduces hot flashes for breast cancer patients.)

"The power of the human mind is amazing," says certified medical hypnotherapist Jeanne

Fournier, who teaches guided imagery workshops in the Stanford Cancer Center's Supportive Care Program. "The benefits I've seen include deep relaxation, an easier experience during chemotherapy, and just feeling more confident. There's a sense of empowerment, of being more open to the healing potential of strong cancer treatments with less fear about the side effects."

A sense of spirituality, regardless of whether or not you follow a particular religion, can bring *strength, hope, and courage* to your battle with cancer.

Mind-Body Techniques

One mind-body technique, the support group, has become such an accepted component of cancer care in hospitals across the United States that it's not even viewed as "alternative" anymore. Other mind-body therapies offered at major integrative cancer care centers include:

Guided imagery. Offered in classes, on audiotapes, and in one-on-one sessions with a guided imagery leader, this therapy uses visualization to create a sense of calm and overcome fears about cancer and cancer treatment. During a guided imagery session, you relax, close your eyes, and listen to a series of "suggestions" such as imagining yourself in a safe, comforting place or imagining your body responding well to cancer treatment. Guided imagery can help subdue anxiety before radiation or chemo. "We have very good antinausea drugs these days, but some people still experience anticipatory nausea before treatment," says Claire Casselman, M.S.W., who provides guided imagery as part of the complementary therapies program at the University of Michigan Comprehensive Cancer Center. "Imagery can also control pain so you need less medication. And some people listen to imagery tapes until just before surgery—and even have family members play tapes to them while they're in the recovery room. Others use guided imagery during potentially painful procedures such as bone marrow biopsies and bronchoscopy, an examination of the throat, larynx, and airways."

Hypnosis. Hypnosis can help ease anxiety and lessen pain. Research suggests that hypnosis may be even more effective than imagery for relieving pain in children with cancer.

Meditation. Meditation can provide deep relaxation that calms fears and eases anxieties at high-stress moments, such as before a procedure or treatment. Once you've learned how to do it, you can meditate anywhere, anytime. Meditation often involves breathing calmly and using one of several techniques, such as paying close attention to your breath or silently repeating a calming word or phrase, to quiet the mind.

How It Can Help

Today integrative-medicine researchers at the nation's major research centers are grappling with one of the mysteries of mind-body therapies: Many seem to improve immunity, though for very brief periods of time—as little as a few seconds. So far, there's no evidence that this can prolong life or directly battle cancer, though one intriguing Ohio State University study suggests that it could keep immunity stronger so that patients can stick with a chemotherapy treatment schedule.

What **You** Should Know

ABOUT MIND-BODY TECHNIQUES

• **Mind-body techniques are not a replacement for conventional cancer care.** Your thoughts and feelings cannot cause cancer—and your mind alone cannot conquer it. That said, taking care of your emotional health can improve your quality of life significantly.

• **For best results, practice relaxation, meditation, or listen to guided-imagery tapes** for a few minutes every day. "This is a tool just like pain medication," says Jeanne Fournier, a hypnotherapist at the Stanford Cancer Center. "You have to do it over and over again. And the more you do it, the better it works."

• **Mind-body techniques may not replace drugs for relieving side effects** such as pain, but they can help you lower the dose and therefore avoid a secondary problem: drug side effects.

• **All mind-body techniques work for someone.** Don't worry about which one is "best"—start with the one that appeals to you the most. If you don't like it, try another.

• **Start with a class or a few one-on-one sessions** with a teacher. "Individual help is more effective than a generic audiotape for getting started with guided imagery, meditation, and relaxation," Fournier says. "After that, tapes are great."

The real value of mind-body techniques? "They can help you cope and find meaning, change your outlook on yourself and the world and your relationships. In the long term, they can help you stay healthy for life," says Lorenzo Cohen of the M. D. Anderson Cancer Center.

Meditation for stress, anxiety, and anger. Stress levels dropped for 90 women with breast cancer and men with prostate cancer who took an eight-week mindfulness meditation class, report researchers at the University of Calgary. They got more—and better—sleep, exercised more frequently, and drank less caffeine. They also showed healthy changes in levels of stress hormones.

In a pilot study at the Dana-Farber Cancer Institute, mindfulness-based stress reduction helped 18 people undergoing stem cell/bone marrow transplantation to feel happier and calmer. Pain diminished, and their heart rates and breathing slowed to more relaxed levels.

Hypnosis for less nausea and pain. Hypnosis helped 54 children reduce nausea and vomiting before and after chemotherapy, report researchers from the University of California School of Medicine, Los Angeles. "Sometimes just anticipating chemotherapy makes children and adults feel very nauseated," Stanford hypnotherapist Fournier comments. "Hypnosis can really help." Hypnosis also reduced pain and anxiety before and after two invasive procedures: bone marrow aspiration and lumbar puncture.

Relaxation and guided imagery for pain reduction. Progressive muscle relaxation (described in Part 2 on page 61) and guided imagery eased cancer pain in studies from Seattle's Fred Hutchinson Cancer Research Center and the University of Sydney. Australian researchers speculate that the techniques may break the pain-muscle-tension-anxiety cycle, allowing mind and body to calm down.

Support groups for mental and physical healing. Women with breast cancer who attended weekly support group meetings for four months not only felt better, they also ate more nutritiously, smoked fewer cigarettes, and showed signs of stronger immunity that allowed them to receive higher doses of chemotherapy than women who didn't go to a group, Ohio State researchers reported.

PART 5

Resources

Integrative Medicine Centers

A Sampling of Integrative Medicine Centers by State

Here is a list of major integrative medicine centers in the United States. For more information you can also check the Web site of the Consortium of Academic Health Centers for Integrative Medicine at www.imconsortium.org/html/about.php.

Arizona

University of Arizona (Tucson)
Program in Integrative Medicine
www.integrativemedicine.arizona.edu

California

University of California, Irvine
Susan Samueli Center for Integrative Medicine
www.ucihs.uci.edu/com/samueli

University of California, Los Angeles
Collaborative Centers for Integrative Medicine
www.uclamindbody.org

University of California, San Francisco
Osher Center for Integrative Medicine
www.ucsf.edu/ocim

Connecticut

University of Connecticut (Farmington)
Health Center
health.uchc.edu/clinicalservices/integrativemed

District of Columbia

Georgetown University Medical Center
School of Medicine, Complementary and Alternative Medicine
www.georgetown.edu/schmed/cam

George Washington University
Center for Integrative Medicine
www.integrativemedicinedc.com

Hawaii

University of Hawaii at Manoa
Program in Integrative Medicine
www.uhm.hawaii.edu

Maryland

University of Maryland (Baltimore)
Center for Integrative Medicine
www.compmed.umm.edu

Massachusetts

Harvard Medical School (Boston)
Osher Institute
www.osher.hms.harvard.edu

University of Massachusetts (North Worcester)
Center for Mindfulness
www.umassmed.edu/cfm

Michigan

University of Michigan (Ann Arbor)
Integrative Medicine
www.med.umich.edu/umim

Minnesota

University of Minnesota (Minneapolis)
Center for Spirituality and Healing
www.csh.umn.edu

New Jersey

University of Medicine and Dentistry of New Jersey (Newark)
Institute for Complementary and Alternative Medicine
www.umdnj.edu/icam

New Mexico

University of New Mexico (Albuquerque)
Section of Integrative Medicine
hsc.unm.edu/medicine/integrative_med

New York

Albert Einstein College of Medicine of Yeshiva University (New York City)
Continuum Center for Health and Healing
www.healthandhealingny.org

Columbia University (New York City)
Richard and Hinda Rosenthal Center for Complementary and Alternative Medicine
www.rosenthal.hs.columbia.edu

North Carolina

Duke University (Durham)
Duke Center for Integrative Medicine
www.dcim.org

University of North Carolina-Chapel Hill School of Medicine
Program on Integrative Medicine
pim.med.unc.edu

Wake Forest University Baptist Medical Center (Winston-Salem)
Program for Holistic and Integrative Medicine
www1.wfubmc.edu/phim

Oregon

Oregon Health and Science University (Portland)
Oregon Center for Complementary and Alternative Medicine in Neurological Disorders
www.ohsu.edu/orccamind

Center for Women's Health, Integrative Medicine Program
www.ohsuwomenshealth.com/services/doctors/integrative.html

Pennsylvania

Thomas Jefferson University (Philadelphia)
Jefferson-Myrna Bird Center of Integrative Medicine
www.jeffersonhospital.org/cim

University of Pennsylvania (Philadelphia)
Complementary/Alternative Medicine, PENN-CAM
www.med.upenn.edu/penncam

University of Pittsburgh
Center for Integrative Medicine
integrativemedicine.upmc.com

Texas

University of Texas Medical Branch (Galveston)
UTMB Integrative Health Care
cam.utmb.edu

Washington

University of Washington (Seattle)
Department of Family Medicine
www.fammed.washington.edu/predoctoral/cam

Integrative Medicine Techniques

Acupuncture

The American Academy of Medical Acupuncture
Toll-free: 800-521-2262
www.medicalacupuncture.org
A professional association of medical doctors who practice acupuncture. You can obtain a referral list of doctors and get general information about acupuncture.

The American Association of Oriental Medicine
Toll-free: 866-455-7999
www.aaom.org
A nonprofit organization that will provide you with the state licensing status of acupuncture practitioners across the United States.

Acupuncture and Oriental Medicine Alliance
253-851-6896
www.acuall.org
A professional society of state-licensed, registered, and certified acupuncturists. It lists thousands of acupuncturists on its Web site and provides the list to people who call its information and referral line.

The National Certification Commission for Acupuncture and Oriental Medicine
703-548-9004
www.nccaom.org
Certifies highly trained acupuncturists with a diplomate in acupuncture. Diplomates are nationally board-certified in acupuncture. The Web site includes a locater service.

Aromatherapy

The National Association for Holistic Aromatherapy
509-325-3419
www.naha.org
A nonprofit organization dedicated to enhancing public awareness of the benefits of aromatherapy.

Biofeedback

Association for Applied Psychophysiology and Biofeedback
Toll-free: 800-477-8892
www.aapb.org
Certifies biofeedback therapists and provides information and education about the therapy.

Guided Imagery

The Academy for Guided Imagery
Toll-free: 800-726-2070
www.academyforguidedimagery.com
Use its locater service to find a practitioner. The AGI also offers audiotapes for coping with pain, relaxing, sleep, and general comforting.

Imagery International
www.imageryinternational.org
Imagery International has an online journal with interesting full-text articles. The site includes a directory of practitioners.

Herbs and Supplements

American Botanical Council
512-926-4900
www.herbalgram.org
A membership organization that publishes a journal as well as a number of reference texts on herbal medicine. Its home page has information including breaking news on herbs.

Bastyr University
425-823-1300
www.bastyr.edu/library/bibliographies/botmcore.htm
Bastyr University is one of the oldest naturopathic universities in the United States. This site contains references from its extensive library collection on herbs. The general university Web site (which you can access from here) has a great deal of information on health and wellness.

Consumer Lab
914-722-9149
www.consumerlab.com
This independent lab tests supplement brands—herbs, vitamins, minerals, and others—for quality, purity, and potency. Test results are published on its free-access Web site. Subscribers ($24/year) can read more details.

Food and Drug Administration Dietary Supplements
www.cfsan.fda.gov/~dms/ds-info.html
Provides general guidelines, warnings, and alerts about the safety of individual supplements.

Herb Research Foundation
303-449-2265
www.herbs.org/index.html
This foundation provides a search service from its specialty research library containing more than 300,000 scientific articles on thousands of herbs.

MedlinePlus-Herbal Medicine
www.nlm.nih.gov/medlineplus/herbalmedicine.html
An excellent consumer source for information on herbal therapies.

National Institutes of Health Office of Dietary Supplements
ods.od.nih.gov
Provides general supplement advice, fact sheets on botanicals, dietary supplements, and vitamins and minerals, plus access to databases on dietary supplement research, such as the International Bibliographic Information on Dietary Supplements database.

Homeopathy

American Institute of Homeopathy
Email: aih@homeopathyusa.org
www.homeopathy.org
A professional organization of licensed homeopaths. Includes a referral service.

National Center for Homeopathy
www.homeopathic.org
Provides general education to the public about homeopathy.

Supplement Buying Guide

You can buy most of the products mentioned in this book in natural food stores. But some products, especially those made in Europe, are harder to find. Below we've listed the manufacturers of some of these products. Contact the company by phone or log onto its Web site to find out how to purchase the supplement.

Bionorica
www.bionoricausa.com
800-264-2325
- Agnucaston/Cyclodynon (chaste tree berry)
- Asalixx (willow bark)
- Bronchipret
- Klimadynon (black cohosh)
- Sinupret

CV Technologies
www.cvtechnologies.com/coldfx/default.aspx
- Cold-fX (American ginseng)

Enzymatic Therapies
www.enzy.com
800-783-2286
- Iberogast
- Esberitox
- Remifemin (black cohosh)

Nature Made (Pharmavite)
www.naturemade.com
800-276-2878
- MoodPlus SAM-e
- TriMune

Nature's Way
www.naturesway.com
801-489-1500
- Ginkgold
- Sambucol (elderberry)

Pharmaton
www.pharmaton-sa.ch/ch_eng
- Venastat (horse chestnut)
- Ginsana (ginseng)

Phytopharmica
www.phytopharmica.com
800-376-7889
- Petadolex (butterbur)

Hypnotherapy

H.E.L.P. Hypnosis Exchange of Licensed Professionals
hypnosishelp.apmha.com
Here you can get referrals to doctors and therapists who use hypnosis.

The International Medical and Dental Hypnotherapy Association
Toll-free: 800-257-5467
www.imdha.com
An organization of health-care professionals trained in hypnotherapy; they use hypnosis to help reduce the stress of medical treatments.

Integrative Medicine

American Holistic Medicine Association
505-292-7788
www.holisticmedicine.org
The Web site includes a practice locator to help you find physicians with training in integrative medicine.

MedlinePlus-General CAM
www.nlm.nih.gov/medlineplus/alternativemedicine.html
Excellent source of authoritative consumer information on complementary and alternative medicine.

National Center for Complementary and Alternative Medicine
nccam.nih.gov
A wealth of information on complementary and alternative medicine from the National Institutes of Health.

Meditation

University of Massachusetts Medical School Center for Mindfulness
www.umassmed.edu/cfm/mbsr
Hundreds of hospitals across the United States offer classes to the public on mindfulness and stress reduction, as do psychologists and social workers trained in mindfulness. To find one nearby, type your ZIP code into the locater service on the Web site. The center also offers guided meditation tapes, including tapes for people with psoriasis and with cancer. Go to www.umassmed.edu/cfm/tapes/other.cfm.

Naturopathy

The American Association of Naturopathic Physicians
Toll-free: 866-538-2267
Local: 202-237-8150
E-mail: member.services@naturopathic.org
www.naturopathic.org
This organization represents naturopathic physicians nationally. Its referral service will help you find an N.D.

Movement and Bodywork

The American Chiropractic Association
Toll-free: 800-986-4636
www.amerchiro.org
Supports standards of professional competency and provides information to the public on chiropractic.

American Massage Therapy Association
Toll-free: 877-905-2700
www.amtamassage.org
Works to promote high professional standards and establish massage as integral to health maintenance.

The Qi Gong Institute
www.qigonginstitute.org
Extensive Web site includes a locater service for qi gong practitioners, a database of research, and more.

The Yoga Alliance
www.yogaalliance.org
Offers lists of yoga teachers who have met stringent registration requirements.

Nutrition

American Dietetic Association
Nutrition Information Line
Toll-free: 800-366-1655
www.eatright.org
Call ADA's Nutrition Information Line for a referral to a registered dietitian in your area.

Food and Nutrition Information Center National Agricultural Library
301-504-5719
www.nal.usda.gov/fnic
A wealth of information on food and nutrition topics.

Additional Resources for Cancer Patients

Herbs

Memorial Sloan-Kettering Cancer Center Information Resource: About Herbs, Botanicals, and Other Products
www.mskcc.org/aboutherbs
Offers consumer and scientific/clinical information about 190 herbs, supplements, and treatments. Updated regularly.

M. D. Anderson Cancer Center Complementary/Integrative Medicine Education Resources
www.mdanderson.org/departments/CIMER
This comprehensive database includes reviews of dietary supplements.

National Cancer Institute PDQ® Cancer Information Summaries
www.cancer.gov/cancertopics/pdq/cam
These are peer-reviewed summaries of cancer treatments and supplements, updated twice a year.

Creative Therapies

The National Coalition of Creative Arts Therapies Associations
www.nccata.org
This is an alliance of professional associations dedicated to the advancement of the arts as therapeutic modalities. NCCATA represents over 8,000 members of six creative arts therapies associations.

American Art Therapy Association
Toll-free: 888-290-0878
E-mail: info@arttherapy.org
www.arttherapy.org
This is a nonprofit organization devoted to promoting the therapeutic use of art. It represents more than 4,500 members.

American Dance Therapy Association
410-997-4040
www.adta.org
This organization works to establish and maintain high standards of professional education and competence in the field of dance/movement therapy.

American Music Therapy Association
301-589-3300
www.musictherapy.org
The mission of the AMTA is to advance public awareness of the benefits of music therapy and increase access to quality music therapy services in a rapidly changing world. The Web site offers information on how to find a music therapist.

Guided Imagery

Health Journeys
www.healthjourneys.com
Audiotapes and books by guided-imagery expert Belleruth Naparstek are available from this Web site. Tapes for cancer patients cover these topics and more: chemotherapy, radiation therapy, successful surgery, bone marrow and stem cell transplantation, chemo-related fatigue, and fighting cancer.

Imagery for Healing
www.imageryforhealing.com
Cancer support through healing imagery, run by guided-imagery practitioner Jeanne Fournier.

Integrative Cancer Care

American Cancer Society
www.cancer.org
Provides extensive reviews of complementary, alternative, and integrative therapies.

The National Cancer Institute Cancer Centers Program

www3.cancer.gov/cancercenters/centerslist.html
Provides contact information for the NCI's comprehensive and clinical cancer care centers—60 high-quality cancer-treatment centers that also perform extensive research.

The National Cancer Institute Office of Cancer Complementary and Alternative Medicine

www3.cancer.gov/occam
Coordinates the NCI's support of rigorous complementary and alternative medicine research. The Web site contains information on clinical trials.

Medline Plus-Cancer Alternative Therapies

www.nlm.nih.gov/medlineplus/canceralternativetherapies.html
Good general site that includes information from a number of government and other authoritative sites.

Annie Appleseed Project

annieappleseedproject.org
This nonprofit organization provides information, education, advocacy, and awareness for people with cancer interested in complementary and alternative medicine and natural therapies. Web site contains lots of useful information and links.

Association of Cancer Online Resources

acor.org
Offers information about treatment options, links for online support groups, and lists of clinical trials.

Cancer Links

cancerlinks.com
Online resources with links, including an integrative medicine section.

Nutrition

American Institute for Cancer Research

www.aicr.org
Web site offers science-based, down-to-earth advice on eating to prevent cancer. You can also call the AICR Nutrition Hotline, 800-843-8114, which is staffed by registered dietitians, from 9 a.m. to 5 p.m. EST, Monday through Friday.

Diana Dyer, M.S., R.D.

www.dianadyermsrd.com
Diana Dyer is a three-time cancer survivor and registered dietitian. Her Web site provides nutritional and general information of importance to cancer survivors.

Natural Medicine Cautions

Just because something is "natural" doesn't necessarily mean it's without risks. Herbs and other supplements are still drugs when it comes to their effects in your body; like any drug, they may have side effects and can interact with over-the-counter or prescription drugs, and even with other herbs and supplements. And techniques from acupuncture to aromatherapy, while generally safe, need to be used properly.

Supplement Cautions

Always tell all your doctors and other health-care practitioners about any herb or supplement you're taking, no matter how benign you think it is. And before adding a new medication, make sure you check with your doctor and/or pharmacist about possible interactions. If you're pregnant or breast-feeding, don't take any herbs or supplements without first talking to your doctor.

Here we've listed cautions for some of the most commonly recommended herbs and supplements in *Best Remedies*.

Acidophilus. May initially increase bloating or gassiness, which disappears after a week or two.

Arnica. Don't apply to broken or bleeding skin.

Black cohosh. May cause gastrointestinal discomfort.

Bromelain. May cause diarrhea. Don't take if you're allergic to pineapple. Rare instances of allergy may occur if you are also allergic to wheat, papain, and other plants.

L-carnitine. Doses above 2 grams may cause diarrhea. Note: Take only L-carnitine. Serious side effects have been reported for the combination of D- and L-carnitine.

Chamomile. Don't take if you're allergic to the plant. If you have a serious ragweed allergy, you may be allergic to this plant as well.

Chasteberry (chaste tree berry). May counteract the effectiveness of birth control pills.

Coenzyme Q$_{10}$. May cause mild gastrointestinal side effects. May decrease the effectiveness of the blood-thinning medication warfarin (Coumadin), although this is not certain.

Deglycyrrhizinated licorice (DGL). If you have high blood pressure or are taking corticosteroids, diuretics, or antiarrhythmia medication, make sure you use only this form of licorice.

Digestive enzymes, proteolytic enzymes. Mild allergic reactions may occur. Swallow enzymes quickly with enough water. Do not hold in mouth. Do not use if you have recently had surgery or have a bleeding problem.

Echinacea. Don't take if you have a chronic immune system disease or autoimmune disease for more than a few days. If you have serious ragweed allergy, you may be allergic to this herb.

Fish oil. Don't take more than 3,000 milligrams a day without checking with your doctor, because it could interfere with blood clotting. Don't take without your doctor's okay if you have blood-clotting disorder or are taking anticoagulants. Some preparations can have a fishy aftertaste. Large doses may cause loosening of the stool.

Flaxseed. May decrease absorption of some medications. Always take with water. Note that heating or cooking will destroy the omega-3 fatty acids in flaxseed oil and create harmful free radicals. Like most sources of fiber, flaxseed can cause bloating, flatulence, etc., if you take too much.

Ginger. Don't use the dried root or powder if you have gallstones. At higher doses, mild heartburn may occur. Use with caution if you're also taking antiplatelet drugs or you're having surgery.

Ginkgo. Consult your doctor before using this with MAO antidepressants, anticoagulants, aspirin or other nonsteroidal anti-inflammatory drugs (NSAIDs), or antiplatelet drugs. Stop this medication at least two weeks before surgery.

Ginseng, American. May affect blood sugar, so use with caution if you have diabetes.

Ginseng, Panax. Consult your doctor if you have a heart condition, high blood pressure, or an anxiety disorder before taking. May cause insomnia and rarely, with higher doses, increases in blood pressure, tachycardia, and agitation. May affect blood sugar, so use with caution if you have diabetes.

Horse chestnut. Theoretically, may interfere with the action of antiplatelet drugs, although problems have not been reported.

Magnesium. Don't take if you have kidney disease or are taking diuretics. May cause loose stools or diarrhea. Don't exceed 350 milligrams a day.

N-acetyl-cysteine (NAC). Can cause allergic reactions. Supplement may have unpleasant odor.

Probiotics. May increase gassiness or bloating at first, a sign the good bacteria are working. Symptoms should disappear within a week or two.

Psyllium. Take with at least 8 ounces of water. May cause bloating or constipation. Take only with your doctor's knowledge if you have any serious intestinal disorder such as Crohn's disease.

St. John's wort. May make you more sensitive to sun. Don't try to treat serious depression on your own; see your doctor. Don't start this medication if you are on other prescription drugs (especially for HIV, organ transplant, or heart disease) without checking with your pharmacist or doctor.

SAMe. May cause mild gastrointestinal symptoms (the most common side effect). In depressed patients, may cause an excessive elevation of mood (mania), although this has not been reported in studies. Take with a B vitamin supplement to improve effectiveness.

Valerian. Use with caution if you're also taking a prescription antianxiety medication such as Valium or Xanax.

Vitamin C. Daily doses over 2,000 milligrams may cause diarrhea. Never take more than 2,500 milligrams a day on your own, and don't take if you have kidney failure or are on dialysis without your doctor's okay. Use with caution if you have a history of kidney stones.

Vitamin E. Limit to 400 IU a day if using on your own, and check with your doctor before taking if you're also taking blood thinners.

Willow bark. Don't use if you're allergic to aspirin or are taking any blood-thinning medicine like warfarin (Coumadin).

Zinc. Do not exceed 30 milligrams a day. Higher doses may cause nausea and vomiting and suppress the immune system. Zinc may also interfere with copper absorption.

Other Cautions

Acupuncture. Make sure you find a qualified, licensed practitioner as described on page 32. Let the practitioner know about any medical conditions you have, or if you're pregnant. People on anticoagulant or antiplatelet drugs should talk to their doctor beforehand, since they may bleed easily despite the thinness of the needles. Electroacupuncture could cause problems for people with pacemakers.

Aromatherapy. Don't take essential oils internally, or use if you're pregnant. If you have a medical condition—especially asthma, sensitive skin, epilepsy, or high blood pressure—or you recently had surgery, seek advice from your doctor before using aromatherapy. Also, try a small amount on a patch of skin first to see if you have any allergic reaction. Only use highly diluted essential oils for babies and children. Never use peppermint oil on a child younger than 30 months. Store these oils in dark bottles, tightly sealed, in a cool, dark place.

Chiropractic. Make sure you find a licensed, qualified practitioner as described on page 32. If you have osteoarthritis of the neck, rheumatoid arthritis, or vascular disease, especially in the carotid arteries, seek advice from your doctor before using chiropractic. Also, tell your chiropractor about these or any other medical conditions. Certain kinds of adjustments would not be indicated with certain medical conditions.

Massage. Make sure you find a licensed, qualified practitioner as described on page 32. Be specific about the reason you're there, and ask for a recommendation on the type of massage that is best for your condition. If you have any health conditions, such as cancer, fibromyalgia, cancer, or herniated disk, or you're pregnant, talk to your doctor before getting a massage, and tell your massage therapist before the session. Avoid massage if you have a high fever, inflammation, an infection, phlebitis (inflammation of a vein), thrombosis (blood clot in a blood vessel), or jaundice. If you have had breast cancer with a lymph node dissection as part of your treatment, do not have massage on that arm.

Index

hemorrhoids, 232
high cholesterol, 285
insulin resistance, 50-51
obesity, 292
reproductive health ailments, 132,
  156, 162, 167
Fibrates, 286
Fibromyalgia, 323-326
Fish, 20, 42, 114, 141, 267
Fish oil. *See* Essential fatty acids
5-alpha reductase inhibitors, 159
5-HTP, 230, 237, 274, 325
Flatulence, 98-99
Flavonoids, 107, 213, 231. *See also
  specific flavonoids*
Flaxseed, flaxseed oil. *See* Essential
  fatty acids
Flomax, 158
Flower pollen, 159
Flu, 29, 86-87
Fluid retention, 265
Folic acid
  prescription drugs and, 191, 308
  as remedy, 115, 253, 282, 304
Follicle-stimulating hormone (FSH)
  drugs, 142-143
Food allergies, effects on
  ADHD, 261
  immune stress, 55, 57
  inflammatory bowel disease, 114
  rheumatoid arthritis, 308
  skin ailments, 200, 202
Food diaries, 67, 294
Free radicals, 37, 44-45, 58
Fried foods, 46, 56
Fruit juice, 226
FSH drugs, 142-143

G

Gallstones, 100-101
Gargles, 82-83, 254
Garlic
  effects on cancer, 343
  as remedy, 56, 81-82, 214-215, 279,
    285-286
Gastroesophageal reflux disease
  (GERD), 102-105
Geranium oil for
  anxiety, 216-217
  nerve pain, 330
  reproductive health ailments, 61,
    147, 154, 163
GERD, 102-105
Ginger
  contraindications for, 369-370

as remedy for
  bad breath, 168
  cancer patients, 343
  digestive and urinary complaints,
    93, 96, 100, 116-117, 120, 122
  migraines, 245
  muscle soreness, 249-250
  reproductive health ailments, 130,
    151-152, 154-155
  rheumatoid arthritis, 307
  sinusitis, 89
Ginkgo
  contraindications for, 187, 370
  as remedy for
    Alzheimer's disease, 256-257
    chronic fatigue syndrome, 321
    depression, 273
    eczema, 199
    eye diseases, 179, 182-183
    fibromyalgia, 325
    hemorrhoids, 231
    memory problems, 242-243
    peripheral vascular disease, 303
    reproductive health ailments, 134,
      149, 155
    tinnitus, 187
Ginseng
  cautions about, 370
  as remedy for
    chronic fatigue syndrome, 321
    fatigue, 223
    fibromyalgia, 324
    flu, 87
    HIV, 289
    memory problems, 243
    reproductive health ailments, 133-
      134, 144
Glaucoma, 178-179
Glucocorticoids, 307
Glucosamine, 255, 333-334
Glucose levels, testing, 50
Glutathione, 127, 179, 183, 299
GnRH agonists, 131, 143, 161-162
Goldenrod, 128
Goldenroot, 223
Goldenseal, 84
Gonadotropin-releasing hormones
  (GnRH agonists), 131, 143, 161-
  162
Gotu kola, 213, 331
Gout, 333
Graded exercise, 322
Grapefruit juice, 266
Grapefruit oil, 122, 154-155
Grapes, 269, 271

Grape seed extract, 89, 196
Gravel root, 120-121
"Green" products, 65
Greens, 42
Green supplements, 224-225,
  320-321
Green tea. *See* Tea
Guarana, 243
Guggul, 286
Guggulipid, 191
Guided imagery, 24, 232, 358-360,
  364, 367
Gum disease, 45, 180-181
Gymnema sylvestre, 277

H

Hand washing, 84, 87, 108, 172
Hangovers, 226-227
Harvey, William, 11
Hawthorn, 264-265, 269
H$_2$ blockers, 102, 105, 124-126,
  202
HCG, 143
Headaches, 29, 228-230. *See also*
  Migraines
Heartburn, 29, 102-105
Heart disease, 39, 44-45, 53, 256
Heat treatments. *See also* Castor oil
  packs
  contraindications for, 136
  as remedy for
    bruises, 194
    chronic pain, 310, 314, 327, 333-
      334
    ear infections, 175
    kidney stones, 120
    muscle soreness, 249
    sore throat, 254
    TMJ, 185
Heimlich maneuver, 109
Hemorrhoids, 231-232
Hepatitis, 106-108
Herbs, 18-19, 29, 364-365, 367. *See
  also specific herbs*
Herb teas. *See specific herbs*
Herpes (genital), 138-140
Hibiscus flower, 282
Hiccups, 109
High blood pressure, 29, 271, 280-
  283, 303
High cholesterol, 179, 256, 259, 271,
  284-287
HIV and AIDS, 288-290
Hives, 202
Hobbies, 61

Lidocaine, 164, 210, 246, 331
Lime, 227
Liquid bandages, 196
Lithium, 206
Lithotripsy, 101, 121
Liver function, 63-64
Lomotil, 94
Lotrimin, 146, 193
Lotronex, 118
Low-glycemic diet, 46-47, 244, 276-277, 279
L-propionylcarnitine, 303-304
L-theanine, 217
Lutein, 182-183
Lycopene, 108
Lyme disease, 240-241
Lysine, 138-140, 170-171

M

Macular degeneration, 182-184
Magnesium
  contraindications for, 370
  as remedy for
    anxiety, 217
    asthma, 79
    chronic fatigue syndrome, 322
    chronic pain, 323-324, 328, 332
    congestive heart failure, 265
    diabetes, 277
    digestive and urinary complaints, 92, 121
    glaucoma, 179
    headaches, 229, 247
    obesity, 293
    osteoporosis, 296
    reproductive ailments, 152, 155
    RLS, 253
    TMJ, 186
Magnet therapy, 111, 336
Makeup, for problem skin, 208
Malnutrition, 53-54
Manganese, 156, 295-296
Manual therapy, 329
MAO inhibitors, 301
Marijuana, 301
Marjoram, 98, 123
Marshmallow, 112-113, 117, 124-125
Massage
  cautions about, 371
  clinical studies of, 25
  practitioners of, 32-33
  as remedy for
    Alzheimer's disease, 258
    anxiety, 219
    cancer patients, 354-357

chronic pain, 313, 326
constipation, 93
depression, 274
gum disease, 181
muscle soreness, 249-250
PMS, 157
respiratory ailments, 74-75, 81
RLS, 253
stress, 61
TMJ, 185
Mast cell stabilizers, 74, 78
McKenzie therapy, 312-313
Meat tenderizer, for bee stings, 220
Medical equipment, 335
Medical errors, 17
Medical food, 112
Medical spa therapy, 302
Medications. *See* Drug side effects; *specific drugs or drug types*
Medicine cabinet, stocking, 28-29
Meditation
  classes in, 366
  described, 24
  as remedy, 60-61, 218, 266, 276, 280, 359-360
Meglitinides, 278-279
Melatonin, 188, 237, 239, 258, 321
Memory problems, 242-244
Menopause, 147-150
Menorrhagia, 136-137
Menstrual bleeding, heavy, 136-137
Menstrual cramps, 29, 151-153
Mental imagery, 57, 60
Mercury exposure, 62
Mesalamine, 97
Metformin, 143, 293
Methotrexate, 205, 308
Methyl sulfonyl methane (MSM), 179
Metronidazole, 208
Migraines, 245-248
Migralief, 247
Milk, 20, 237
Milk of magnesia, 169
Milk thistle for
  gallstones, 100
  hangover, 227
  hepatitis, 106
  nicotine addiction, 252
  reproductive health ailments, 131, 161
  toxin exposure, 65
Mind-body medicine, 24-25, 357-360. *See also* Stress management; *specific therapies*
Mineral deficiencies, 51

Moisturizers, 201, 206
Motion sickness, 122
Mouth splints, 91, 186, 189
MSM, 179
Mucuna pruriens, 301
Multivitamins, effects on
  canker sores, 169
  coronary artery disease, 271
  diabetes, 277
  flu, 87
  gum disease, 181
  HIV, 288-289
  infertility, 141-142
  stress, 47, 57
  toxin exposure, 65
Muscle relaxants for
  chronic pain, 311-312, 325, 328
  digestive and urinary complaints, 109, 118
  migraines, 246
Muscle soreness, 249-250
Mushrooms, 56
Music, as remedy, 61, 187, 202, 216-217, 275

N

N-acetyl-cysteine (NAC), 107, 142, 179, 288-289, 370
Namenda, 256-257
Naproxen. *See* NSAIDs
Naps, 222
Nasal irrigation, 72, 88
Nasal sprays, 74, 84
Nasal strips, 90
Natural medicine, 10-12, 14, 17-19. *See also specific treatments*
Naturopathic physicians (N.D.'s), 33, 366
Nausea, 122-123
Neck braces, 91
Neck pain, 326-329
Neck stretches, 228, 247
Nerve conduction studies, 318
Nerve pain, 330-332
Nettle
  NSAIDs and, 336
  as remedy, 72-73, 154-155, 159, 202-203
Neurofeedback, 218, 263
Niacin, 285-286
Nicotine, as remedy, 114
Nicotine addiction, 251-252. *See also* Smoking
Nishino Breathing Method, 57
Nitrates, 266, 270

Toxin exposure, 37, 62-65, 145
Traditional Chinese Medicine (TCM)
  clinical studies of, 22-23
  practitioners of, 31-32
  as remedy for
    digestive and urinary complaints, 104, 107-108, 113, 126
    fatigue, 225
    reproductive health ailments, 131, 139, 161
Tramadol, 325
Transcutaneous electrical nerve stimulation (TENS), 132, 153
Trans fats, 41-42, 46, 67. *See also* Diet and eating habits
Traumeel, 194, 314
Triamcinolone, 169
Triphala, 98, 117
Triptans, 245-246
Tulsi, 123
Tumor necrosis factor (TNF) inhibitors, 308
Turmeric, 18, 125-126, 343
Tylenol. *See* Acetaminophen

U

Ulcers, 124-127
Ultrasound, 315, 318
Underwear, 144, 167
Urinalysis, 223
Urinary incontinence, 110-111
Urinary tract infections (UTIs), 128
Uterine fibroids, 160-162
UTIs, 128-129

V

Vaccines, 87, 108, 177
Vacuum constriction devices, 135
Vaginal lubricants, 141-142, 163-164
Vaginal pain, 163-165
Valerian root
  contraindications for, 370
  as remedy for
    anxiety, 217
    chronic fatigue syndrome, 320
    digestive and urinary complaints, 112, 116, 120
    fibromyalgia, 324
    insomnia, 235-236
    jet lag, 239
    reproductive health ailments, 130, 151, 160-161
    rheumatoid arthritis, 307
    RLS, 253
    TMJ, 185

Vanilla extract, 189
Varicose veins, 212-213
Vegetable oils, 42, 114
Vegetables, 20. *See also* Diet and eating habits
Viagra, 133-134
Vinegar, 197
Vinpocetine, 187, 243, 258
Visualization, 187
Vitamin A, 192, 288. *See also* Retinoids
Vitamin B_2, 247
Vitamin B_6, 123, 156, 227
Vitamin B_{12}, 144, 224, 311
Vitamin C
  contraindications for, 370
  as remedy for
    Alzheimer's disease, 257, 259
    asthma, 77
    chronic pain, 315, 336
    diabetes, 277
    eye diseases, 179, 182-183
    gallstones, 101
    HIV, 288-289
    oxidative stress, 47
    Parkinson's disease, 299-300
    reproductive health ailments, 137-140, 145
    skin ailments, 194, 196
  UTIs and, 129
Vitamin D
  insulin resistance and, 51
  as remedy, 156, 205, 293, 295, 307
Vitamin E
  contraindications for, 370
  as remedy for
    Alzheimer's disease, 257, 259
    coronary artery disease, 271
    diabetes, 277
    HIV, 288-289
    macular degeneration, 182-183
    Parkinson's disease, 299-300
    reproductive health ailments, 137, 139, 145, 152
Vitamin K, 107

W

Walking. *See* Exercise
Warts, 214-215
Water intake. *See* Hydration
Weil, Andrew, 13
Wheat bran, 121
Wheat germ, 56
Wheatgrass juice, 113
WHI, 16

Wild yam cream, 148, 163-164
Willow bark, 306, 317, 328, 334, 370
Wine, 20, 43, 46, 121, 184
Wintergreen oil, 80, 84
Witch hazel, 211, 231
Women's Health Initiative (WHI), 16
Wrist-pressure bands, 122

X

Xylitol gum, 168, 181

Y

Yarrow, 131, 161
Yeast infections, 164, 166-167
Yoga
  clinical studies of, 23-24
  as remedy for
    anxiety, 218
    asthma, 79
    cancer patients, 352-353
    chronic pain, 310-311, 318, 329, 332
    diabetes, 279
    reproductive health ailments, 147, 153
    stress, 61
Yogurt, 56, 65, 167, 211

Z

Zeaxanthin, 182-183
Zelnorm, 93, 118
Zicam, 82
Zinc
  contraindications for, 370
  as remedy for
    ADHD, 261-262
    canker sores, 169
    cold sores, 171
    depression, 273-274
    diabetes, 277
    macular degeneration, 182-183
    osteoporosis, 296
    reproductive health ailments, 140, 145
    respiratory ailments, 73, 82
    rheumatoid arthritis, 307
    tinnitus, 188

About the Authors

Mary L. Hardy, M.D.

Dr. Mary Hardy, a fifth-generation physician, trained initially as an internist, but has been integrating complementary therapies and alternative practitioners into her practice for more than 15 years. She is the founding medical director of the Integrative Medicine Program at Cedars-Sinai Medical Center in Los Angeles and has been the associate director of the UCLA Botanical Center. Currently she is starting the Integrative Medicine Service in Oncology at the UCLA Ted Mann Family Resource Center and codirecting the development of integrative medicine and wellness programming at the Venice Family Clinic, the largest free clinic in the United States. She has been recognized as an expert in integrative medicine by the California Board of Medicine, and serves on the newly founded Advisory Council for the Naturopathic Medical Board of California.

She has had advanced training in herbal medicine and has consulted with traditional healers all over the world, including Peru, China, Kenya, and South Africa. Her current research interests include performing systematic reviews of the scientific literature on herbal therapies and dietary supplements as well as other projects at the Evidence-Based Practice Center of the nonprofit RAND Corporation. She is also involved in conducting clinical research using natural products.

Debra L. Gordon

A health writer for nearly two decades, Debra Gordon has witnessed the changing landscape of medicine. She recalls when hormone therapy was considered a miracle cure, when ulcers were blamed on stress instead of the *H. pylori* bacterium, when doctors were so averse to nutritional supplements that most wouldn't even recommend a daily multivitamin, and when the best advice for back pain was bed rest—something no doctor would recommend today. After interviewing hundreds of doctors and patients, observing dozens of surgeries, reading thousands of medical journal articles, and writing and editing numerous consumer health books, she's come to the conclusion that medicine is as dynamic as the individuals it serves. She believes *Best Remedies* represents another giant step forward in its evolution.

When she's not researching and writing about health, Debra is trying to keep her own family healthy—her three sons, Jonathan, Callum, and Iain, her husband, Keith, and her office mate and dog, Tyler. The family lives in northeastern Pennsylvania, where Southern-born Debra has learned to operate a snow blower. She is also the author of several other Reader's Digest books, including *Cut Your Cholesterol*, *Stealth Health*, and *Allergy and Asthma Relief*.